Perspectives in Cancer Prevention – Translational Cancer Research

Perumana R. Sudhakaran
Editor

Perspectives in Cancer Prevention – Translational Cancer Research

Co-Edited by
Oommen V. Oommen
M. Radhakrishna Pillai

Springer

Editor
Perumana R. Sudhakaran
Computational Biology
& Bioinformatics
University of Kerala
Kariavattom, Trivandrum
Kerala, India

Co-Editors
Oommen V. Oommen
Kerala State Biodiversity Board
Pallimukku, Trivandrum
Kerala, India

M. Radhakrishna Pillai
Rajiv Gandhi Centre
for Biotechnology
Thiruvananthapuram
Kerala, India

ISBN 978-81-322-3481-4 ISBN 978-81-322-1533-2 (eBook)
DOI 10.1007/978-81-322-1533-2
Springer New Delhi Heidelberg New York Dordrecht London

Softcover reprint of the hardcover 1st edition 2014

Printed on acid-free paper

Springer is part of Springer Science+Business Media (www.springer.com)

Preface

Over 7.5 million people worldwide are reported to die of cancer each year. Nearly 70 % of the cancer deaths occur in low and middle income countries. Further, there is a progressive increase in the number of persons who have undergone treatment against cancer and there are chances of recurrence of the disease. About one third of cancers are known to be preventable, and prevention offers the most cost-effective long-term strategy for control of cancer. A number of factors can affect a person's risk of developing cancer. These range from the use of tobacco, alcohol consumption, dietary factors, obesity, infections, environmental pollutants, occupational carcinogens and radiation.

Extensive research suggests that several methods can be employed for the prevention of specific types of cancers. Results of several studies have shown that biologically active phytochemicals and antioxidants present in several plant foods protect cells from damage caused by free radicals. Vaccines that prevent infection by human papilloma virus or hepatitis B virus are being tested to prevent cancers with viral aetiology, such as certain types of cervical or liver cancers. Dietary supplements such as curcumin, vitamins etc. are believed to lower risk for several cancers including colorectal and skin cancers.

The IV International Symposium on Translational Cancer Research held in Udaipur, India, in December 2011, was an opportunity to update the major advances in the area of cancer prevention. A few contributions from the meeting are presented in this book entitled *Perspectives in Cancer Prevention*. Comprising of 13 chapters, it provides in-depth analysis of data on biological process in cancer cells, cancer therapeutics and approaches to cancer prevention. These contributions are either critical reviews or research reports containing the views of the contributors, and cover most relevant and recent topics related to molecular aspects of cancer prevention and recommendations for cancer prevention.

We would like to acknowledge the efforts of all the contributors and the referees who critically reviewed the manuscripts. We are also grateful to Springer (India) and to Dr. (Mrs.) Mamta Kapila (Springer, India) for publishing the book. The technical support received from Ms. Vijayasree A.S. is gratefully acknowledged. Our thanks are also due to scientists and authorities of M. D. Anderson Cancer Centre, USA, Jai Sukhlal Suhadia University, Udaipur, Rajasthan, Central University of Kerala and Society for Translational Cancer Research for the support in bringing together a group of scientists, physicians and other experts in this area.

Computational Biology & Bioinformatics
University of Kerala, Kariavattom
Trivandrum, Kerala, India
Perumana R. Sudhakaran

Kerala State Biodiversity Board,
Thiruvananthapuram, Kerala, India
Oommen V. Oommen

Rajiv Gandhi Centre for Biotechnology,
Thiruvananthapuram, Kerala, India
M. Radhakrishna Pillai

Contents

1 **Nutrition in Cancer: Evidence-Based Nutrition Recommendations in Cancer Patients and Survivors** 1
Anis Rashid

2 **Tumour Stem Cell Enrichment by Anticancer Drugs: A Potential Mechanism of Tumour Recurrence** 9
T.R. Santhosh Kumar and M. Radhakrishna Pillai

3 **Curcumin: A Potent Candidate to be Evaluated as a Chemosensitizer in Paclitaxel Chemotherapy Against Cervical Cancer** 21
Chanickal N. Sreekanth, Smitha V. Bava, Arun Kumar T. Thulasidasan, Nikhil P. Anto, Vino T. Cheriyan, Vineshkumar T. Puliyappadamba, Sajna G. Menon, Santhosh D. Ravichandran, and Ruby John Anto

4 ***Azadirachta indica*** **(Neem) and Neem Limonoids as Anticancer Agents: Molecular Mechanisms and Targets** 45
Siddavaram Nagini and Ramamurthi Vidya Priyadarsini

5 **In Vitro Studies on the Antioxidant/Antigenotoxic Potential of Aqueous Fraction from *Anthocephalus cadamba* Bark** 61
Madhu Chandel, Upendra Sharma, Neeraj Kumar, Bikram Singh, and Satwinderjeet Kaur

6 **Possible Involvement of Signal Transducer and Activator of Transcription-3 (STAT3) Signaling Pathway in the Initiation and Progression of Hepatocellular Carcinoma** 73
Aruljothi Subramaniam, Muthu K. Shanmugam, Ekambaram Perumal, Feng Li, Alamelu Nachiyappan, Alan P. Kumar, Benny K.H. Tan, and Gautam Sethi

7 **Simple Sequence Repeats in 5′ and 3′ Flanking Sequences of Cell Cycle Genes** 89
Seema Trivedi

8 **Mechanisms of Chemopreventive Activity of Sulforaphane** ... 103
Yogesh C. Awasthi, Shailesh Jaiswal, Mukesh Sahu, Abha Sharma, and Rajendra Sharma

9 Reciprocal Relationship Between VE-Cadherin and Matrix Metalloproteinases Expression in Endothelial Cells and Its Implications to Angiogenesis 113
A.P. Athira, M.S. Kiran, and P.R. Sudhakaran

10 Androgen Receptor Expression in Human Thyroid Cancer Tissues: A Potential Mechanism Underlying the Gender Bias in the Incidence of Thyroid Cancers 121
Jone A. Stanley, Ramalingam Neelamohan, Esakky Suthagar, Kannan Annapoorna, Sridharan Sharmila, Jayaraman Jayakumar, Narasimhan Srinivasan, Sakhila K. Banu, Maharajan Chandrasekaran, and Michael M. Aruldhas

11 Novel Coordination Complexes of a Few Essential Trace Metals: Cytotoxic Properties and Lead Identification for Drug Development for Cancer 133
Anvarbatcha Riyasdeen, Rangasamy Loganathan, Mallayan Palaniandavar, and Mohammad A. Akbarsha

12 Why Is Gallbladder Cancer Common in the Gangetic Belt? ... 145
Ruhi Dixit and V.K. Shukla

13 Stress and Cancer Risk: The Possible Role of Work Stress 153
Marcus James Fila

About the Editors 163

Author Index 165

Subject Index 167

Contributors

Mohammad A. Akbarsha Mahatma Gandhi-Doerenkamp Center, Bharathidasan University, Tiruchirappalli, Tamil Nadu, India

Kannan Annapoorna Department of Endocrinology, Dr. ALM. Post Graduate Institute of Basic Medical Sciences, University of Madras, Chennai, TN, India

Nikhil P. Anto Integrated Cancer Research Program, Division of Cancer Research, Rajiv Gandhi Centre for Biotechnology, Thiruvananthapuram, Kerala, India

Ruby John Anto Integrated Cancer Research Program, Division of Cancer Research, Rajiv Gandhi Centre for Biotechnology, Thiruvananthapuram, Kerala, India

Michael M. Aruldhas Department of Endocrinology, Dr. ALM. Post Graduate Institute of Basic Medical Sciences, University of Madras, Chennai, TN, India

A.P. Athira Department of Biochemistry, University of Kerala, Kariavattom, Thiruvananthapuram, Kerala, India

Yogesh C. Awasthi Department of Molecular Biology and Immunology, University of North Texas Health Science Center, Fort Worth, TX, USA

Sakhila K. Banu Department Integrative Biosciences, College of Veterinary Medicine & Biomedical Sciences, Texas A&M University, College Station, TX, USA

Smitha V. Bava Integrated Cancer Research Program, Division of Cancer Research, Rajiv Gandhi Centre for Biotechnology, Thiruvananthapuram, Kerala, India

Madhu Chandel Department of Botanical and Environmental Sciences, Guru Nanak Dev University, Amritsar, India

Maharajan Chandrasekaran Department of Endocrine Surgery, Madras Medical College, Chennai, TN, India

Vino T. Cheriyan Integrated Cancer Research Program, Division of Cancer Research, Rajiv Gandhi Centre for Biotechnology, Thiruvananthapuram, Kerala, India

Ruhi Dixit Department of General Surgery, Institute of Medical Sciences, Banaras Hindu University, Varanasi, India

Marcus James Fila Department of Economics, Management, and Accounting, Hope College, Holland, Michigan, USA

Shailesh Jaiswal Department of Molecular Biology and Immunology, University of North Texas Health Science Center, Fort Worth, TX, USA

Jayaraman Jayakumar Department of Endocrine Surgery, Madras Medical College, Chennai, TN, India

Satwinderjeet Kaur Department of Botanical and Environmental Sciences, Guru Nanak Dev University, Amritsar, India

M.S. Kiran Department of Biochemistry, University of Kerala, Kariavattom, Thiruvananthapuram, Kerala, India

Biomaterials Division, Central Leather Research Institute, Adyar, Chennai, Tamil Nadu, India

Alan P. Kumar Department of Pharmacology, Yong Loo Lin School of Medicine, National University of Singapore, Singapore, Singapore

Cancer Science Institute of Singapore, National University of Singapore, Centre for Translational Medicine, Singapore, Singapore

Neeraj Kumar Natural Plant Products Division, CSIR-Institute of Himalayan Bioresource Technology, Palampur, HP, India

Feng Li Department of Pharmacology, Yong Loo Lin School of Medicine, National University of Singapore, Singapore, Singapore

Rangasamy Loganathan Department of Chemistry, Central University of Tamil Nadu, Thiruvarur, Tamil Nadu, India

Sajna G. Menon Integrated Cancer Research Program, Division of Cancer Research, Rajiv Gandhi Centre for Biotechnology, Thiruvananthapuram, Kerala, India

Alamelu Nachiyappan Department of Pharmacology, Yong Loo Lin School of Medicine, National University of Singapore, Singapore, Singapore

Siddavaram Nagini Department of Biochemistry and Biotechnology, Faculty of Science, Annamalai University, Annamalainagar, Tamil Nadu, India

Ramalingam Neelamohan Department of Endocrinology, Dr. ALM. Post Graduate Institute of Basic Medical Sciences, University of Madras, Chennai, TN, India

Mallayan Palaniandavar Department of Chemistry, Central University of Tamil Nadu, Thiruvarur, Tamil Nadu, India

Ekambaram Perumal Molecular Toxicology Lab, Department of Biotechnology, Bharathiar University, Coimbatore, 641046, Tamil Nadu, India

Vineshkumar T. Puliyappadamba Integrated Cancer Research Program, Division of Cancer Research, Rajiv Gandhi Centre for Biotechnology, Thiruvananthapuram, Kerala, India

M. Radhakrishna Pillai Cancer Research Program, Rajiv Gandhi Centre for Biotechnology, Thiruvananthapuram, Kerala, India

Department of Surgical Oncology, Regional Cancer Centre, Thiruvananthapuram, Kerala, India

Anis Rashid MD Anderson Cancer Center, Houston, TX, USA

Santhosh D. Ravichandran Integrated Cancer Research Program, Division of Cancer Research, Rajiv Gandhi Centre for Biotechnology, Thiruvananthapuram, Kerala, India

Anvarbatcha Riyasdeen Department of Animal Science, Bharathidasan University, Tiruchirappalli, Tamil Nadu, India

Mukesh Sahu Department of Molecular Biology and Immunology, University of North Texas Health Science Center, Fort Worth, TX, USA

T.R. Santhosh Kumar Cancer Research Program, Rajiv Gandhi Centre for Biotechnology, Thiruvananthapuram, Kerala, India

Seema Trivedi Department of Zoology, JN Vyas University, Jodhpur, Rajasthan, India

Gautam Sethi Department of Pharmacology, Yong Loo Lin School of Medicine, National University of Singapore, Singapore, Singapore

Cancer Science Institute of Singapore, National University of Singapore, Centre for Translational Medicine, Singapore, Singapore

Muthu K. Shanmugam Department of Pharmacology, Yong Loo Lin School of Medicine, National University of Singapore, Singapore, Singapore

Abha Sharma Department of Molecular Biology and Immunology, University of North Texas Health Science Center, Fort Worth, TX, USA

Rajendra Sharma Department of Molecular Biology and Immunology, University of North Texas Health Science Center, Fort Worth, TX, USA

Upendra Sharma Natural Plant Products Division, CSIR-Institute of Himalayan Bioresource Technology, Palampur, HP, India

Sridharan Sharmila Department of Endocrinology, Dr. ALM. Post Graduate Institute of Basic Medical Sciences, University of Madras, Chennai, TN, India

V.K. Shukla Department of General Surgery, Institute of Medical Sciences, Banaras Hindu University, Varanasi, India

Bikram Singh Natural Plant Products Division, CSIR-Institute of Himalayan Bioresource Technology, Palampur, HP, India

Chanickal N. Sreekanth Integrated Cancer Research Program, Division of Cancer Research, Rajiv Gandhi Centre for Biotechnology, Thiruvananthapuram, Kerala, India

Narashiman Srinivasan Department of Endocrinology, Dr. ALM. Post Graduate Institute of Basic Medical Sciences, University of Madras, Chennai, TN, India

Jone A. Stanley Department of Endocrinology, Dr. ALM. Post Graduate Institute of Basic Medical Sciences, University of Madras, Chennai, TN, India

Department Integrative Biosciences, College of Veterinary Medicine & Biomedical Sciences, Texas A&M University, College Station, TX, USA

Aruljothi Subramaniam Department of Pharmacology, Yong Loo Lin School of Medicine, National University of Singapore, Singapore, Singapore

Molecular Toxicology Lab, Department of Biotechnology, Bharathiar University, Coimbatore, Tamil Nadu, India

P.R. Sudhakaran Computational Biology & Bioinformatics, University of Kerala, Kariavattom, Thiruvananthapuram, Kerala, India

Esakky Suthagar Department of Endocrinology, Dr. ALM. Post Graduate Institute of Basic Medical Sciences, University of Madras, Chennai, TN, India

Benny K.H. Tan Department of Pharmacology, Yong Loo Lin School of Medicine, National University of Singapore, Singapore, Singapore

Arun Kumar T. Thulasidasan Integrated Cancer Research Program, Division of Cancer Research, Rajiv Gandhi Centre for Biotechnology, Thiruvananthapuram, Kerala, India

Ramamurthi Vidya Priyadarsini Department of Biochemistry and Biotechnology, Faculty of Science, Annamalai University, Annamalainagar, Tamil Nadu, India

Nutrition in Cancer: Evidence-Based Nutrition Recommendations in Cancer Patients and Survivors

1

Anis Rashid

Abstract

Decades of research have revealed a direct association between diet and cancer. In fact, it is suggested that at least one third of all cancers are directly related to diet, and this number goes up when other factors such as sedentary lifestyle, obesity, and addictive behaviors (e.g., smoking and drinking) are taken into consideration. Interactions between dietary constituents and gene function that lead to cancer prevention or development have been identified. For example, dietary constituents modulate genes involved in DNA repair, apoptosis, and enzyme induction. An integrative approach to modify diet and lifestyle will support cancer patients during active treatment and potentially prevent cancer recurrence during survivorship. Additionally, changes in diet are likely to improve the patient's quality of life and prolong survivorship.

Keywords

NF-kappa B • Nutrition • Phytochemicals • Soy isoflavones • Carotenoids • Breast cancer

1.1 Objective

The purpose of this chapter is to increase awareness among clinicians, cancer patients, and the general population of dietary factors that promote carcinogenesis and to promote diets rich in antioxidants and phytochemicals that enhance the immune system and prevent cancer.

A. Rashid, M.D. (✉)
MD Anderson Cancer Center, Houston, TX, USA
e-mail: anrashid@mdanderson.org

1.2 Introduction

Carcinogenesis is a long process that takes years to develop. It involves an inefficient and incomplete repair or removal process within the body, and hundreds and thousands of such failures occur over a period of 10–30 years before a cancerous lesion is identified. Hence, there is enough time to act and reverse this change by dietary and lifestyle modifications (University of Arizona: Integrative Medicine Program 2011). Interactions between dietary constituents and gene function that lead to cancer prevention or development

P.R. Sudhakaran (ed.), *Perspectives in Cancer Prevention – Translational Cancer Research*, DOI 10.1007/978-81-322-1533-2_1, © Springer India 2014

have been identified. Dietary constituents also modulate genes involved in DNA repair, apoptosis, and enzyme induction (University of Arizona: Integrative Medicine Program 2011).

Decades of research have shown that dietary choices may affect development of cancer, its progression and relapse, and overall survival. In fact, one third of all cancers are due to unhealthy dietary choices, and plant-based diets are associated with reduced risk of cancer (Cancer 2012). According to statistics published by the World Health Organization (WHO), about 30 % of cancer deaths are due to five behavioral and dietary factors. These include low fruit and vegetable intake, lack of physical activity, high body mass index, and tobacco and alcohol use. Cancer is the leading cause of death worldwide accounting for 7.6 million deaths in 2008 (World Health Organization 2012). Does this mean that about 2.5 million lives could have been saved by good dietary choices? To get the scientific evidence and best approach toward nutrition and physical activity, the American Cancer Society arranged a group of experts in nutrition, physical activity, and cancer survivorship to study the effects of lifestyle changes on cancer and to identify the best clinical practices for cancer patients and survivors (Rock et al. 2012). In the past few years, nutrition has been the focus of many scientific studies. Multiple research studies from epidemiological to human intervention have been conducted to find the optimal anticancer diet.

This paper will highlight foods that have anticancer, antioxidant, and immune-boosting properties, as well as foods that can increase inflammation, suppress immunity, and may enhance tumor progression. Evidence has also shown that certain micronutrients and phytochemicals can enhance immune system and prevent cancer. This paper also will cover topics of macronutrients, micronutrients, and the role of phytochemicals in cancer prevention. Finally, this paper will also provide dietary recommendations and guidelines for lifestyle changes for certain types of cancers.

1.3 Method

A literature review will be conducted on evidenced-based dietary recommendations for cancer patients during treatment and survivorship. In addition, a review of nutritional guidelines for healthy individuals will be discussed as a means to enhance the immune system functioning which will ultimately prevent cancer.

1.3.1 Macronutrients

Macronutrients are food macromolecules that when absorbed and digested by animals/humans yield energy which is utilized by the individuals for cell functions.

These include:

1. Fats
2. Proteins
3. Carbohydrates
4. Fibers

1.3.2 Micronutrients

Micronutrients are minerals or vitamins that are needed in small quantity but are essential to the body and must be obtained from an outside source.

These include:

1. Vitamins A, C, E, and D
2. Calcium
3. Selenium
4. Folic acid
5. Zinc

1.3.3 Fats

Fatty acids are carboxylic acid with aliphatic chains with even number of carbon atoms. About 90 % of dietary fats consist of triglycerides. These are three fatty acid chains linked to glycerol molecule with a number of arrangements of double bonds. It is the number and the position of double bond that is responsible for specific biochemical characteristics of the fat and its effects on health and disease. It is a common concept that a high-fat diet is a risk factor for cancer development. In fact, not only the total amount of fat but also the type of fat consumed is equally important in cancer development.

Fats can be classified as saturated fats and unsaturated fats. Saturated fatty acids, often classified as "bad fats," contain no double bonds in their fatty acid chain. Examples of saturated fats are red meat, coconut oil, and fats in dairy products. Another category of "bad fats" is trans fats, in which naturally occurring cis-isomer is replaced by trans-isomer. This is due to the industrial hydrogenation of unsaturated fatty acids. Examples of food containing trans fats are margarine, shortening, commercially fried foods, and commercially baked cookies and doughnuts.

Unsaturated fats can be classified into monounsaturated fatty acids and polyunsaturated fatty acids. Monounsaturated fatty acids are heart healthy. One example is the omega-9 family which includes olive oil, canola oil, olives, and avocados. Polyunsaturated fatty acids include omega-3 and omega-6 fatty acids. The essential compound in omega-3 fatty acids is alpha-linolenic acid. Sources of alpha-linolenic acids are flax seeds, walnuts, pumpkin seeds, and leafy green vegetables. More bioavailable forms of alpha-linolenic acids are eicosapentaenoic acid and docosahexaenoic acid which can be obtained from animal sources such as fish, fish oil, eggs, and sea foods. The essential compound in omega-6 fatty acids is linoleic acid. As a part of the western diet, we already consume an excess of omega-6 fatty acids. Foods rich in omega-6 fatty acids include meat, milk, and refined oils. Excess of omega-6 fatty acid leads to chronic diseases as it promotes inflammation, platelet aggregation, thrombosis, and vasospasm.

1.3.3.1 Dietary Recommendations for Fats

- Total daily calorie intake from fats 25–30 %.
- Up to 20 % of the intake should be from monounsaturated fats.
- Up to 7–10 % should be from polyunsaturated fats.
- Less than 1 % of the fat intake should be from trans fats.

1.3.4 Proteins

Proteins are biochemical compounds with one or more polypeptides, facilitating biological function. Amino acid compounds of proteins may be classified as essential and non essential. Non essential proteins are those that the body can synthesize. Essential proteins are those that the body cannot synthesize, and these compounds need to be obtained from outside sources. There are nine essential amino acids, and complete proteins provide all nine essential amino acids. Animal-based proteins that provide all essential amino acids are meat, milk cheese, and eggs. Soy is the only plant that provides all essential amino acids. Hence, products from grains and nuts alone may be incomplete in proteins; combining them with other plant-based proteins will make a complete food.

1.3.4.1 Essential Amino Acids

Leucine	Isoleucine	Valine
Lysine	Methionine	Phenylalanine
Threonine	Tryptophan	Histidine

1.3.4.2 Protein: Risk Factors

- Three ounces of red meat for men and 2 oz for women over a period of 10 years.
- One ounce of processed meat for 5–6 days for men and 2–3 days for women.
- Higher red meat intake in estrogen and progesterone receptor-positive breast cancer among premenopausal women.
- High-temperature cooking and grilling is a risk as compared to steaming, stewing, or poaching.

1.3.5 Carbohydrate

The primary function of carbohydrate is to provide energy for metabolism as glucose is the main fuel source of all cells. Carbohydrates are also the essential part of the composition of RNA, DNA, and glycoproteins. Carbohydrates are classified as monosaccharides, disaccharides, oligosaccharides, fructooligosaccharides, and polysaccharides. It is important to note that the type of carbohydrate consumed affects glucose and insulin levels differently. Natural resources of fructo-oligosaccharides include bananas, barley, onions, tomatoes, and artichokes.

1.3.6 Fibers

Fibers are plant polysaccharides and lignins which are resistant to hydrolysis by human digestive enzymes. Fibers minimize constipation and slow the absorption of glucose and cholesterol from the gut. Sources of fiber include apples, citrus, strawberries, and carrots.

1.3.7 Micronutrients

Micronutrients are vitamins or a mineral that is either a component of an enzyme or acts as coenzyme. These are essential and must be obtained. These compounds are needed in small amounts. These include vitamins, minerals, and herbs.

1.3.7.1 Micronutrients that Increase Immunity and Decrease Inflammation

- Vitamin A: High concentration of beta-carotene.
- Vitamin C: Reduces risk of gastric cancer.
- Vitamin E: Major antioxidant in cell membrane.
- Vitamin D: Inhibits proliferation, DNA synthesis, and angiogenesis and promotes apoptosis.
- Calcium: Calcium inhibits glucuronidase which releases carcinogens.
- Selenium: Glutathione peroxidase in selenium removes organic peroxides.
- Folic acid: Reduces risks of neural tube defect (Omenn 1996).
- Zinc: Antioxidant and prevents angiogenesis (Prasad and Kucuk 2002).

1.3.8 Phytochemicals

Phytochemicals are plant-based substances that have antioxidant properties. These include fruits, vegetables, herbs, and spices. They protect plants from ultraviolet light, and in humans, they prevent certain diseases.

Phytochemicals can be classified as follows:

- Polyphenols
  - Flavonoids
  - Non-flavonoids
- Terpenoids
  - Carotenoids
  - Non-carotenoids
- Glucosinolate
- Thiosulfonates
- Capsaicin
- Piperine (Ben Best, 2005)

1.3.9 Polyphenols

(a) *Flavonoids*

The best-defined flavonoids are water-soluble compounds found in fruits, vegetables, leaves, grains, and bark. Examples include the following:

- Tea and cranberries: The active ingredient is epigallocatechin gallate, which is an antioxidant that inhibits nuclear transcription factor kappa B (NF-kappa B), reduces prostaglandin E2, and hence may reduce the risk of colorectal cancer.
- Onion: The active ingredient is quercetin, which promotes apoptosis and is a blood thinner and vasodilator.
- Berries: The active ingredient is cyanidin, which protects cells from oxidative damage.
- Soy isoflavones are found in soy and parsley. Active ingredient in soy is Genistein which interacts with estrogen- and androgen-mediated signaling pathways. Genistein is a phytoestrogen, and this estrogen-like substance may actually promote tumor proliferation in breast cancer patients (Sarkar and Li 2003). Soy inhibits tyrosine kinase activity. Studies have shown the protective effects of soy in young females, but there is little

evidence to show its benefit in postmenopausal female patients (Cassileth and Vickers 2003). It has strong antioxidant properties, prevents osteoporosis, reduces menopausal symptoms, reduces low-density lipoproteins and increases high-density lipoproteins.

(b) *Non-flavonoids*:

- Turmeric: The active ingredient is curcumin, which is anti-inflammatory and antioxidant. It also inhibits NF-kappa B, cyclooxygenase-2, activating protein-1, and tumor necrosis factor-alpha.
- Red grapes: The active ingredient is resveratrol, which inhibits nuclear transcription factor kappa B (NF-kappa B).

1.3.10 Carotenoids

- Carotenoids include red, yellow, and orange pigments synthesized by plants.
- Beta-carotene: Orange carotenoids are found in orange peel, papaya, mangoes, carrots, and eggs. They repair damaged DNA, inhibit NF-kappa B, angiogenesis, and boost the activity of natural killer cells.
- Alpha-carotene: Also orange carotenoids found in sweet potato, pumpkin, squash, green beans, spinach, and broccoli. Alpha carotenoids are ten times more anticarcinogenic than beta-carotenoids. They enhance the release of interleukin-1 and tumor necrosis factor-alpha.
- Lycopene: Lycopene is found in tomato, watermelon, guava, papaya, and grapefruits. It is an antioxidant and provides protection against UV light and also suppresses insulin-like growth factor-1 (Barber and Barber 2002).
- Lutein: Kale, corn, avocado, spinach, and parsley may protect eyes from macular degeneration and protects against colon cancer (Best 2012).

1.3.11 Organosulfur Compounds

These compounds belong to thiosulfonates, which include *Alliums* such as garlic, onion, leeks, chives, and scallions. Garlic has more sulfur than onions. Garlic's active ingredient is alliin which converts to allicin by enzyme alliinase when crushed. This gives odor to garlic. It inhibits *Helicobacter pylori* and reduces the risk in gastric cancer. Organosulfur compounds also lower lipids. Allicin inhibits mammary cell proliferation and endometrial and colon cell proliferation (Univ. of Arizona). Garlic can lower blood pressure and blood cholesterol.

1.3.12 Capsaicin

It makes chili pepper hot, relieves chemotherapy-induced neuropathy, promotes apoptosis in pancreatic cancer, and inhibits NF-kappa B transcription.

1.4 Results

The results will include reviews of nutritional guidelines published by the American Cancer Society and American Institute of Cancer Research, as well as data from multiple studies conducted at independent institutions worldwide showing that diet plays a critical role in cancer development and prevention.

1.4.1 Recommendations for Breast Cancer Patients (National Cancer Institute; Nutrition in Cancer (PDQ R), China Study; Hidden Diabetic Cures www.hidden-diabetes-cures.com)

- Low-fat diet with 20 % calories from fat to reduce sarcopenic obesity. Reduce saturated fats.
- Dietary fat intake from nuts, avocado, and olive oil.
- Omega-3 fatty acid from legumes, green leafy vegetable, and marine fish.
- Cruciferous vegetables and flax seeds.
- Avoid alcohol and soy.
- Regular physical activity (University of Arizona: Integrative Medicine Program 2011).

1.4.2 Recommendations for Prostate Cancer Patients (University of Arizona; Program in Integrative Medicine 2011)

- High-fat diet may increase testosterone level, which may promote tumor growth.
- Low-fat diet, high in fruits and vegetables.
- Lycopene (tomato, watermelon, papaya, grapefruit, and guava) lowers prostate cancer incidence (Clinton et al. 1996).
- Selenium (garlic, walnuts, raisins, brown rice, mushrooms, and shellfish) has protective effect against prostate cancer (Clark et al. 1996).
- Avoid calcium as it reduces vitamin D level which reduces growth of prostate cancer.

1.4.3 Recommendations for Lung Cancer Patients (University of Arizona; Program in Integrative Medicine 2011)

- Reduced risk of lung cancer in smokers and nonsmokers who eat at least 5 servings of fruits and vegetables a day (ACS Guidelines on Nutrition and Physical Activity for Cancer Prevention 2012).
- Lycopene-rich diet including tomatoes and tomato-based foods.
- Lutein-rich diet including avocado, corn, and carotenoids are recommended.
- Avoid beta-carotene as it may increase mortality.
- No benefits with vitamin supplementation.
- Chemotherapy- and radiation-induced dysphagia and esophagitis demand small, frequent easy to swallow, nutrient dense meals.

1.4.4 Recommendations for Colorectal Cancer (University of Arizona; Program in Integrative Medicine 2011)

- Dietary fiber recommendations for men 30 g/day and for women 21 g/day (University of Arizona: Integrative Medicine Program 2011).
- Therapeutic doses of selenium (200 mcg/day) after completion of treatment (University of Arizona: Integrative Medicine Program 2011).
- Calcium is recommended. Colon cancer is associated with inadequate intake of calcium (McCullough et al. 2003).
- Avoid red meats.
- Avoid charcoal grilled meat and fish.
- Alpha-carotene and vitamin A is protective in colon cancer recurrence (Steck-Scott et al. 2004).

1.4.5 American Institute for Cancer Research Guidelines for Cancer Survivors

- Choose predominantly plant-based diets rich in fruits and vegetables.
- If eaten at all, limit intake of red meat to less than 3 oz a day.
- Limit consumption of fatty foods, particularly those of animal origin.
- Limit consumption of salted foods and use of cooking and table salt.
- Use herbs and spices to season foods.
- Limit alcoholic drinks to two drinks a day for men and one for women.
- Avoid charred food and cured or smoked meats. Only occasionally eat meat and fish grilled in direct flame.
- Avoid being overweight and limit weight gaining during adulthood.
- Take an hour's brisk walk or similar exercise daily.

1.5 Research

Identification of damage to DNA and an understanding of diet-gene interactions have enabled clinicians to intervene and prevent cancer development. Further research will improve our understanding in this field as we better understand the mechanisms through which various foods impact health, eventually allowing us to develop an optimal cancer prevention diet.

1.6 Conclusion

Once diagnosed with cancer, a patient is challenged from every conceivable angle. He experiences emotional turmoil, low motivation, sleep difficulties, poor appetite, fatigue, and extreme stress. Managing a cancer patient is a challenge, as the physicians have to focus on all aspects of patient care. One area that needs special attention is stress, extreme anxiety, and depression. Prolonged stress may play a key role in immune suppression which may lead to increased inflammatory response and tumor progression. A study of 10,000 women in Finland has shown that loss of important relationships doubles the risk of breast cancer (Servan-Schreiber 2009). Hence, physicians need to focus not only on nutrition but other areas of concern as well. Eastern traditions such as yoga, meditation, and tai chi bring harmony and stimulate the body's natural defenses. A balanced diet, healthy sleep habits, regular exercise, and a positive attitude also play major roles in health and in healing.

References

ACS Guidelines on Nutrition and Physical Activity for Cancer Prevention (2012) Diet and activity factors that affect risks for certain cancers. http://www.cancer.org/Healthy/EatHealthyGetActive/ACSGuidelinesonNutritionPhysicalActivityforCancerPrevention/acs-guidelines-on-nutrition-and-physical-activity-for-cancer-prevention-diet-and-activity

Barber NJ, Barber J (2002) Lycopene and prostate cancer. Prostate Cancer Prostatic Dis 5(1):6–12. doi:10.1038/sj.pcan.4500560

Best B (2012) Phytochemicals as nutraceuticals. http://www.benbest.com/nutrceut/phytochemicals.html

Cancer C (2012) Overview: nutrition and cancer prevention. https://www.caring4cancer.com/go/cancer/nutrition/eating-well-nutrition/overview-nutrition-and-cancer-prevention.htm

Cassileth BR, Vickers AJ (2003) Soy: an anticancer agent in wide use despite some troubling data. Cancer Invest 21(5):817–818

Clark LC et al (1996) Effects of selenium supplementation for cancer prevention in patients with carcinoma of the skin: a randomized controlled trial. JAMA 276(24):1957–1963. doi:10.1001/jama.1996.03540240035027

Clinton SK, Emenhiser C, Schwartz SJ, Bostwick DG, Williams AW, Moore BJ, Erdman JW Jr (1996) cis-trans lycopene isomers, carotenoids, and retinol in the human prostate. Cancer Epidemiol Biomarkers Prev 5(10):823–833

McCullough ML, Robertson AS, Chao A, Jacobs EJ, Stampfer MJ, Jacobs DR, Diver WR, Calle EE, Thun MJ (2003) A prospective study of whole grains, fruits, vegetables and colon cancer risk. Cancer Causes Control 14(10):959–970

Omenn GS (1996) Micronutrients (vitamins and minerals) as cancer-preventive agents. IARC Sci Publ 139: 33–45

Prasad AS, Kucuk O (2002) Zinc in cancer prevention. Cancer Metastasis Rev 21(3–4):291–295

Rock CL, Doyle C, Demark-Wahnefried W, Meyerhardt J, Courneya KS, Schwartz AL, Bandera EV, Hamilton KK, Grant B, McCullough M, Byers T, Gansler T (2012) Nutrition and physical activity guidelines for cancer survivors. CA Cancer J Clin 62(4):243–274. doi:10.3322/caac.21142

Sarkar FH, Li Y (2003) Soy isoflavones and cancer prevention. Cancer Invest 21(5):744–757

Servan-Schreiber D (2009) Anticancer: a new way of life. J Altern Complement Med 15(7):805–806

Steck-Scott S, Forman MR, Sowell A, Borkowf CB, Albert PS, Slattery M, Brewer B, Caan B, Paskett E, Iber F, Kikendall W, Marshall J, Shike M, Weissfeld J, Snyder K, Schatzkin A, Lanza E (2004) Carotenoids, vitamin A and risk of adenomatous polyp recurrence in the polyp prevention trial. Int J Cancer (Journal international du cancer) 112(2):295–305. doi:10.1002/ijc.20364

University of Arizona: Program in Integrative Medicine (2011) Nutrition and cancer.

World Health Organization (2012) World health statistics. World Health Organization. http://www.who.int/mediacentre/factsheets/fs297/en/index.html

Tumour Stem Cell Enrichment by Anticancer Drugs: A Potential Mechanism of Tumour Recurrence

2

T.R. Santhosh Kumar and M. Radhakrishna Pillai

Abstract

Tumour recurrence after chemotherapy is a serious clinical problem. An emerging concept in tumour biology is the cancer stem cell hypothesis, which emphasises the importance of rare tumour stem cell-like cells to reinitiate the tumour even after a successful elimination of the primary tumour mass by surgery, chemotherapy or radiotherapy. We employed live cell tools to monitor caspase-mediated cell death or survival after in vitro drug treatment to investigate events associated with enrichment of CSCs in breast and colon cancer cells. We provide evidence for rare escape of cells from drug-induced caspase activation that enriches cells with stem cell-like cells. Interestingly, an intermediate senescent-dominating population was evident during the transition and the post-senescent; drug-surviving cells were enriched with dye efflux cells with embryonic stem cell markers. Since senescence-escaped stable colonies generated are enriched with stem cell-like phenotype from natural tumour cell models and also stably express sensitive caspase sensor, in the future they can be utilised for screening compounds that target them.

Keywords

Tumour stem cells • Anticancer drugs • Drug resistance • Side population cells • Senescence • Apoptosis

2.1 Introduction

Most chemotherapeutics or target-specific drugs used for the treatment of cancer are capable of reducing tumour burden with immediate promising tumour-free survival. However, this initial successful treatment outcome is most often followed by tumour recurrence in a subset of tumours. The accumulating evidence attributes quiescent tumour stem cell-like cells within the heterogeneous tumour population as the cellular origin for tumour recurrence (Gangemi et al. 2009; Milas and Hittelman 2009). This theory is further strengthened by the recent reports suggesting that tumour stem cell-like cells are inherently resistant to conventional antitumour agents (Singh and

T.R. Santhosh Kumar • M. Radhakrishna Pillai (✉)
Cancer Research Program, Rajiv Gandhi Centre for Biotechnology, Thycaud P O, Thiruvananthapuram 695014, Kerala, India
e-mail: mrpillai@rgcb.res.in

P.R. Sudhakaran (ed.), *Perspectives in Cancer Prevention – Translational Cancer Research*, DOI 10.1007/978-81-322-1533-2_2, © Springer India 2014

Settleman 2010; Ribatti 2012). The concept of tumour stem cells, even though known for many years, experimentally proved for its existence first time in leukaemia (Lapidot et al. 1994). Subsequently both surface marker and functional trait-based identification of this rare population were documented in a variety of solid tumours including breast, colon and CNS (Korkaya et al. 2011; Lathia et al. 2011). Cancer stem cells, just like normal stem cells, exist as quiescent phenotype that renders them resistant to conventional cytotoxic agents that often exerts more damage to proliferating cells in the bulk tumour. However, several recent studies indicate that cancer stem cell phenotype can be induced by a variety of stimuli. Epithelial–mesenchymal transition by TGF-β treatment or by ectopically expressed transcription factors like Twist and Snail and overexpression of pluripotency-inducing factors also contributes for the induction of stem cell phenotype (Ksiazkiewicz et al. 2012; Zhu et al. 2012; Krantz et al. 2012; Kong et al. 2011; Floor et al. 2011). In addition, several reports attribute a role for certain drugs to induce EMT as well as tumour stem cell phenotype as a potential mechanism for drug failure. We have recently showed evidence for rare escape of tumour cells from drug-induced cell death, after an intermediate stay in a noncycling senescent stage followed by unstable multiplication often characterised with spontaneous cell death (Achuthan et al. 2011). The cells which escaped from drug-induced toxicity showed increased resistance to cell death by caspase activation and tumour stem cell-like phenotype such as CD133 and Oct4 expression. Extensive functional characterisation of the drug-escaped cells revealed that their drug resistance phenotype is closely related to low levels of intracellular reactive oxygen species (ROS) subsequent to reactivation of antioxidant enzymes (Achuthan et al. 2011). The drug-induced tumour stem cell enrichment, even though not well defined, carries tremendous implications in the understanding of drug failure, tumour recurrence and metastasis and also provides opportunities for drug intervention. Here, we further provide evidence for the existence of rare tumour stem cell-like cells in multiple tumour cells and their enrichment after drug exposure. The colon cancer cells used in the current study also showed evidence for intermediate senescent stage and indication for rare entry into cell cycle from drug-induced senescence. Currently, it is not clear whether the enrichment is due to the escape of rare cells from drug treatment or it is induced by the drugs either by genetic or epigenetic signalling. However, the drug-escaped population remains as a potential cell source to identify agents that target physiologically relevant drug-resistant cells with stem cell-like property. Since tumour stem cell-like cells are very rare and difficult to identify from natural cancer cell models, it remains as a challenge to develop cell-based assays to identify compounds that target them (Gupta et al. 2009). Since the methods described here enrich the cells with stem cell-like phenotype from natural tumour cell models, that can be utilised for screening compounds that targeting them.

2.2 Materials and Methods

2.2.1 Cell Lines

Human breast tumour cell lines MCF-7; colon cancer cell lines SW480, SW620 and HCT11; and cervical cancer cell lines SiHa, HeLa and C3AA were obtained from ATCC, USA. All cancer cell lines were maintained in RPMI medium supplemented with 1 % penicillin–streptomycin and 10 % foetal bovine serum. All cell lines were incubated in a humidified incubator at 37 °C supplied with 5 % carbon dioxide.

2.2.2 Side Population (SP) Analysis

The cell suspensions were labelled with Hoechst 33342 dye (Invitrogen, USA) using methods as previously described (Sobhan et al. 2012; Bleau et al. 2009). Briefly, cells were resuspended at 1×10^6/mL in prewarmed RPMI with 2 % FBS and 10 mM HEPES buffer containing 5 μg/mL of Hoechst 33342 in the presence or absence of verapamil at 37 °C for 90 min. Then, the cells were washed and resuspended in ice-cold HBSS containing 2 % FBS and 10 mM HEPES. Propidium iodide at a final concentration of 2 μg/mL was added to the cells to gate viable cells. Side population analyses were done on FACSAria I (BD, USA).

2.2.3 Drug Treatment

Cells were seeded at a density of 2×10^5 cells/well in 12-well plates containing DMEM supplemented with 10 % FBS. After overnight incubation, different drugs were added to each cell line and maintained at 37 °C in a water-saturated atmosphere containing 5 % CO_2. Medium replacement was done every fourth day with fresh drug-containing medium. The duration of exposure to each drug was about 3–6 weeks.

2.2.4 Live Cell Visualisation of Cell Death and Survival Using Cells Expressing Caspase-3 Fluorescence Resonance Energy Transfer (FRET) Probe

We have previously employed caspase sensor expression vector, SCAT 3.1, which consists of ECFP and EYFP (Venus), separated by caspase cleavage site – DEVD – to generate stable clones in breast cancer cell lines (Joseph et al. 2011). This approach enabled us to visualise immediate cell death by caspase activation upon drug treatment and also tracking of the surviving cells. Since the surviving clones were enriched with cells with tumour stem cell-like properties including surface phenotype of CD133 and CD44 as well as functional traits low ROS, Oct4 induction and reactivation of antioxidant machinery, we hypothesised that if proved in more cells, the emerging cell population may form a better tool for identifying agents that target them. Keeping this in mind, a new-generation FRET probe for caspase activation was employed to generate stable clones. This vector consists of Ametrine as the donor fluorescent protein and Tomato as the acceptor protein linked in-between the sequence, DEVD, with a nuclear exclusion signal (NES).

Stable clones were generated with this vector both in MCF-7 and colon cancer cell line SW480 by transfections followed by flow sorting to get cells that are enriched with high FRET efficiency using FACSAria I (BD, USA). For FRET imaging by microscopy, cells were seeded on a chambered cover glass (Nunc International, NY) and maintained in live cell incubation chamber (Tokai-Hit, Japan) at 37 °C with 5 % CO_2 for indicated time periods. Images were collected using an Epi fluorescent microscope TE-2000E (Nikon, Japan) at regular intervals. Single excitations of pmAmetrine at 387/11 and dual emission at 535/30 and 585/29 were collected using automated excitation and emission filter wheel controlled by NIS software (Nikon, Tokyo) as described (Ai et al. 2008).

2.2.5 Assessment of Cell Cycle Progression in Live Cells

For live cell visualisation of cell cycle progression, G1-specific fluorescent component of FUCCI, Cdt1–Kusabira Orange fusion construct and G2-specific green fluorescent marker Geminin–Azami Green were employed to generate stable clones (Sakaue-Sawano et al. 2008). Cells were transfected with the expression vector Cdt1–KO and Geminin–Azami Green followed by selection in G418. The cell expressing both red and green fluorescent proteins was isolated by flow sorting. Stable integration and cell cycle-specific fluorescence were evaluated by live cell imaging. The cells were seeded on chambered cover glass for live cell imaging as described above.

2.3 Results

2.3.1 Side Population Cells in Established Cancer Cell Lines

Despite increasing number of reports substantiating the existence of tumour stem cell-like cells in multiple tumour types, their identification remains as a challenge due to lack of a common surface marker. In the last decade, contributions from several laboratories revealed importance of several phenotypes to identify them from multiple tumour cell models. $CD44^{+}/CD24^{low}$ and Aldefluor-high and CD133-high fractions were reported as enriched with cells with tumour-initiating potential in breast, colon, neural and prostate cancers (Scheel and Weinberg 2011; Fang et al. 2012; Singh and Dirks 2007). Functional features like low reactive oxygen species and drug efflux were also explored as valuable marker of tumour stem cell-like cells (Wang et al. 2010). Another widely used method, side population analysis utilises the ability of cells to exclude the fluorescent dye Hoechst, owing to the preferred expression of p-glycoprotein in stem cell-like compartment (Bleau et al. 2009; Sobhan et al. 2012; Engelmann et al. 2008). In an effort to characterise side population cells, we have employed multiple tumour cells of different tissue origin to determine the steady-state level of side population cells by flow cytometry. A typical scatter plot of side population analysis in the colon cancer cell line SW620 is shown in Fig. 2.1a. The percentage of cells gated as side population in the scatter plot is diminished in verapamil- treated cell population substantiating their dependence on drug efflux transporters. The histogram shown in Fig. 2.1b is the quantitative representation of the average percentage of side population cells in multiple tumour cells as determined by FACS ($n = 3$).

The results shown above indicate that cancer cells maintained continuously in culture will retain a small fraction of cells with drug efflux property that can be identified by FACS. As shown in the histogram, most cells retain a small fraction of SP irrespective of the tissue origin and that varies significantly between cells. Several reports as well as our previous studies substantiated the drug-resistant nature of side population cells compared to the main population (Sobhan et al. 2012; Achuthan et al. 2011; Gangemi et al. 2009).

2.3.2 Side Population Cells Are Enriched in Drug-Evaded Cells

In a previous study, we have shown that exposure of breast cancer cells to multiple antitumour agents generates drug-resistant clonal expansion in a delayed manner (Achuthan et al. 2011). Currently, it is not clear whether this phenomenon is unique to breast cancer cells or general in nature. So we have employed colon cancer cells SW480, SW620 and HCT 116 and exposed them to camptothecin and doxorubicin for two cycles with an interval of 3 days. Then the plates were maintained in drug-free medium to allow expansion of colonies as described previously. At the end of 30–45 days, the emerging colonies were trypsinised and analysed side population by FACS. Both the drugs significantly increased the percentage of cells with drug efflux property in all the cells. The results from SW480 are shown on the graph in Fig. 2.2a. A representative scatter plot of SW480 cells generated after treatment with doxorubicin is also shown (Fig. 2.2b). The results shown above prove that side population cells are enriched after multiple cycles of drug exposure in colon cancer cells. This is consistent with similar observation noticed in breast cancer cells (Achuthan et al. 2011). Overall, these results indicate for a possible unique general signalling in cancer cells that enriches cells with considerable phenotype transition, rendering them resistant to drugs during exposure to cytotoxic agents.

2.3.3 A FRET-Based Caspase Sensor to Track the Emergence of Drug-Resistant Colonies

Since most antitumour agents kill cancer cells by apoptosis involving activation of caspases, we have previously employed stable breast cancer cell lines expressing caspase-specific FRET probe ECFP–DEVD–EYFP to track caspase-evading cells in breast cancer cell line (Joseph

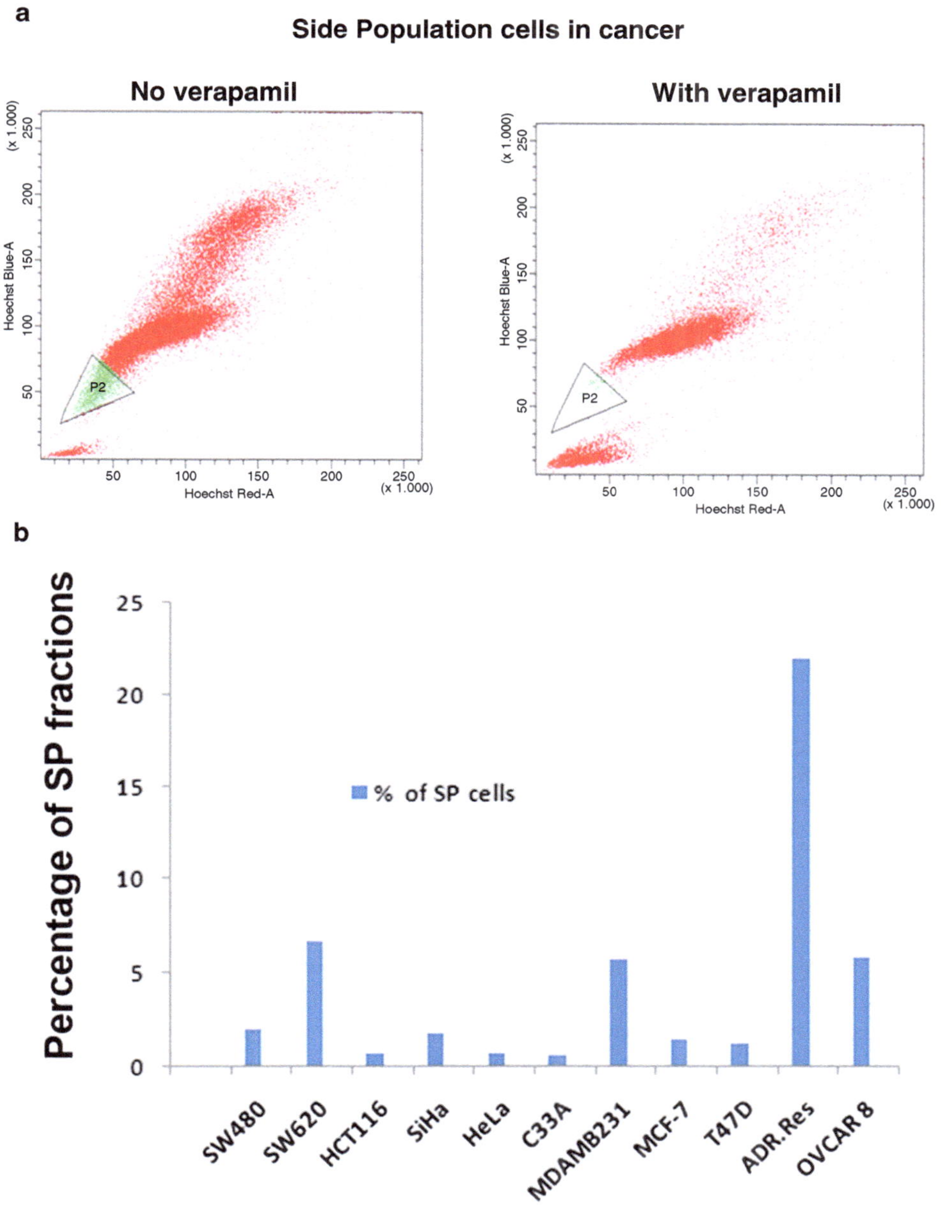

Fig. 2.1 *Side population cells were present in established cancer cell lines.* (**a**) SW620 cells were stained with Hoechst 33342 dye in the presence (*right*) or absence (*left*) of 50 μmol/L verapamil and analysed by flow cytometry. (**b**) Indicated cell lines were stained with Hoechst for side population analysis as described in materials and methods. Average percentage of SP cells gated in multiple cancer cells is shown as *bar diagram*

et al. 2011). This model was quite useful to visualise the emerging colonies and also to study their drug response. The results shown above from the colon cancer cell lines indicate that drug-escaped cells are enriched with high fraction of side population cells, a population with stem cell-like properties. So, we hypothesised that since the drug treatment enriches cells with stem

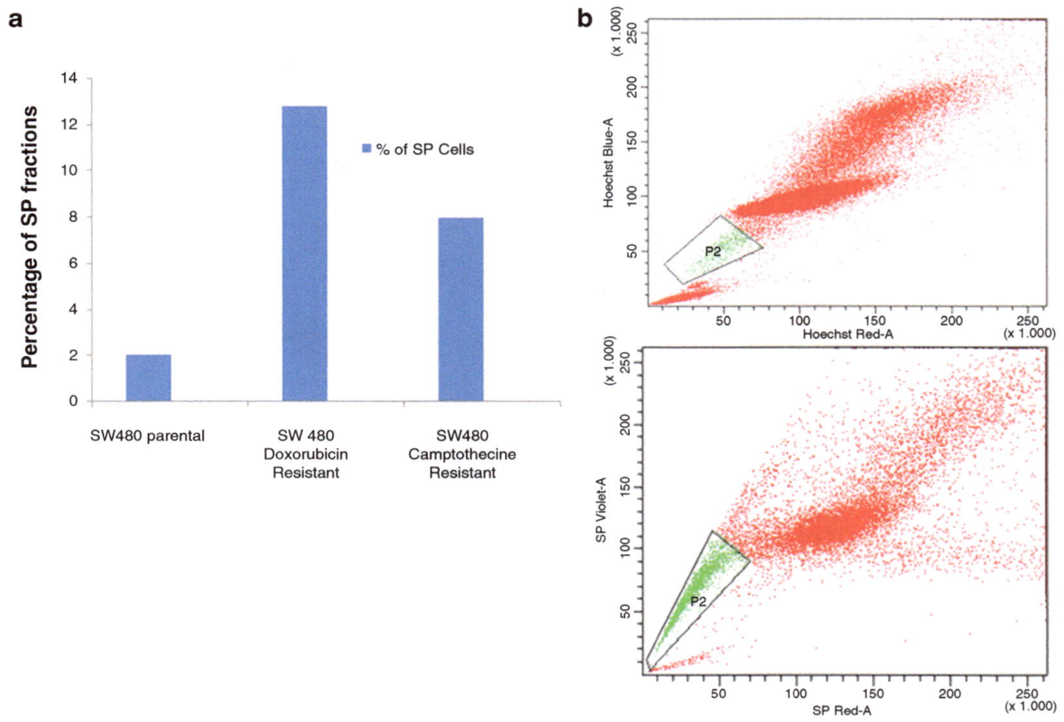

Fig. 2.2 *Drug-induced enrichment of side population cells*. (**a**) SW480 cells were exposed to doxorubicin and camptothecin and drug-escaped cells were generated as described. The side population analysis was done as described. (**b**) A representative scatter plot of SW480 cells generated after treatment with doxorubicin and the parental SW480 is shown

cell-like properties, this enriched fraction may form a better cell source for screening drugs that specifically target them. The FRET-based caspase sensor cell system is highly adaptable for high-throughput image-based drug screening (Joseph et al. 2011). So we have employed a sensitive system of FRET-based caspase activation tool Ametrine–DEVD–Tomato (Ai et al. 2008). Initially, we developed breast cancer cell line, MCF-7, expressing Ametrine–DEVD–Tomato stable cell line as described. The colon cancer SW480 was also employed to study the generation of drug-tolerant cells.

Consistent with our earlier results in breast cancer cells, it was seen that after an initial phase of massive cell death by caspase activation, few cells enter into noncycling quiescent-like state with large, flattened morphology, a characteristic feature of senescent cells in SW480 cells also. A representative live cell image of senescent cells generated after doxorubicin treatment in MCF-7 and SW480 cells expressing Ametrine–DEVD–Tomato is given in Fig. 2.3a, b. As evident from the figure, few cells with flattened senescent morphology are flanked by small dividing cells indicating occasional cell cycle entry during the transition.

2.3.4 Senescence and Delayed Cell Cycle Entry in Drug-Treated Cells

Even though late outgrowth colonies were known to emerge from the drug-treated population after an intermediate senescent-dominating cell population, currently it is not clear whether the cells were generated from senescent cells. Cellular senescence is a general response of normal cells undergoing limited replication before

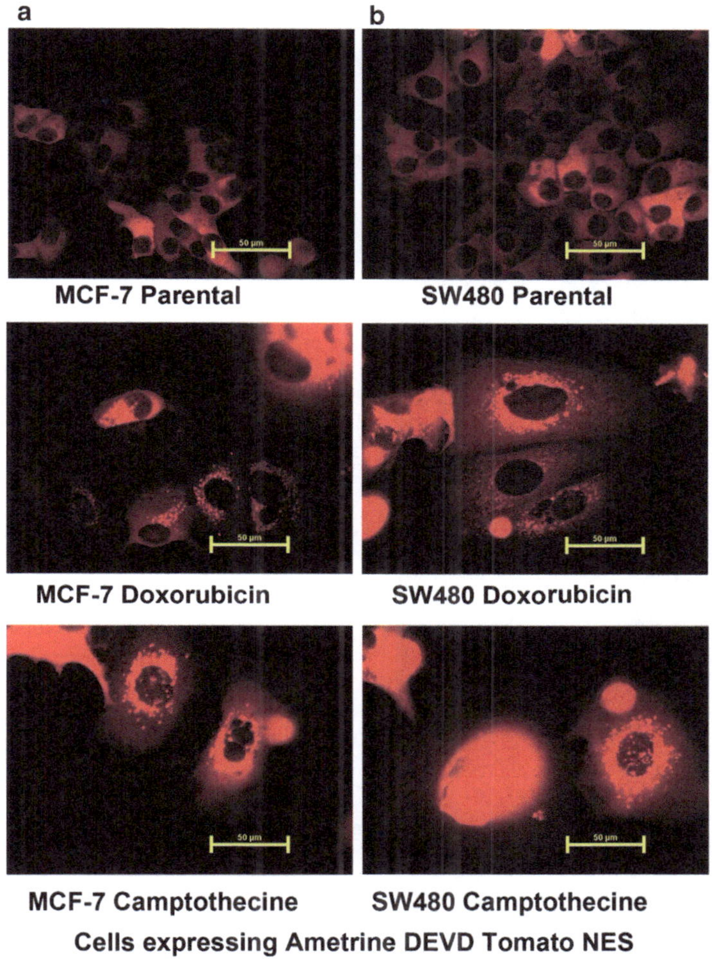

Fig. 2.3 *Drug-induced senescence and cell cycle entry*. (**a**) A representative live cell image of senescent cells generated after doxorubicin treatment in MCF-7 expressing Ametrine–DEVD–Tomato. (**b**) A representative live cell image of senescent cells generated after doxorubicin treatment in SW480 cells expressing Ametrine–DEVD–Tomato NES

entering into a terminally growth-arrested state attributed to telomere attrition. Tumour cells, though considered as immortal, also retain the capacity to undergo senescence in response to genotoxic stress, radiotherapy and chemotherapy. Senescent cells are generally resistant to apoptosis and can serve as reservoirs of secreted factors for mitogenic and angiogenic activity; however, the evidence for their entry into cell cycle is not well established. In order to prove cell cycle entry, we have employed the cell cycle indicator in live cell, FUCCI, as described (Sakaue-Sawano et al. 2008). The SW480 cells stably expressing cytochrome c-EGFP were stably transfected with cdt–KO and Geminin–Azami Green. Cells in the G1 phase show red cdt fluorescence in the nucleus and the G2 phase with Geminin–Green fluorescence as described (Sakaue-Sawano et al. 2008). The S-phase cells expressed both cdt and Geminin in the nucleus. This approach helped to identify the S-phase fractions during the course of drug treatment. Close observation of multiple wells revealed rare S-phase entry by few cells with senescent morphology. A representative image is shown in Fig. 2.4. As seen from the figure around senescent cells, few cells show expression of both cdt and Azami Green substantiating S-phase entry.

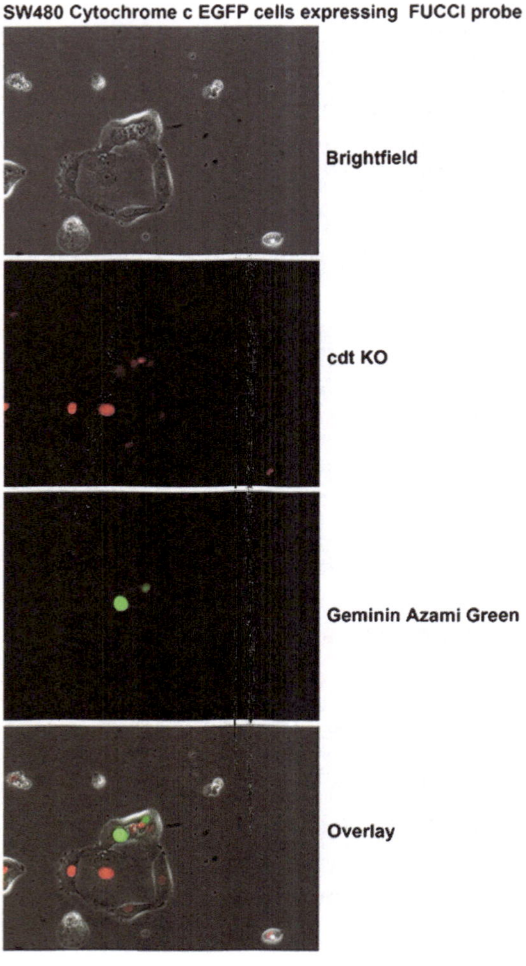

Fig. 2.4 *Evidence for cell cycle entry from senescence.* The SW480 cells stably expressing cytochrome c-EGFP were stably transfected with cdt–KO and Geminin–Azami Green. The cells were exposed to three cycles of doxorubicin and allowed to recover in drug-free medium. As seen from the figure around senescent cells, few cells show both cdt and Azami Green indicating they are in S phase

2.3.5 Drug-Surviving Cells Are Resistant to Drugs and Enriched with Tumour Stem Cell-Like Properties: Potential Applications in Drug Screening

Results from the above studies indicate possible generation of drug-resistant cells from senescent cells by occasional reentry into cell cycle. Moreover, the drug-escaped populations were highly enriched in side population cells as well as cells with stem cell properties. To examine whether drug-surviving cells displayed resistance to drugs, the cells expressing the FRET probes were exposed to drugs, and drug-tolerant cells were generated as described. Both parental and drug-tolerant cells were exposed to different anticancer agents, and caspase activation was analysed by ratio imaging as described in the materials and methods. A representative ratio imaging of doxorubicin-resistant and parental cells to three different drugs is shown in Fig. 2.5a–c. Compared to parental cells, drug-escaped cell showed marked resistance to caspase activation. Most cells failed to change the ratio of Ametrine–Tomato compared to the parental cells.

Our results again indicate a role for drug-induced senescence in tumour recurrence through clonal expansion of multidrug-resistant cells both in breast and colon cancer cells. The ratio imaging described here using the Ametrine–DEVD–Tomato NES-stable cells is highly adaptable for high-throughput imaging, and the drug-escaped cell model has potential applications in drug screening, specially to identify compounds that target cells with tumour stem cell-like properties.

2.4 Discussion

Treatment failure and tumour recurrence after chemo- or radiotherapy remain as the major challenge in successful cancer treatment. It has been increasingly realised that the conventional treatment modalities are not enough to ensure complete eradication of tumour cells even with targeted therapies. In general, cancer that relapses after treatment remains resistant to most chemotherapeutic agents even to the different chemical compounds than used for initial treatment. Multiple hypotheses were put forwarded to explain tumour recurrence and their resistance. Cancer has been viewed as a highly heterogeneous population, and this heterogeneity also brings differential response to drugs. This heterogeneity of response may allow some cells to escape drug-induced cytotoxic stimuli to ensure

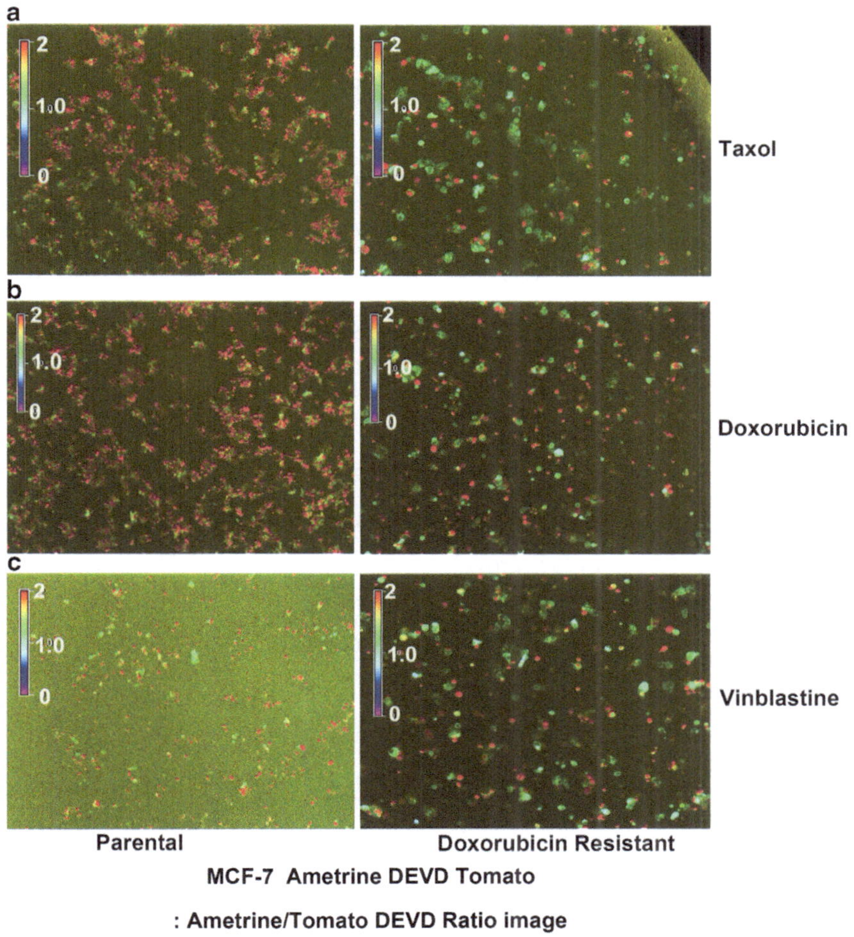

Fig. 2.5 *Apoptosis resistance in drug-escaped cells.* MCF-7 Ametrine–DEVD–Tomato NES-stable cells were treated with doxorubicin for three cycles as described. The drug-escaped cells were further treated with Taxol (**a**), doxorubicin (**b**) and vinblastine (**c**) for 48 h. The ratio of pmAmetrine and tdTomato is shown. The parental cells were also treated with the same drug and shown for comparison

population maintenance. Another emerging concept of tumour stem cells also supports the tumour recurrence after chemotherapy, emphasising that a small fraction of cells within a tumour is responsible for the tumour initiation, and they are resistant than the bulk tumour cells. This hypothesis explains the immediate response to drugs as revealed by the death of the bulk cells; however, the small fraction remaining after chemotherapy reinitiates the tumour later. Previously, several studies have reported the generation of drug-resistant cells with or without stem cell characteristics after initial drug treatment. Sharma et al. (2010) showed induction of reversible drug-tolerant state in non-small cell lung cancer cells to a lethal exposure of EGFR–TKI (Sharma et al. 2010). They also observed that the drug-tolerant cells were enriched with putative progenitor marker CD133. Similarly, we have recently employed an in vitro model system where breast cancer cell lines were exposed to diverse antitumour agents that generated drug-tolerant cells. We have employed breast cancer cell lines expressing live cell caspase detection FRET probe involving ECFP–EYFP linked with DEVD sequence, a preferred site for activated caspases. This system helped us to visualise and track the fate of these cells for a long time using high-throughput imaging. Even though the system substantiated the immediate death of the cell by caspase activation, few cells that resisted the initial drug treatment remained sensitive to apoptosis by spontaneous caspase activation. Even after removal of the drug, most cells succumbed to cell death slowly upon entering into division or remained quiescent with replicative senescence. This senescent-dominating phase is followed by rare emergence of growing colonies that repopulate the tumour. Interestingly, our studies using the emerging colonies indicate that drug-escaped cells are enriched with drug-resistant cells, drug efflux side population cells and cells with low reactive oxygen species subsequent to reactivation of antioxidant systems. Here, we further provide evidence that drug escape is general in nature and not restricted only to breast cancer cells. The colon cancer cells treated with multiple drugs also generate drug-tolerant cells that are enriched in tumour stem cell-like cells. Here, we also provide evidence for rare entry of senescent cells to cell cycle using the sensitive live cell cycle indicator FUCCI in SW480 cells. Even though the molecular switch that drives senescent cells to enter into cell cycle is not clear, it plays a critical role in the emergence of drug-tolerant cells both in breast and colon cancer cells. In this report, we have used a highly sensitive cellular system of live cell caspase activation Ametrine–DEVD–Tomato. Ratio imaging by microscopy utilising these cells is a powerful and sensitive tool for drug screening that is also adaptable for high-throughput image-based systems. Since our earlier studies substantiate that the drug-escaped cells are highly enriched with tumour stem cell markers like CD133, OCT4 expression, low ROS and high-invasion potential, they are the ideal cell source for identification of compounds that specifically target them. Even though tumour stem cells are now considered as the best target for drug development, because of their rarity and difficulty to characterise, it remains as a challenge for drug screening. Since the cell system employed here expresses a sensitive probe for caspase activation and is also enriched with drug-resistant tumour stem cell-like cells, they will form better tools for drug screening in future.

Acknowledgement We thank the Department of Bio technology, Government of India (grant no: BT/PR/7793/MED/14/1112/2006 to MRP and IYBA grant to TRSK), and Flow Cytometry Technical Support Team, Rajiv Gandhi Centre for Biotechnology, Trivandrum. We also thank Dr. Atsushi Miyawaki, RIKEN, for the generous gift of the expression vectors cdt–KO and Geminin–Azami Green and Dr. Campbell, RE, for pmAmetrine–DEVD–tdTomato NES vector.

References

Achuthan S, Santhoshkumar TR, Prabhakar J, Nair SA, Pillai MR (2011) Drug-induced senescence generates chemoresistant stemlike cells with low reactive oxygen species. J Biol Chem 286:37813–37829

Ai HW, Hazelwood KL, Davidson MW, Campbell RE (2008) Fluorescent protein FRET pairs for ratiometric imaging of dual biosensors. Nat Methods 5:401–403

Bleau AM, Hambardzumyan D, Ozawa T, Fomchenko EI, Huse JT, Brennan CW, Holland EC (2009) PTEN/PI3K/Akt pathway regulates the side population phenotype and ABCG2 activity in glioma tumor stem-like cells. Cell Stem Cell 4:226–235

Engelmann K, Shen H, Finn OJ (2008) MCF7 side population cells with characteristics of cancer stem/progenitor cells express the tumor antigen MUC1. Cancer Res 68:2419–2426

Fang DD, Wen D, Xu Y (2012) Identification of cancer stem cells provides novel tumor models for drug discovery. Front Med 6:112–121

Floor S, van Staveren WC, Larsimont D, Dumont JE, Maenhaut C (2011) Cancer cells in epithelial-to-mesenchymal transition and tumor-propagating-cancer stem cells: distinct, overlapping or same populations. Oncogene 30:4609–4621

Gangemi R, Paleari L, Orengo AM, Cesario A, Chessa L, Ferrini S, Russo P (2009) Cancer stem cells: a new paradigm for understanding tumor growth and progression and drug resistance. Curr Med Chem 16:1688–1703

Gupta PB, Onder TT, Jiang G, Tao K, Kuperwasser C, Weinberg RA, Lander ES (2009) Identification of selective inhibitors of cancer stem cells by high-throughput screening. Cell 138:645–659

Joseph J, Seervi M, Sobhan PK, Retnabai ST (2011) High throughput ratio imaging to profile caspase activity: potential application in multiparameter high content apoptosis analysis and drug screening. PLoS One 6:e20114

Kong D, Li Y, Wang Z, Sarkar FH (2011) Cancer stem cells and Epithelial-to-Mesenchymal Transition (EMT)-phenotypic cells: are they cousins or twins? Cancers (Basel) 3:716–729

Korkaya H, Liu S, Wicha MS (2011) Breast cancer stem cells, cytokine networks, and the tumor microenvironment. J Clin Invest 121:3804–3809

Krantz SB, Shields MA, Dangi-Garimella S, Munshi HG, Bentrem DJ (2012) Contribution of epithelial-to-mesenchymal transition and cancer stem cells to pancreatic cancer progression. J Surg Res 173:105–112

Ksiazkiewicz M, Markiewicz A, Zaczek AJ (2012) Epithelial-mesenchymal transition: a hallmark in metastasis formation linking circulating tumor cells and cancer stem cells. Pathobiology 79:195–208

Lapidot T, Sirard C, Vormoor J, Murdoch B, Hoang T, Caceres-Cortes J, Minden M, Paterson B, Caligiuri MA, Dick JE (1994) A cell initiating human acute myeloid leukaemia after transplantation into SCID mice. Nature 367:645–648

Lathia JD, Heddleston JM, Venere M, Rich JN (2011) Deadly teamwork: neural cancer stem cells and the tumor microenvironment. Cell Stem Cell 8:482–485

Milas L, Hittelman WN (2009) Cancer stem cells and tumor response to therapy: current problems and future prospects. Semin Radiat Oncol 19:96–105

Ribatti D (2012) Cancer stem cells and tumor angiogenesis. Cancer Lett 321:13–17

Sakaue-Sawano A, Kurokawa H, Morimura T, Hanyu A, Hama H, Osawa H, Kashiwagi S, Fukami S, Miyata T, Miyoshi H, Imamura T, Ogawa M, Masai H, Miyawaki A (2008) Visualizing spatiotemporal dynamics of multicellular cell-cycle progression. Cell 132:487–498

Scheel C, Weinberg RA (2011) Phenotypic plasticity and epithelial-mesenchymal transitions in cancer and normal stem cells? Int J Cancer 129:2310–2314

Sharma SV, Lee DY, Li B, Quinlan MP, Takahashi F, Maheswaran S, McDermott U, Azizian N, Zou L, Fischbach MA, Wong KK, Brandstetter K, Wittner B, Ramaswamy S, Classon M, Settleman J (2010) A chromatin-mediated reversible drug-tolerant state in cancer cell subpopulations. Cell 141:69–80

Singh S, Dirks PB (2007) Brain tumor stem cells: identification and concepts. Neurosurg Clin N Am 18: 31–38, viii

Singh A, Settleman J (2010) EMT, cancer stem cells and drug resistance: an emerging axis of evil in the war on cancer. Oncogene 29:4741–4751

Sobhan PK, Seervi M, Joseph J, Chandrika BB, Varghese S, Santhoshkumar TR, Radhakrishna Pillai M (2012) Identification of heat shock protein 90 inhibitors to sensitize drug resistant side population tumor cells using a cell based assay platform. Cancer Lett 317:78–88

Wang Z, Li Y, Sarkar FH (2010) Signaling mechanism(s) of reactive oxygen species in Epithelial-Mesenchymal Transition reminiscent of cancer stem cells in tumor progression. Curr Stem Cell Res Ther 5:74–80

Zhu LF, Hu Y, Yang CC, Xu XH, Ning TY, Wang ZL, Ye JH, Liu LK (2012) Snail overexpression induces an epithelial to mesenchymal transition and cancer stem cell-like properties in SCC9 cells. Lab Invest 92:744–752

Curcumin: A Potent Candidate to be Evaluated as a Chemosensitizer in Paclitaxel Chemotherapy Against Cervical Cancer

3

Chanickal N. Sreekanth, Smitha V. Bava, Arun Kumar T. Thulasidasan, Nikhil P. Anto, Vino T. Cheriyan, Vineshkumar T. Puliyappadamba, Sajna G. Menon, Santhosh D. Ravichandran, and Ruby John Anto

Abstract

Rigorous efforts in searching for novel chemosensitizers and unraveling their molecular mechanism have identified curcumin as one of the promising candidates. Our earlier report has shown that cervical cancer cells can be sensitized by curcumin to paclitaxel-induced apoptosis through down-regulation of NF-κB and Akt. The present study is an attempt to decipher the signaling pathways regulating the synergism of paclitaxel and curcumin and to determine whether the synergism exists in vivo. The study has clearly proved that Akt and NF-κB function successively in the sequence of paclitaxel-induced signaling events where Akt is up-stream of NF-κB. Inactivation of NF-κB did not affect the activation of Akt and survivin, while that of Akt significantly inhibited NF-κB and completely inhibited up-regulation of survivin. Up-regulation of cyclin-D1, COX-2, XIAP, and c-IAP1 and phosphorylation of MAPKs were completely inhibited on inactivation of NF-κB assigning a key regulatory role to NF-κB in the synergism. While up-regulation of survivin by paclitaxel is regulated by Akt, independent of NF-κB, inactivation of neither Akt nor NF-κB produced any change in Bcl-2 level suggesting a distinct pathway for its action. Mouse cervical multistage squamous cell carcinoma model using 3-methylcholanthrene and a xenograft model of human cervical cancer in NOD-SCID mice using HeLa cells were used to evaluate the synergism

C.N. Sreekanth • S.V. Bava • A.K.T. Thulasidasan
N.P. Anto • V.T. Cheriyan • V.T. Puliyappadamba
S.G. Menon • S.D. Ravichandran • R.J. Anto, Ph.D. (✉)
Integrated Cancer Research Program, Division of Cancer Research, Rajiv Gandhi Centre for Biotechnology, Thiruvananthapuram, Kerala 695014, India
e-mail: rjanto@rgcb.res.in

P.R. Sudhakaran (ed.), *Perspectives in Cancer Prevention – Translational Cancer Research*, DOI 10.1007/978-81-322-1533-2_3, in vivo. The results suggest that curcumin augments the antitumor action of paclitaxel by down-regulating the activation and down-stream signaling of antiapoptotic factors and survival signals such as NF-κB, Akt, and MAPKs.

Keywords
Paclitaxel • Curcumin • NF-κB • Akt • MAPKs • Synergism

3.1 Introduction

In parallel to the identification of chemotherapeutic agents, a great deal of effort is put in for the identification of phytochemicals known as chemosensitizers, which can enhance the efficacy of conventional chemotherapy. Paclitaxel, isolated from *Taxus brevifolia*, is one of the commonly prescribed chemotherapeutic drugs against a wide spectrum of epithelial cancers. However, administration of lower doses of this drug has been shown to activate various survival signals, leading to chemoresistance (Aggarwal et al. 2005; Mabuchi et al. 2004). Earlier studies, including ours, have shown that curcumin, the active principle of *Curcuma longa*, has synergistic effect with paclitaxel in inducing apoptosis in cancer cells and reducing tumorigenesis (Bava et al. 2005; Aggarwal et al. 2006), and this has been correlated with the down-regulation of various survival signals by curcumin (Aggarwal et al. 2006; Anto et al. 2000; Chen and Tan 1998).

Studies from our laboratory as well as that of others have clearly established that paclitaxel activates NF-κB and Akt in several cell systems, inhibition of which sensitizes cancer cells to paclitaxel (Bava et al. 2005; Mabuchi et al. 2004; Aggarwal et al. 2005). However, no study has yet explored whether these two molecules act independently or interdependently in the synergism of paclitaxel and curcumin. Moreover, the regulatory role of other survival signals such as mitogen-activated protein kinases (MAPKs), AP-1, Bcl-2, COX-2, cyclin D1, and IAPs have never been correlated to this synergism. Hence, this study investigates the major signaling molecules regulating the synergism.

Moreover, apart from a xenograft study using human breast cancer cells (Aggarwal et al. 2005), the combination of paclitaxel and curcumin has not been tested in vivo. Based on our earlier in vitro observations on the synergistic anticancer activity of curcumin and paclitaxel in cervical cancer cells (Bava et al. 2005), we carried out two preclinical studies: one a carcinogen-induced multistage tumor model that better reflects the architectural and cellular complexity of patient-derived tumor specimens and the other a human cervical cancer xenograft model in NOD-SCID mice. We have identified for the first time that activation of NF-κB is associated with 3-methylcholanthrene-induced tumorigenesis in *Swiss albino* mice and the suppression of NF-κB activation and other survival signals by curcumin leads to the augmentation of paclitaxel-induced apoptosis, thereby enhancing the therapeutic outcome of paclitaxel in vivo.

3.2 Materials and Methods

3.2.1 Reagents

All the cell culture reagents were purchased from Life Technologies Inc. Radiolabeled (γ-^{32}P) ATP was purchased from Bhabha Atomic Research Centre, India. The primers used in the PCR studies and the oligos for electrophoretic mobility shift assay (EMSA) were custom synthesized by Genosys, Sigma. Antibodies against β-actin and IκBα and all secondary antibodies were purchased from Sigma. Paclitaxel, U0126, SP600125, SB203580, and LY294002 were purchased from Calbiochem (San Diego, CA). Antibodies against phospho-ERK1/2, phospho-p38, phospho-Akt, Akt, c-Jun, cyclin D1, PCNA, caspase-3, caspase-7, caspase-8, caspase-9, c-IAP1, phospho-p38, phospho-SAPK/JNK, and survivin- and rhodamine-conjugated secondary antibody were obtained from Cell Signaling Technology (Beverly, MA) and those against Bcl-2, MDR-1, MMP-2, MMP-9, VEGF, p50, RelA, Bcl-2, c-IAP, XIAP, survivin, COX-2, phospho-JNK, ERK-2, JNK-1, p38 DAPI, and Annexin V apoptosis detection kit were purchased from Santa Cruz Biotechnology (Santa Cruz, CA). Mouse monoclonal anti-XIAP was procured from BD Biosciences (San Diego, CA). All other reagents and antibodies were obtained from Sigma.

3.2.2 Cell Culture

HeLa cells were purchased from the National Centre for Cell Sciences (NCCS), Pune, India. For immunoblotting, FACS, and electrophoretic mobility shift assay (EMSA), 1×10^6 cells were seeded/60 mm plate and for MTT assay 5,000 cells/well were seeded/96-well plate.

3.2.3 Western Blot Analysis

Cell/tissue samples were lysed in ice-cold RIPA buffer with protease inhibitors and Western blotting was performed as described (Bava et al. 2005).

3.2.4 MTT Assay

Proliferative/cytotoxic effect of paclitaxel and/or curcumin was determined by MTT assay as described earlier (Anto et al. 2002).

3.2.5 Drug Treatment

In all combination treatments, curcumin (5 μM) was added 2 h before adding paclitaxel (5 nM). Inhibitors of MAPKs and Akt were added 1 h before the addition of paclitaxel.

3.2.6 Stable Transfection

HeLa cells were stably transfected with IκBα DM-pcDNA3, Akt-DNpcDNA3, and Akt WT-pcDNA3 vector using the calcium phosphate transfection kit (Invitrogen) according to manufacturer's protocol. Stable clones were isolated using G418. Reverse Transcription Polymerase Chain Reaction (RT-PCR) – Total RNA isolated was reverse transcribed to cDNA using MMLV reverse transcriptase. The PCR products were resolved by electrophoresis.

3.2.7 Annexin V-Propidium Iodide Staining

The membrane flip-flop induced by paclitaxel and/or curcumin was assessed as described earlier (Anto et al. 2003) according to manufacturer's protocol.

3.2.8 Electrophoretic Mobility Shift Assay (EMSA)

Nuclear extract was isolated from cells after drug treatment and nuclear translocation of NF-κB and AP-1 was detected by EMSA and the specificity of the bands was confirmed by supershift and cold competition as described earlier (Anto et al. 2002; Amato et al. 1998). Nuclear extracts from tissue samples were prepared and EMSA was performed to evaluate DNA-binding activity of NF-κB or AP-1 as described elsewhere (Banerjee et al. 2002; Chaturvedi et al. 2000).

3.2.9 Immunocytochemical Analysis

For immunocytochemical localization of intracellular proteins, the cells were grown on glass cover slips and exposed to various concentrations of the drugs for the desired time. The cells were then washed with PBS, fixed with 4 % paraformaldehyde, permeabilized with 0.4 % Triton X-100 for 20 min at room temperature, and blocked with 3 % normal goat serum in PBS for 1 h. Antibody (anti-p65) diluted 1:100 in PBS containing 3 % normal goat serum was added to cover the cells and incubated overnight at 4 °C. Unbound antibody was washed off with PBS, and the cells were incubated with 2 μg/ml rhodamine-conjugated secondary antibody for 1 h at room temperature. The unbound secondary antibody was washed off and the cells were covered with 1 μg/ml 4′,6-diamidino-2-phenylindole (DAPI) for 10 min. The cover slips with cells were mounted in glycerol, examined, and photographed under a fluorescence microscope.

3.2.10 Animal Experiments

All animal studies were done in accordance with Institute Animal Ethics Committee-approved protocols. Murphy's string method (Hussain and Rao 1991; Murphy 1961) was followed for tumor induction in the uterine cervices of 6-week-old, virgin female *Swiss albino* mice. Carcinogen (∽600 μg)-impregnated cotton threads or similar cotton threads without carcinogen were inserted into the canal of the uterine cervix of *Swiss albino* mice. Tumor development was checked by palpation thrice a week, starting from the 15th day of tumor induction. After 30 days, the 3-MC-treated animals were randomized into four groups ($n = 12$) to yield even distribution of tumor sizes and control animals into two groups ($n = 12$), and drug administration was started the same day as indicated in Fig. 3.1a. Curcumin was encapsulated into a uni-lamellar liposome formulation containing phosphatidyl choline and cholesterol (Kuttan et al. 1985) and injected intraperitoneally on alternate days at the dose of 25 mg/kg body weight. Paclitaxel was dissolved in Cremophor vehicle (Cremophor EL/ethanol 1:1, diluted 1:4 with PBS) and injected i.p. at 10 mg/kg doses twice weekly. The control animals were injected with empty liposomes and/or Cremophor vehicle. The drug treatment was continued until the animals were sacrificed on the 120th day and the cervical tumors or the normal cervices were excised. Tumor volume was calculated as (length × width^2)/2.

The xenograft studies to evaluate the efficacy of paclitaxel and curcumin, either alone or in combination against human cervical cancer cells in vivo, were carried out in female, 6-week-old, nulliparous non-obese diabetic severe combined immunodeficient (NOD-SCID) mice. HeLa cells (5×10^6) were injected subcutaneously in the flank of a NOD-SCID female mouse, and after 4 weeks, when the xenograft tumor reached a volume of ∽2.5 cm^3, the tumor was excised, cut into small pieces (∽0.5 mm × 0.5 mm), and these tumor fragments were subcutaneously transplanted into the left flank of 24 NOD-SCID mice using an 11-gauge trocar. Six animals each were randomly assigned to four study cohorts including a positive control group where the animals were left untreated, a paclitaxel-alone group, a curcumin-alone group, and the combination group where the animals received both paclitaxel and curcumin. Drug administration was started when the tumors reached the volume of ∽50 mm^3. The route and dose of drug administration were exactly the same as that followed in the carcinogen-induced cervical tumor model in *Swiss albino* mice and continued up to 6 weeks, after which the animals were sacrificed and the tissue samples were collected for further analyses.

3.2.11 Histology and Immunohistochemistry

For histopathologic examination, 5 μm sections cut from the formalin-fixed, paraffin-embedded tissues were deparaffinized, rehydrated, stained with hematoxylin and eosin, and mounted with DPX. Immunolocalization of specific proteins in the tissue sections was done using the Iso-IHC kit (Biogenex) following manufacturer's instructions. Photomicrographs were captured using a Nikon Eclipse E600 microscope.

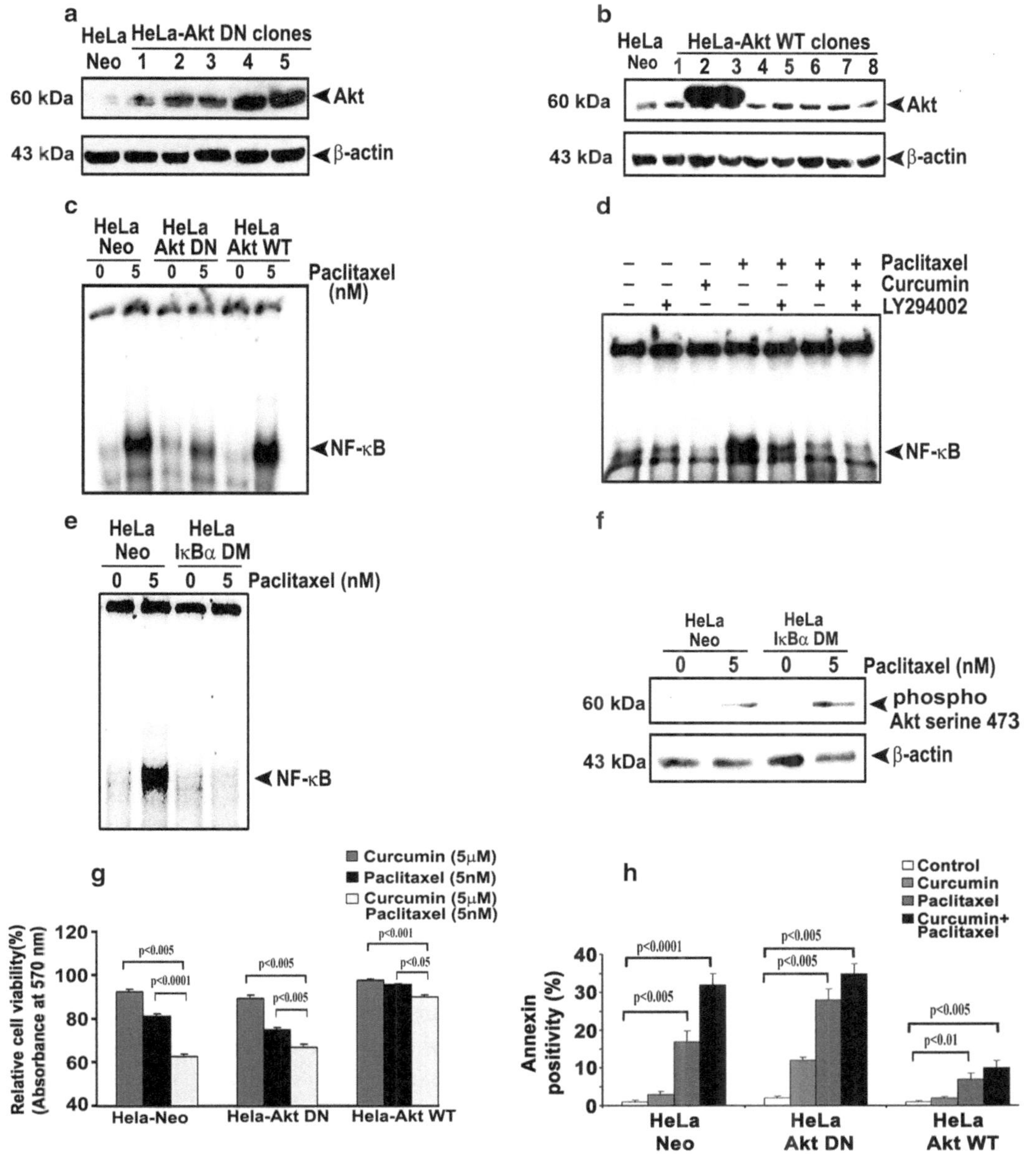

Fig. 3.1 *Dependence of NF-κB and Akt in paclitaxel-mediated signaling events and on the synergistic effect of paclitaxel and curcumin.* (**a-b**) HeLa cells were transfected with pcDNA3-vector or pcDNA3-AktDN or pcDNA3-Akt WT construct by calcium phosphate transfection method, G418-resistant clones were selected, and expression level of Akt was detected by Western blot. (**c**) HeLa-Neo, HeLa-AktDN, and HeLa-Akt WT cells were treated with paclitaxel for 1 h. Nuclear extracts were prepared and EMSA was done to detect NF-κB activation in response to paclitaxel. (**d**) HeLa cells pre-treated with curcumin or LY294002 (5 μM) were treated with paclitaxel for 1 h, nuclear extracts were prepared, and EMSA was done to study NF-κB status in response to paclitaxel treated with the Akt inhibitor, LY294002, and/or curcumin. (**e**) HeLa-Neo and Hela-IkBα DM cells were treated with paclitaxel for 1 h and nuclear extracts were prepared to do EMSA using γ-32P labeled NF-κB oligonucleotide. (**f**) HeLa-Neo and Hela-IkBα DM cells were treated with paclitaxel for 1 h whole cell lysates were prepared for immunoblotting against p-Akt serine 473. (**g**) HeLa-Neo, HeLa-Akt DN, and HeLa-Akt WT cells were treated with paclitaxel and/or curcumin as indicated, incubated for 72 h and the cell viability was assessed by MTT assay (**h**) HeLa cells were treated with paclitaxel and/or curcumin for 16 h and stained for Annexin V-PI positivity. Annexin V-positive cells in five different fields were counted, and the average was taken

3.2.12 RNA Extraction and Real-Time Q-PCR

Total RNA was extracted from tissue samples using TRIZOL reagent (Invitrogen Corporation). Five microgram of RNA was used for cDNA synthesis using MMLV reverse transcriptase and random hexamers (Promega). Real-time quantitative PCR analysis was performed on an ABI 7500 real-time PCR system (Applied Biosystems) with 2 μL of cDNA in a total reaction volume of 20 μL using the SYBR Green PCR mix (Eurogentec, Belgium). Fold change in expression levels between normal and other treatment groups was calculated relative to the endogenous gene β-actin using the 2-ΔΔCt method (Livak and Schmittgen 2001).

3.2.13 Annexin Staining

To identify phosphatidylserine externalization, cells were stained with FITC-conjugated Annexin V (Santa Cruz Biotechnology) according to the manufacturer's instructions followed by flow cytometry.

3.2.14 Terminal Deoxynucleotidyl Transferase-Mediated Nick End Labeling (TUNEL) Assay

TUNEL assay was performed to detect apoptosis in formalin-fixed, paraffin-embedded xenograft tumor tissue sections using DeadEnd™ Colorimetric TUNEL System (Promega) following manufacturer's instructions.

3.2.15 Statistical Analysis

Data are presented as mean ± SE of three independent experiments. Two-tailed Student's *t*-test was used for statistical analysis. *P* value <0.05 was considered statistically significant.

3.3 Results

3.3.1 NF-κB and Akt Act Sequentially in the Synergism of Paclitaxel and Curcumin, and Inactivation and Over-expression of Akt in HeLa Cells Lead to Partial Inhibition of the Synergistic Effect of Paclitaxel and Curcumin

Based on our earlier finding that NF-κB and Akt have a critical role in regulating the chemosensitization of HeLa cells by curcumin (Bava et al. 2005), we investigated whether these two important pathways work independently or concurrently in the synergism of paclitaxel and curcumin. To explore this, stable clones of DN Akt, WT Akt, and HeLa-Neo were developed.

Clones with maximum expression were selected for further studies (clone 5 in the case of DNAkt and clone 2 in the case of wild-type Akt) (Fig. 3.1a–b). Interestingly, compared to HeLa-Neo cells, paclitaxel-induced NF-κB DNA binding was much less in HeLa-Akt DN cells, while in HeLa-Akt WT cells it was much higher confirming that Akt mediates paclitaxel-induced NF-κB activation (Fig. 3.1c). It was noteworthy that inactivation of Akt either by transfection of DN Akt or by using the inhibitor LY294002 did not completely inhibit NF-κB DNA-binding ability by paclitaxel (Fig. 3.1d), indicating that paclitaxel-induced NF-κB activation is only partially regulated by Akt. Earlier studies from our laboratory have shown that paclitaxel activates NF-κB and Akt in HeLa cells, while curcumin down-regulates both of these (Bava et al. 2005). The extent of NF-κB inhibition by LY294002 was less than that of curcumin (Fig. 3.1d), suggesting that curcumin acts not only by inhibiting Akt but has other mediators through which it down-regulates NF-κB. Further, the pretreatment with LY294002 and then curcumin, synergistically reduced the paclitaxel-induced NF-κB activation (Fig. 3.1d). To examine whether NF-κB has any role in regulating the activation of Akt, we used HeLa-IkBα DM cells (Bava et al. 2005) and confirmed the activity of IkBα DM cells by EMSA (Fig. 3.1e). However, in these cells paclitaxel did not produce any difference in the phosphorylation status of Akt (Fig. 3.1f), thereby proving that paclitaxel-induced phosphorylation of Akt is independent of NF-κB.

While pretreatment with curcumin brought down the viability of paclitaxel-treated HeLa-Neo cells from 80 to 62 %, the synergistic effect was significantly reduced ($p < 0.0001$), though not completely inhibited in HeLa-Akt DN cells, even though the inactivation of Akt itself sensitized the cells to paclitaxel and curcumin (Fig. 3.1g). Moreover, the over-expression of WT Akt abolished the effect of paclitaxel and curcumin either alone or in combination (Fig. 3.1g). Over-expression of WT Akt increased the resistance to paclitaxel producing negligible synergistic effect with curcumin (Fig. 3.1g). It was remarkable to note that neither inhibition nor over-expression of Akt completely inhibited the synergistic effect of paclitaxel and curcumin, suggesting that Akt has only a partial role in regulating the synergism.

The apoptotic status of the cells was evaluated by Annexin V/PI staining. The results were in concordance with that of the MTT assay. In HeLa-Neo cells, synergism of paclitaxel and curcumin was evident (Fig. 3.1h). But when Akt was shut down, the synergistic effect was significantly reduced ($p < 0.005$) even though the inactivation of Akt itself sensitized the cells to paclitaxel- and curcumin-induced externalization of phosphatidylserine (Fig. 3.1h) highlighting the role of Akt in paclitaxel-induced signaling. Supporting this observation, Akt over-expression significantly inhibited paclitaxel-induced apoptosis ($p < 0.01$), which was not appreciably affected by curcumin (Fig. 3.1h).

3.3.2 COX-2 and Cyclin D1 Play Regulatory Roles in the Synergistic Effect of Paclitaxel and Curcumin in an NF-κB-Dependent Manner, and Among the IAPs that Play Regulatory Roles in the Synergistic Effect of Paclitaxel and Curcumin, Survivin Alone is Independent of NF-κB

As reported earlier (Aggarwal et al. 2005), we observed that paclitaxel induced the expression of COX-2, which is an immediate early gene regulated by NF-κB. In our study, we observed a down-regulation of paclitaxel-induced COX-2 expression by curcumin in HeLa cells both in the protein level (data not shown) as well as in the RNA level (Fig. 3.2a). We observed a complete inhibition of COX-2 expression in HeLa-IκBα DM cells (Fig. 3.2a) and a partial inhibition of the same in HeLa-Akt DN cells (Fig. 3.2a), whereas in the HeLa-Akt WT cells, COX-2 expression was found to be higher than that of HeLa-Neo cells (Fig. 3.2a). Collectively, these data indicate that paclitaxel-induced COX-2 expression is completely regulated by NF-κB and partly by Akt. It is also evident that paclitaxel can induce NF-κB independent of Akt confirming the hypothesis that NF-κB is the key regulator of paclitaxel-induced signaling events.

As several studies have reported that NF-κB is the key regulator of cyclin D1, we investigated whether cyclin D1 has any role in the synergism of paclitaxel and curcumin. We observed a significant down-regulation of paclitaxel-induced cyclin D1 expression by curcumin (Fig. 3.2b), and as expected, inactivation of NF-κB by transfection of IκBα DM completely inhibited the up-regulation of cyclin D1 expression by paclitaxel (Fig. 3.2b). However, the basal expression of cyclin D1 was significantly higher in IκBα DM cells compared to control.

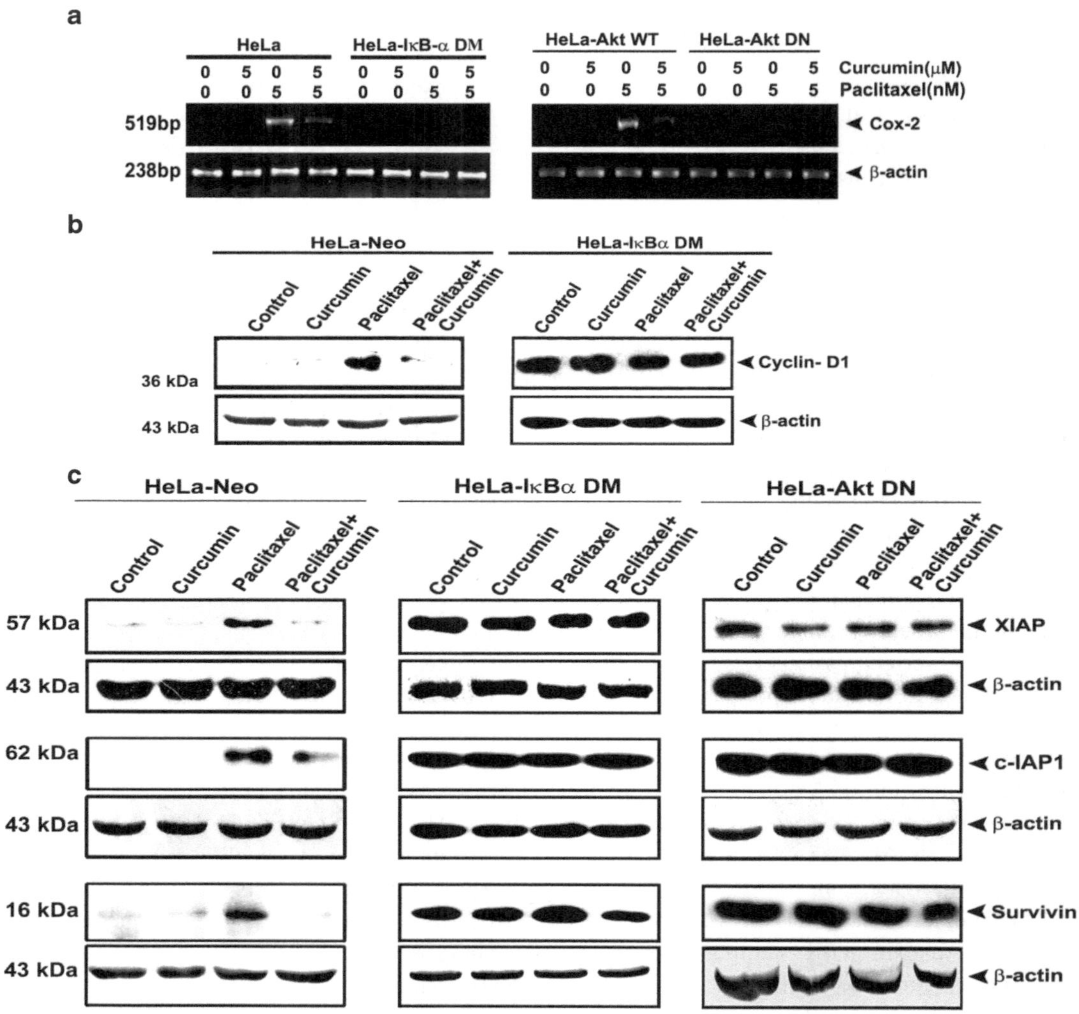

Fig. 3.2 *Regulatory role of NF-κB and Akt in paclitaxel-induced expression of COX-2, cyclin D1, and IAPs.* (**a**) HeLa, HeLa-IkBα DM, HeLa-Akt DN, and HeLa-Akt WT cells were treated with paclitaxel and/or curcumin for 24 h and total RNA was isolated. The RT-PCR products were then resolved by agarose gel electrophoresis. β-actin was used as the internal control. (**b**) HeLa and HeLa-IkBα DM cells were treated with paclitaxel and/or curcumin for 24 h and whole cell lysate was immunoblotted against anti-cyclin D1. β-actin was used as the internal control. (**c**) HeLa-Neo, HeLa-IkBα DM, and HeLa-Akt DN cells were treated with paclitaxel and/or curcumin for 24 h and the whole cell lysate was immunoblotted using antibodies against XIAP, c-IAP1, and survivin and detected by ECL. β-actin was used as the loading control

IAPs are a family of proteins that function as ubiquitin ligases and promote the degradation of caspases and are considered to be regulated by NF-κB. We observed that paclitaxel induced the up-regulation of XIAP, c-IAP1, and survivin in HeLa cells which are significantly down-regulated by curcumin (Fig. 3.2c). Another interesting observation was that the up-regulation of XIAP and c-IAP1 by paclitaxel was completely inhibited when NF-κB was shut down, while that of survivin remained unaffected (Fig. 3.2c). Though survivin is generally considered as an NF-κB-dependent gene, recent reports have clearly demonstrated regulation of survivin by PI3K/Akt pathway (Zhao et al. 2010). This made us to check the status of all the IAPs in response to paclitaxel in HeLa-Akt DN cells. Supporting the observation of Zhao et al. (2010), we observed a complete inhibition in the up-regulation of survivin as well as that of XIAP and c-IAP1 (Fig. 3.2c) indicating that paclitaxel-induced up-regulation of survivin is regulated by Akt in an NF-κB-independent manner. However, as in the case of cyclin D1, the basal expressions of all the IAPs were significantly higher in IκBα DM cells as well as Akt DN cells compared to control.

3.3.3 MAPKs and AP-1 Contribute to the Synergism of Curcumin and Paclitaxel in an NF-κB-Dependent Manner, While Bcl-2 Regulates the Synergism, Independent of NF-κB and Akt

We also investigated the involvement of MAPKs, another set of survival signals induced by lower concentrations of paclitaxel. Our study revealed a transient phosphorylation of ERK1/2, JNK, and p38 that started within 5 min of the paclitaxel treatment, peaked at 15 min, and then receded by 30 min (Fig. 3.3a). Interestingly, curcumin significantly reduced this phosphorylation of MAPKs, signifying a possible role for MAPKs in regulating the synergism (Fig. 3.3b). Further, we also evaluated the role of NF-κB in paclitaxel-induced phosphorylation of MAPKs. Interestingly, we found that inhibition of NF-κB pathway by IκBα-DM transfection completely inhibited the phosphorylation of all the three MAPKs by paclitaxel (Fig. 3.3c) clearly indicating that NF-κB is regulating the phosphorylation of MAPK pathway by paclitaxel.

AP-1 transcription factors are complexes of DNA-binding proteins made up of homodimers of Jun family members or heterodimers of Jun and Fos family members. We observed a dose-dependent increase in the DNA-binding activity of AP-1 in response to paclitaxel in HeLa cells (data not shown). It was also found that pretreatment with curcumin significantly down-regulated the AP-1 activation induced by paclitaxel (Fig. 3.3d). We also examined whether ERK1/2, JNK, or p38 phosphorylation in response to paclitaxel contributes to the activation of AP-1 by treating HeLa cells with paclitaxel and/or U0126 (10 μM), SP600125 (50 μM), and SB203580 (40 μM) which are inhibitors of ERK1/2, JNK, and p38, respectively. As expected the inhibitors of all the MAPKs especially that of p38 and JNK significantly inhibited the AP-1 DNA-binding activity induced by the paclitaxel, suggesting the involvement of ERK1/2, JNK, and p38 in the activation of AP-1 induced by paclitaxel (Fig. 3.3e). Hence, the study demonstrates that the partial down-regulation of the AP-1 DNA binding by curcumin may be due to the inhibition of these MAPKs which acts up-stream of AP-1.

We also explored whether ERK1/2, p38, and JNK can regulate the NF-κB signaling events induced by paclitaxel. It was noteworthy that none of the inhibitors produced a significant downregulation to paclitaxel-induced NF-κB activation (Fig. 3.3f), strongly correlating with our previous observation that NF-κB is up-stream of MAPK pathway in the regulation of paclitaxel signaling.

Deregulated expression of the antiapoptotic protein Bcl-2 plays an important role in cell death as well as in the nonsensitiveness of cancer cells to chemotherapy. Several studies have demonstrated that NF-κB and Akt have regulatory roles in endogenous Bcl-2 protein expression. We observed a dose-dependent up-regulation of Bcl-2 protein by paclitaxel in HeLa cells (data not shown), which was significantly abrogated by curcumin (Fig. 3.3g). However, we observed up-regulation of Bcl-2 protein in HeLa-IκBα DM as well as HeLa-Akt DN cells, indicating that paclitaxel is inducing Bcl-2 in HeLa cells independent of NF-κB as well as Akt (Fig. 3.3g).

3.3.4 Curcumin Potentiates the Antitumor Effects of Paclitaxel in 3-MC-Induced Cervical Tumors in Mice

The schematic representation of various groups employed in the study is depicted in Fig. 3.4A.

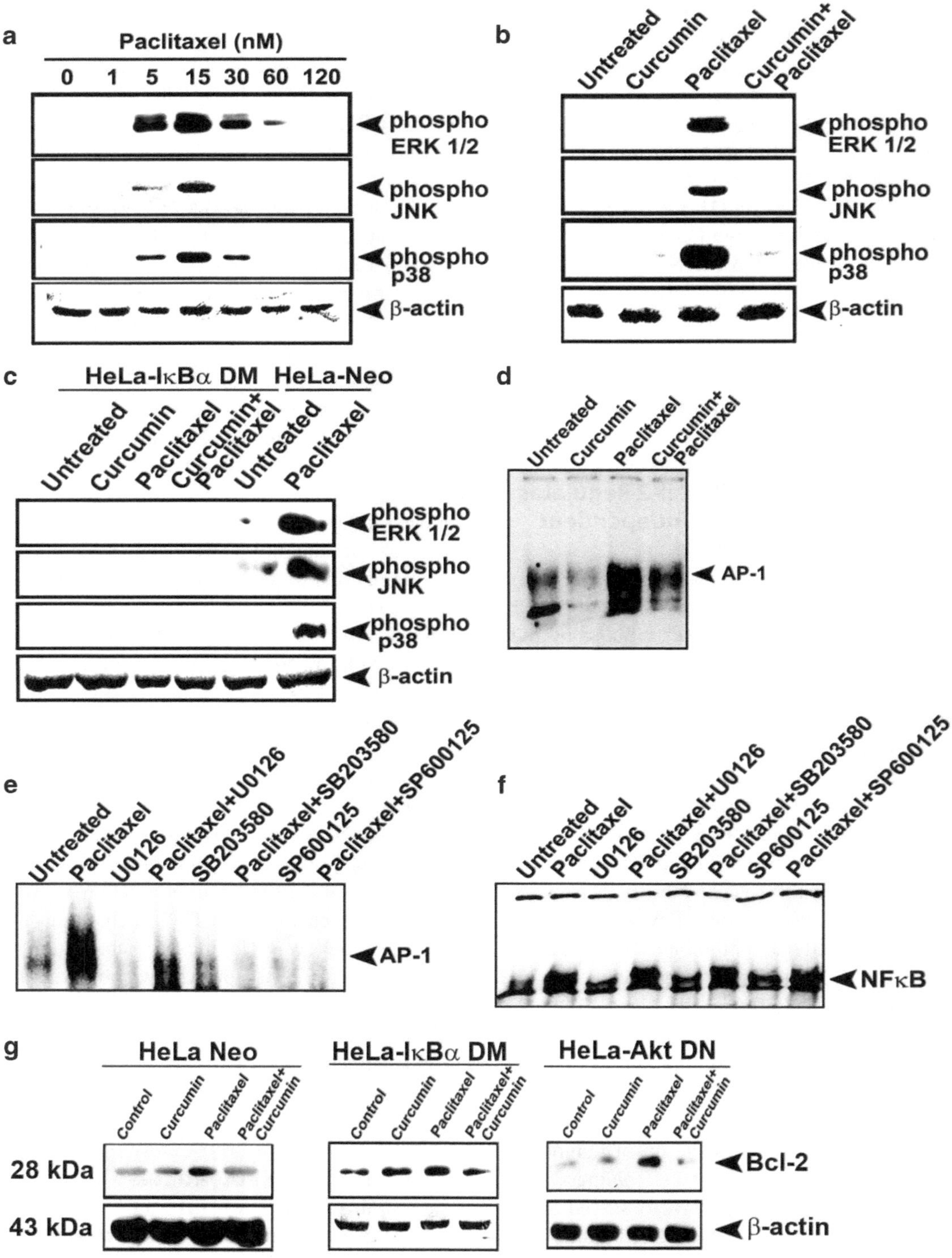
a
Paclitaxel (nM)
0 1 5 15 30 60 120
phospho ERK 1/2
phospho JNK
phospho p38
β-actin
b
Untreated
Curcumin
Paclitaxel
Curcumin+ Paclitaxel
phospho ERK 1/2
phospho JNK
phospho p38
β-actin
c
HeLa-IκBα DM
HeLa-Neo
Untreated
Curcumin
Paclitaxel
Curcumin+ Paclitaxel
Untreated
Paclitaxel
phospho ERK 1/2
phospho JNK
phospho p38
β-actin
d
Untreated
Curcumin
Paclitaxel
Curcumin+ Paclitaxel
AP-1
e
Untreated
Paclitaxel
U0126
Paclitaxel+U0126
SB203580
Paclitaxel+SB203580
SP600125
Paclitaxel+SP600125
AP-1
f
Untreated
Paclitaxel
U0126
Paclitaxel+U0126
SB203580
Paclitaxel+SB203580
SP600125
Paclitaxel+SP600125
NFκB
g
HeLa Neo
HeLa-IκBα DM
HeLa-Akt DN
Control
Curcumin
Paclitaxel
Paclitaxel+ Curcumin
28 kDa
43 kDa
Bcl-2
β-actin

Following tumor induction with 3-MC, palpable tumors began to appear within 20–25 days. Tumors developed in the group I and curcumin-alone-treated group III animals continued to grow during the span of the experiment and reached the maximum volume up to 5,500 mm^3, whereas >60 % of the tumors in the paclitaxel-alone group and >85 % of the combination-treated tumors did not grow beyond a volume of ~3,200 mm^3. The final tumor incidence percentage (Fig. 3.4B) and the mean tumor volume (Fig. 3.4C) among different groups were determined after sacrificing the animals on day 120. In group I, 66 % of the animals treated with 3-MC (positive control) developed tumors with a mean tumor volume of 1,613 mm^3. In group II and group III, where the animals received either paclitaxel or curcumin, respectively, the tumor incidence percentages were 44 and 60, and the mean tumor volume among these groups were 965 and 1,294 mm^3, respectively. Mice of group IV, which received both paclitaxel and curcumin, showed a tumor incidence of only 24 %, and the mean tumor volume was reduced to 656 mm^3. None of the animals from group V and group VI (negative controls) show any signs of tumor development during the span of the study. Moreover, 3-MC treatment or administration of paclitaxel and/or curcumin had no adverse effects on the tumor-bearing animals or normal controls (group VI) as assessed by body weight observation and liver function tests (data not shown). Microscopic analysis of the formalin-fixed paraffin-embedded tissue sections showed different grades of squamous cell carcinoma, and this observation was verified by a histopathologist. Representative photomicrographs of H&E-stained tissue sections showing 3-MC-induced multi-stage squamous cell carcinogenesis are given in Fig. 3.4D.

3.3.5 Curcumin Inhibits Constitutively Active and Paclitaxel-Induced NF-κB in 3-MC-Induced Cervical Tumors and Down-regulates the Transcription of NF-κB Target Genes

Since most of the carcinogens and infectious agents linked with cancer have been shown to activate the NF-κB pathway, we investigated whether NF-κB is associated with 3-MC-induced cervical tumorigenesis. While constitutive activation of NF-κB and higher levels of nuclear DNA-binding activity were observed in 3-MC-induced cervical tumors and 3-MC+ paclitaxel-treated animals, administration of curcumin abolished the constitutively activated as well as paclitaxel-induced NF-κB. Incubation of DNA-protein complexes with p65 antibody resulted in the supershift of active band (Fig. 3.5A). To further confirm the activation of NF-κB by 3-MC and paclitaxel, we examined the NF-κB DNA-binding activity in 10 tissue samples each from the six

Fig. 3.3 *Involvement of MAPK Pathway and Bcl-2 in regulating the synergism of paclitaxel and curcumin.* (**a**) Kinetics of paclitaxel-induced phosphorylation of MAPKs-ERK1/2, JNK, and p38 in HeLa cells were studied by treating them with paclitaxel for different time intervals (0–120 min). The whole cell lysate was immunoblotted against phospho-ERK1/2, phospho-JNK, and phospho-p38 antibodies and detected by ECL. β-actin was used as the loading control. (**b**) The effect of curcumin on phosphorylation of MAPKs was detected by pretreating HeLa cells with curcumin and then with paclitaxel for 15 min and immunoblotting the whole cell lysate against phospho-ERK1/2, phospho-JNK, and phospho-p38 antibodies. (**c**) HeLa-IkBα DM cells were treated with paclitaxel and/or curcumin for 15 min and the whole cell lysate was immunoblotted against phospho-ERK1/2, phospho-JNK, and phospho-p38 antibodies. HeLa-Neo cells treated with and without paclitaxel were used as controls. (**d**) HeLa cells were pretreated with curcumin and then with paclitaxel (5nM) for 30 min, nuclear extracts were prepared, and EMSA was done to study the effect of curcumin on activation of AP-1. The arrowhead shown indicates the position of the active DNA-binding complex of AP-1. (**e–f**) HeLa cells pretreated with U0126 (10 μM), SP600125 (50 μM), or SB203580 (40 μM) were treated with paclitaxel for 30 min. Nuclear extracts were prepared and EMSA was done using radiolabeled AP-1 primer to detect the AP-1 status and radiolabeled NF-κB primer to detect the NF-κB status. (**g**) HeLa-Neo, HeLa-IkBα DM, and HeLa-Akt DN cells were treated with paclitaxel and/or curcumin for 24 h and the whole cell lysate was immunoblotted against Bcl-2 antibody

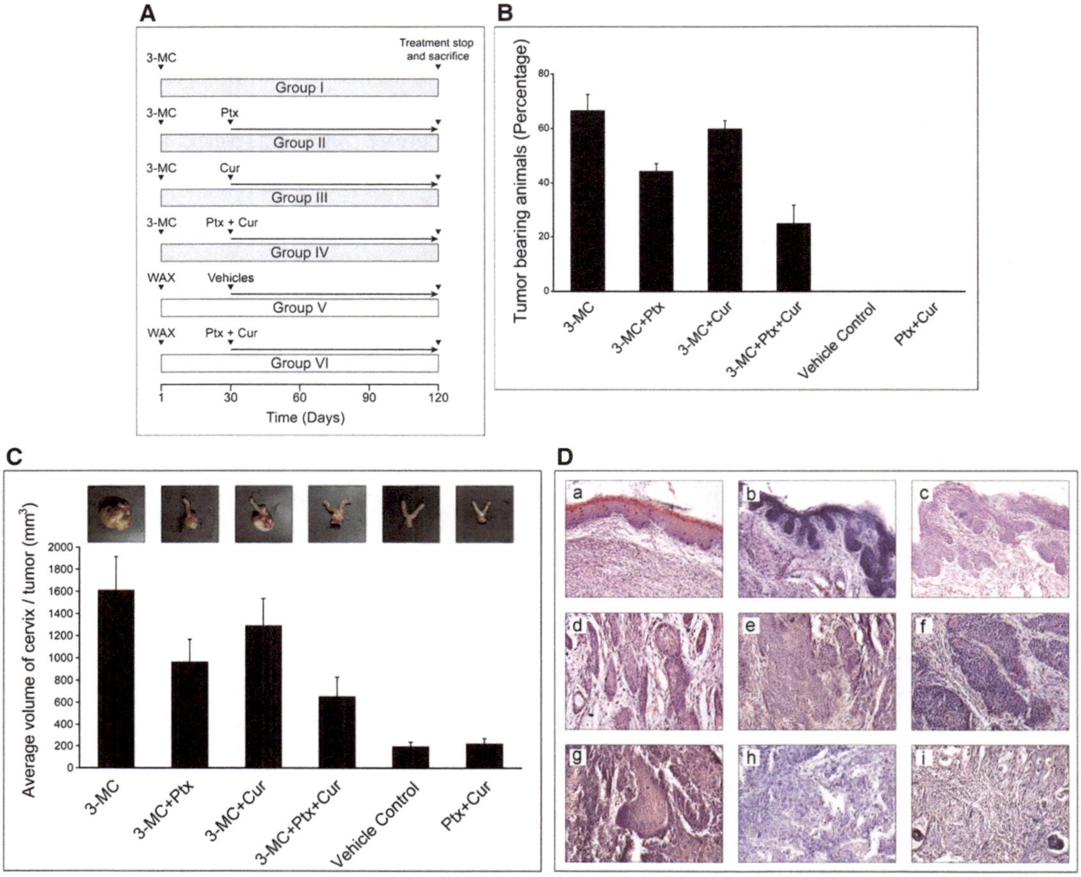

Fig. 3.4 *Combination of paclitaxel and curcumin reduces tumor incidence and tumor volume in cervical tumor model.* (**A**) Schematic representation of experimental protocols for evaluating the anticancer properties of paclitaxel and curcumin against 3-MC-induced carcinogenesis in *Swiss albino* mice. (**B**) Effect of paclitaxel and curcumin, alone or in combination, on 3-MC-induced cervical tumors. The tumors were distinguished from normal cervices based on size as well as histopathology, and the percentage of tumor-bearing animals per group is shown. Data represents three sets of experiments carried out independently. (**C**) The mean tumor volume and representative photographs of cervix samples from different experimental groups are shown. (**D**) Histological changes induced by 3-MC treatment in the cervical epithelium of *Swiss albino* mice. Formalin-fixed, paraffin-embedded tissue sections were stained with hematoxylin and eosin. The representative photomicrographs show progressive stages of squamous cell carcinoma. The panels depict (**a**) normal epithelium, (**b–c**) squamous hyperplasia, (**d–f**) dysplastic epithelium, and (**g–i**) SCC with characteristic keratin pearl formation

experimental groups. But in a few (<10 %) of the tumor-bearing mice, curcumin was unable to inhibit the NF-κB activity, probably because of the need for a higher dose or any genetic variability among animals (Fig. 3.5B). Immunohistochemical analysis of tissue samples harvested from 3-MC-alone and 3-MC+ paclitaxel-treated animals revealed increased expression and prominent nuclear localization of the p65 subunit of NF-κB in comparison with normal cervical epithelium (Fig. 3.5C). Consistent with the results obtained from EMSA, curcumin could down-regulate the expression and nuclear localization of p65 in tissue samples derived from curcumin and curcumin + paclitaxel-treated mice. Having established the association between NF-κB activation and 3-MC-induced tumor progression, we analyzed the functional status of NF-κB activation by assessing the mRNA expression levels of NF-κB target genes such as COX-2, cyclin D1, ICAM-1, VEGF, MMP-2, and MMP-9 by real-time quantitative RT-PCR. Tissue samples from groups I and II showed high mRNA expression levels of these genes, whereas low levels were detected in the tumor samples collected from animals treated with curcumin either alone or in combination with paclitaxel (Fig. 3.5D). Curcumin in combination with paclitaxel could not down-regulate the transactivation of these target genes in a few of the highly aggressive cervical tumors (indicated with "*").

3.3.6 Curcumin Represses NF-κB-Dependent Gene Products, Potentiates the Antiproliferative Effect of Paclitaxel, and Enhances Paclitaxel-Induced Caspase Activation

Western blot analyses revealed that paclitaxel either further induced or did not down-regulate 3-MC-induced activity of various NF-κB-regulated gene products COX-2, cyclin D1, MMP-2, MMP-9, and VEGF that are directly involved in tumor cell proliferation, angiogenesis, and metastasis (Fig. 3.6A). Immunohistochemical analysis for the cell proliferation marker PCNA in the tissue samples revealed that curcumin significantly enhanced paclitaxel-induced inhibition of proliferation as evidenced by reduced PCNA immunoreactivity compared with the positive control group (Fig. 3.6B). Diverse antiapoptotic proteins such as Bcl-2, c-IAP1, survivin, and XIAP which are reported to be transactivated by NF-κB were also found to be up-regulated in most of the tumor samples collected from 3-MC-alone and 3-MC+paclitaxel groups (Fig. 3.6C). The expression levels of these molecules were significantly down-regulated by curcumin. We also observed the cleavage and activation of procaspases 8, 9, 3, and 7 in paclitaxel-treated cervical tumors of mice, which was significantly up-regulated when curcumin was co-administered (Fig. 3.6D).

3.3.7 Curcumin-Mediated Augmentation of Antitumor Effects of Paclitaxel in 3-MC-Induced Cervical Tumors Involves the Down-regulation of MDR1, Akt, MAPK, and AP-1 Pathways

3-MC-induced tumors as well as those treated with paclitaxel exhibited a strong over-expression of MDR1, which was significantly down-regulated by curcumin (Fig. 3.7a). Immunoblotting with a phospho-specific antibody against Akt at Ser473 points toward the hyperactivation of Akt by phosphorylation in 3-MC-induced tumors compared to normal controls. More interestingly, the animals that were administered with curcumin either alone or in combination with paclitaxel showed relatively low levels of phospho-Akt in comparison with the carcinogen-alone- or paclitaxel-treated groups. But, over-expression and hyperactivation of Akt was observed in well-developed tumors from curcumin-treated animals (Fig. 3.7b). We also found hyperphosphorylation at Ser136 of Bad, a well-known direct target of phosphorylation and inactivation by Akt, indicating a possible antiapoptotic effect of activated Akt. The expression and activation status of the three important MAP kinases – extracellular signal-regulated protein kinase (ERK), c-Jun-NH2 kinase (JNK), and p38 – were analyzed by Western blotting, and extensively high phosphorylation of ERK-1/2 and JNK was observed in most of the 3-MC-induced tumor samples when compared to normal controls. Paclitaxel treatment alone did not alter the phosphorylation levels of ERK-1/2 and JNK in the tumor tissues, whereas administration of curcumin, alone or in combination with paclitaxel, inhibited the phosphorylation of these molecules significantly. On the other hand, the phosphorylation and expression status of p38 was not found to significantly vary among the experimental groups, indicating a lesser role of p38 in mediating the carcinogenic action of 3-MC as well as in the chemotherapeutic action of paclitaxel and curcumin (Fig. 3.7c) though we observed a

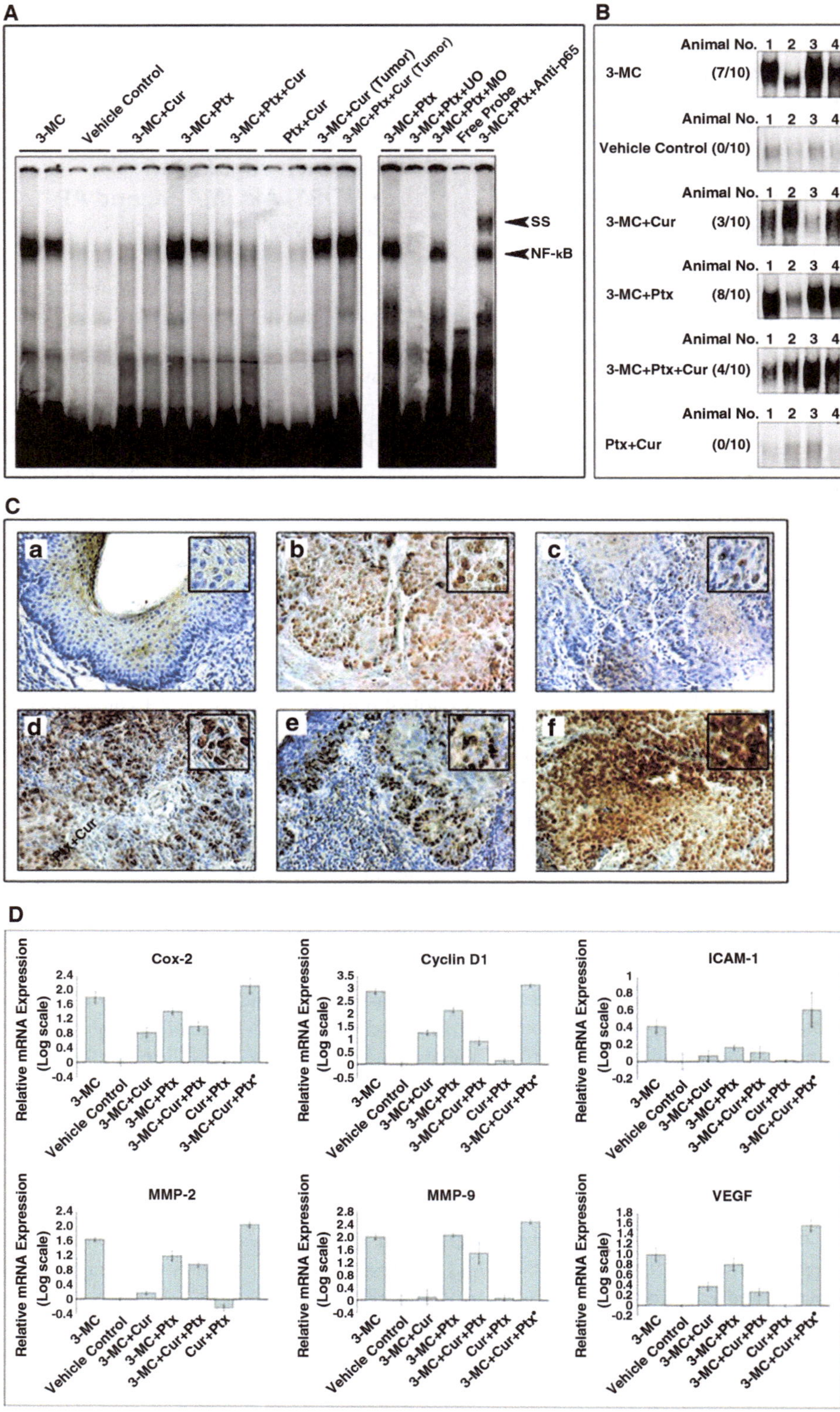
A
3-MC
Vehicle Control
3-MC+Cur
3-MC+Ptx
3-MC+Ptx+Cur
Ptx+Cur
3-MC+Cur (Tumor)
3-MC+Ptx+Cur (Tumor)
3-MC+Ptx
3-MC+Ptx+UO
3-MC+Ptx+MO
Free Probe
3-MC+Ptx+Anti-p65
SS
NF-κB
B
Animal No. 1 2 3 4 5 6 7 8 9 10
3-MC (7/10)
Vehicle Control (0/10)
3-MC+Cur (3/10)
3-MC+Ptx (8/10)
3-MC+Ptx+Cur (4/10)
Ptx+Cur (0/10)
C
a
b
c
d
e
f
D
Cox-2
Cyclin D1
ICAM-1
MMP-2
MMP-9
VEGF
Relative mRNA Expression (Log scale)
3-MC
Vehicle Control
3-MC+Cur
3-MC+Ptx
3-MC+Cur+Ptx
Cur+Ptx
3-MC+Cur+Ptx*

downregulation of paclitaxel-induced activation of p38 by curcumin in the human cervical cancer cell line, HeLa (Fig. 3.3b). The expression of phospho-c-Jun, a proto-oncogene which is the direct target of both JNK and ERK-1/2, and the central component of all activator protein-1 (AP-1) complexes, was found elevated in those samples with high levels of phospho-JNK and phospho-ERK1/2 (Fig. 3.7c). Moreover, the significantly higher levels of nuclear DNA-binding activity of AP-1 detected in 3-MC-induced tumor samples were suppressed by curcumin alone or in combination with paclitaxel (Fig. 3.7d).

3.3.8 Combined Treatment of Paclitaxel and Curcumin Decreases the Tumor Volume, Down-regulates NF-κB, and Enhances Apoptosis in Human Cervical Cancer Xenografts Compared to Individual Treatments, in NOD-SCID Mice

The mean tumor volume at the time of necropsy in the untreated control group was 2.66 cm^3, and administration of curcumin alone did not show any significant effect on the xenograft tumor growth, and the mean tumor volume was 2.47 cm^3. Paclitaxel treatment alone suppressed the growth of HeLa xenograft tumors and reduced the final mean tumor volume to 1.83 cm^3, whereas curcumin considerably enhanced the antitumor activity of paclitaxel, and the remarkable synergistic antitumor efficacy of these compounds resulted in a mean tumor volume of 1.32 cm^3 at the time of necropsy (Fig. 3.8a, b). Nuclear extracts prepared using tumor samples were used for electrophoretic mobility shift assay, and higher NF-κB activation levels were observed in the untreated tumors while paclitaxel treatment resulted in a further up-regulation of NF-κB activation levels. On the contrary, curcumin treatment either alone or in combination with paclitaxel significantly down-regulated the nuclear DNA-binding activity of NF-κB, in vivo (Fig. 3.8c). These results confirmed that suppression of paclitaxel-induced NF-κB activation by curcumin is an important molecular mechanism by which this compound sensitizes HeLa xenograft tumors in NOD-SCID mice to paclitaxel therapy. The in vivo apoptotic effects of curcumin and/or paclitaxel in ectopically implanted human cervical cancer xenografts in NOD-SCID mice were assessed by TUNEL staining. As shown in Fig. 3.8d, tumor sections from control and curcumin-alone-treated groups did not show any considerable positivity for apoptotic cells, while paclitaxel-treated samples showed substantial amount of TUNEL staining. More interestingly, in tumor samples collected from animals treated with both the agents, curcumin could significantly enhance the apoptotic effects of paclitaxel in comparison with the individual treatment.

3.4 Discussion

Tumor cells often escape apoptosis by overexpressing antiapoptotic proteins which give them survival advantage (Gagnon et al. 2008). Some conventional chemotherapeutic drugs in

Fig. 3.5 *Curcumin reduces the activation of NF-κB and its downstream targets induced by paclitaxel and 3-MC.* (**A**) Individual and combined effects of paclitaxel and curcumin on NF-κB activation in 3-MC-induced cervical tumors and normal controls are shown. Equal concentrations of nuclear extracts prepared from tissue samples were analyzed by EMSA. Supershift analysis using anti-p65 antibody is also done as described in "Materials and Methods." (**B**) EMSA results showing NF-κB activation status in ten different animals from each of the six experimental groups. (**C**) Immunohistochemical localization of the p65 subunit of NF-κB in the tissue sections correlates with EMSA results. The different panels indicate (**a**) the cytoplasmic localization of p65 in normal cervical epithelium, increased nuclear localization of p65 in (**b**) 3-MC-alone-treated (**c**) or 3-MC+paclitaxel-treated groups, inhibition of nuclear translocation of p65 in (**d**) 3-MC+curcumin or in (**e**) 3-MC+paclitaxel+curcumin, and (**f**) a highly aggressive tumor from paclitaxel+curcumin group shows strong nuclear positivity for p65. (**D**) Effect of paclitaxel and/or curcumin on transactivation of NF-κB-dependent genes in 3MC-induced cervical tumors and control tissues. Relative mRNA expression levels of target genes were determined by quantitative RT-PCR

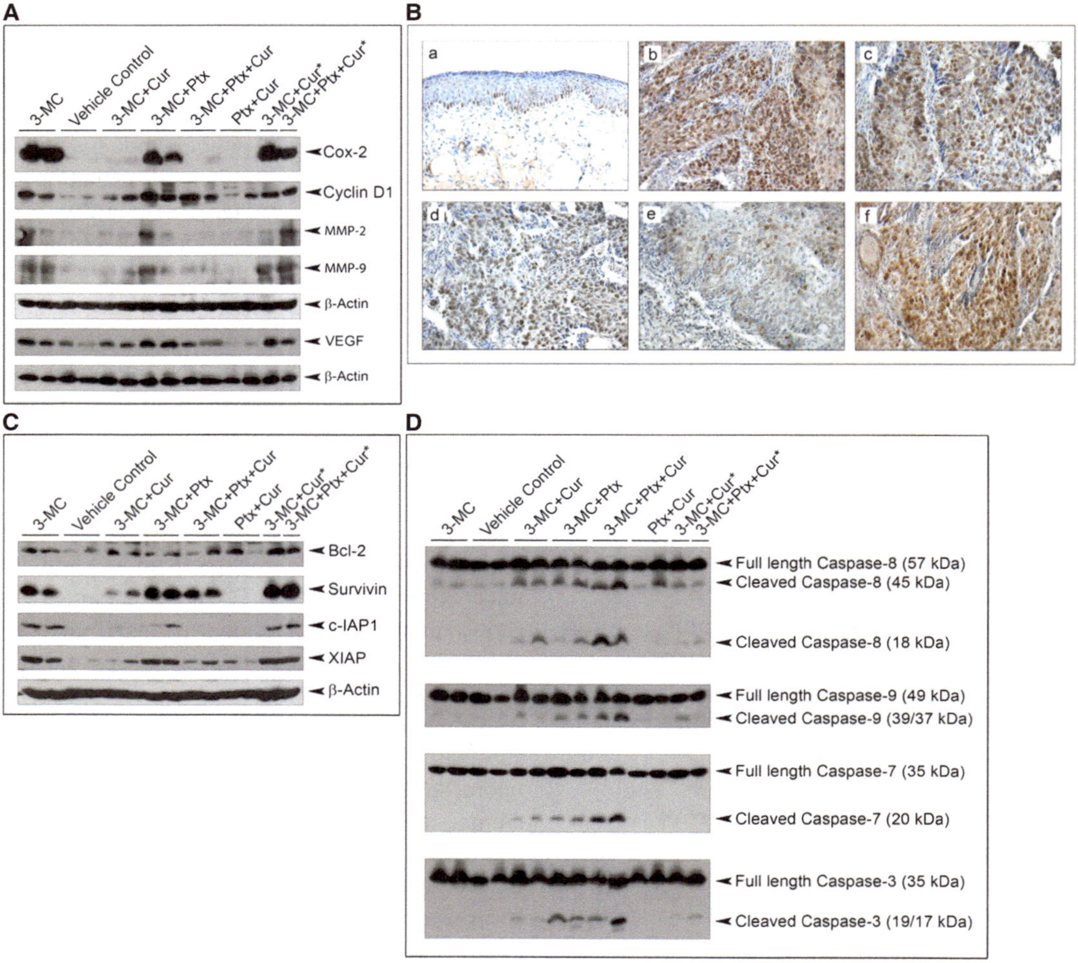

Fig. 3.6 *Curcumin inhibits NF-κB-dependent genes and the proliferative effect of paclitaxel and augments paclitaxel-induced caspase activation.* (**A**) Western blot analysis for different NF-κB-regulated gene products in 3-MC-induced tumors or control tissue samples harvested from mice of different treatment groups. At least six samples per group were analyzed, and representative data of two randomly selected animals from each group is shown. (**B**) Immunohistochemical analysis on tissue sections using PCNA antibody. Representative staining patterns in mouse cervical epithelium of (**a**) normal control, (**b**) 3-MC-treated, (**c**) 3-MC+Cur-treated, (**d**) 3-MC+Ptx-treated, (**e**) 3-MC+Cur+Ptx-treated, and (**f**) a very aggressive tumor from 3-MC+Cur+Ptx-treated group are shown. (**C**) Effect of curcumin and/or paclitaxel on the expression levels of various NF-κB-regulated antiapoptotic proteins in 3-MC-induced cervical tumors was detected by Western blotting. (**D**) Western blots showing curcumin-mediated enhancement of paclitaxel-induced caspase activation in the tumor tissue samples

low concentrations cause up-regulation of survival signals, thereby necessitating increment of the effective dose of treatment. Several studies including ours have shown that paclitaxel activates NF-κB and Akt, which have critical roles in regulating cell survival, proliferation, invasion, and metastasis (Huang and Fan 2002; Bava et al. 2005). On the contrary, curcumin, the natural polyphenolic compound, promotes apoptosis by interfering in various cell survival signaling pathways including NF-κB and Akt (Anto et al. 2002; Aggarwal et al. 2006). Our earlier findings (Bava et al. 2005) have clearly shown that paclitaxel-induced activation of NF-κB and

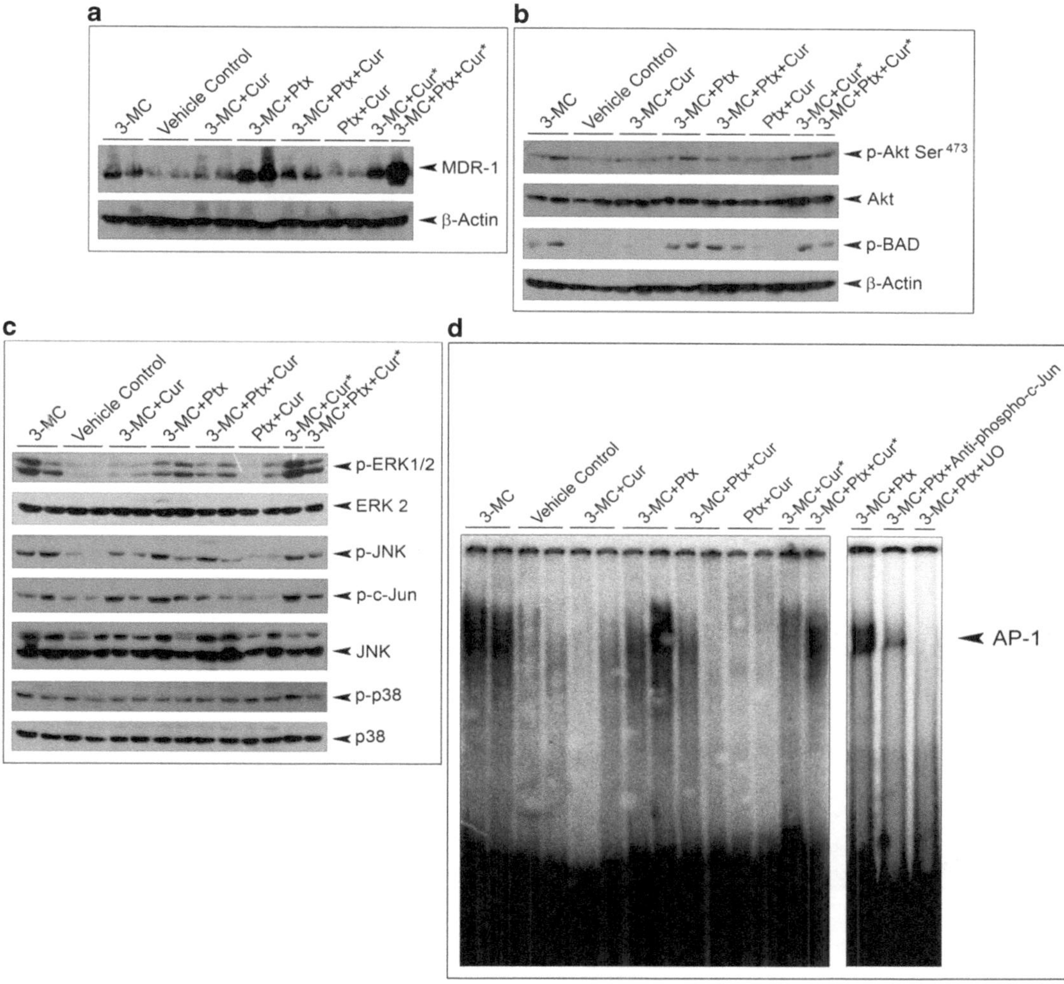

Fig. 3.7 *Curcumin enhances paclitaxel-induced chemotherapy by downregulating Akt, MAPK, and AP-1 pathways in 3-MC-induced cervical tumors*. (**a**) Expression of MDR-1 protein in tissue samples collected from different experimental groups. Western blot analysis was carried out with anti-MDR-1 and β-actin levels are shown as loading control. (**b**) Down-regulation of Akt activation in 3-MC-induced cervical tumors by curcumin. Western blot analyses were performed with anti-phospho-Akt, anti-Akt, and anti-phospho-Bad on tissue lysates. (**c**) Inhibition of MAPK phosphorylation by curcumin in 3-MC-induced tumors. Activation status of various MAPKs in tissue samples was detected by Western blotting using phosphorylation-specific antibodies against ERK1/2, JNK, phospho-c-jun, and p38. The expression levels of total MAPKs are shown as loading control. (**d**) 3-MC-induced cervical carcinogenesis in mice is associated with constitutive activation of AP-1. Curcumin inhibits the constitutive activation of AP-1 when given alone or along with paclitaxel. Nuclear extracts prepared from tumor or control tissue samples were assayed for AP-1 activation by EMSA. The *arrowhead* denotes active AP-1-DNA complex

Akt in HeLa cells involves phosphorylation of IKK, and its down-regulation by curcumin which contributes to the sensitization of HeLa cells to the paclitaxel-induced apoptosis involves inhibition of the same. Here we have tried to dissect out the pathways contributing to the synergism of paclitaxel and curcumin.

In the current study, we observed a significant down-regulation of paclitaxel-induced NF-κB activation upon Akt inactivation. While

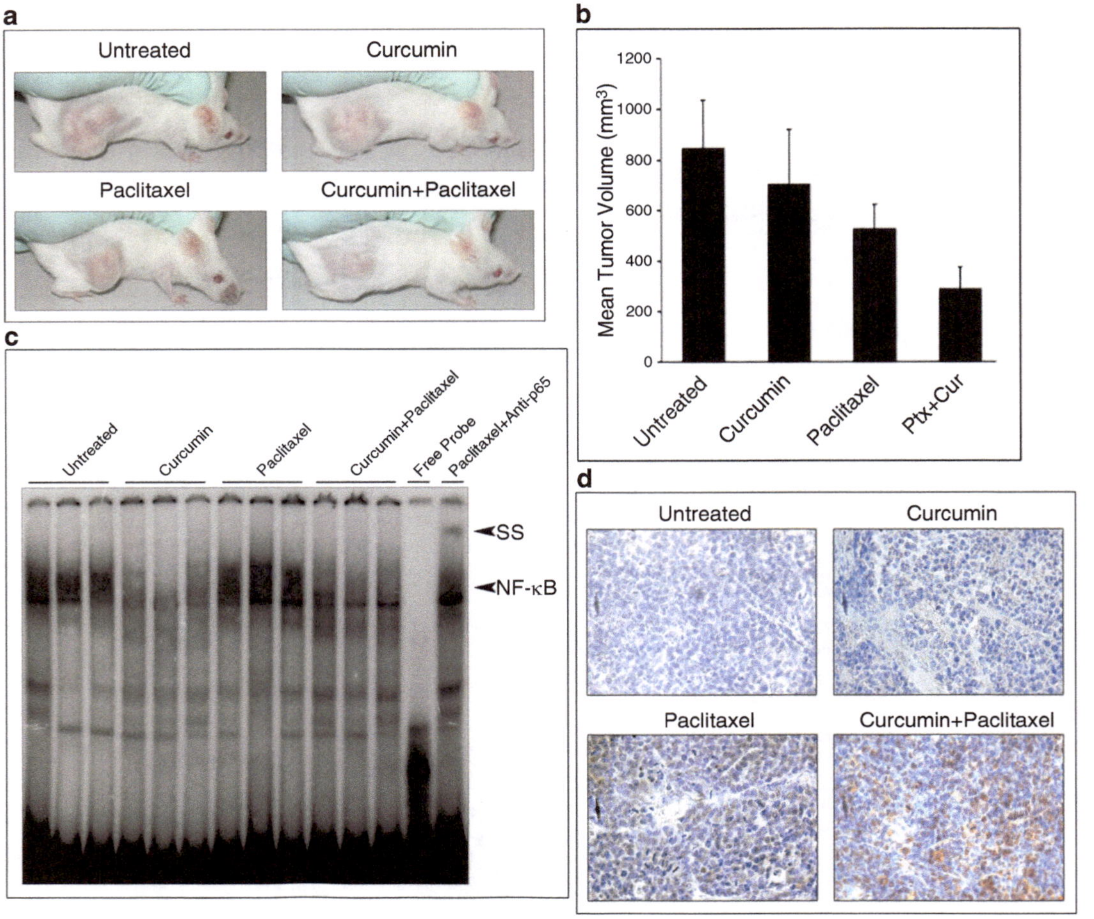

Fig. 3.8 *Curcumin enhances the antitumor activity of paclitaxel against human cervical cancer xenografts in NOD-SCID mice*. (**a**) Representative gross images of mice bearing subcutaneous tumors with or without drug treatment after 6 weeks. (**b**) The mean tumor volumes in different treatment groups after 6 weeks of drug treatment. Individual tumor volume was calculated by the standard formula $a \times b2/2$, where a is the longest diameter and b is the shortest diameter. Data is represented as mean tumor volume + standard error ($P < 0.05$). (**c**) Effect of curcumin treatment, alone or in combination with paclitaxel, on NF-κB activation in HeLa xenograft tumors in SCID mice. Equal concentrations of nuclear extracts prepared from tumor samples or normal controls were analyzed by EMSA as described under "Materials and Methods." Tumor samples from five animals per group were analyzed individually and representative data from three randomly selected tumors from each group is shown. (**d**) Representative photomicrographs showing TUNEL staining pattern in formalin-fixed, paraffin-embedded xenograft tumor sections from different treatment groups. Dark brown staining is indicative of nuclei with fragmented DNA. Cell nuclei were counterstained with hematoxylin. *NOTE*: All error bars indicate standard deviation between three independent experiments

over-expression of Akt resulted in an increase in paclitaxel-mediated NF-κB activation, no change in Akt activation was observed when NF-κB was shut down, clearly indicating that Akt is up-stream of NF-κB in the paclitaxel-mediated signaling events in HeLa cells. Furthermore, analysis of paclitaxel-induced COX-2 expression in the HeLa-Akt WT cells and the HeLa-Akt DN cells shows that the expression of COX-2, an NF-κB-dependent gene, is also regulated by Akt. While inactivation of Akt reduced COX-2 expression, over-expression of Akt resulted in the up-regulation of COX-2. Supporting this observation, a reduction in the synergistic effect of paclitaxel and curcumin was noted in the cell viability and apoptotic studies using the Akt DN-transfected HeLa cells. Over-expression of Akt made the cells resistant to paclitaxel as well as to the synergistic effect. Up-regulation of cyclin D1, another NF-κB-dependent gene, was also completely inhibited when NF-κB was shut down, implicating the key regulatory role of NF-κB in paclitaxel signaling.

Interestingly a marked difference was noted in the synergism in the case of HeLa-Akt DN and HeLa-IκBα DM cells. While a complete inhibition in synergism was observed in the case of HeLa-IκBα DM cells, only partial inhibition was noted in HeLa-Akt DN cells suggesting that inhibition of Akt by curcumin is not the only pathway by which curcumin inhibits NF-κB.

While expression of XIAP and c-IAP1 was dependent on NF-κB, that of survivin was independent though curcumin effectively down-regulated paclitaxel-induced expression of all these. However, we observed a complete inhibition of survivin up-regulation in HeLa-Akt DN cells confirming that Akt is regulating survivin signaling independent of NF-κB as observed by other investigators (Zhao et al. 2010; Zhu et al. 2008). Our study also indicates that paclitaxel-mediated up-regulation of Bcl-2 is independent of NF-κB and Akt even though contradictory reports exist (Catz and Johnson 2003).

Paclitaxel-induced activation of MAPK signaling pathway is already reported (Bacus et al. 2001). Among these three kinases, ERK1/2 module has most often been implicated in cell proliferation (Cobb 1999) while the biological effects of JNK and p38 activation are highly conflicting and, depending on the cellular context and stimuli, they exert both protective as well as proapoptotic functions (Lee et al. 1998; Seidman et al. 2001). Even though JNK signaling is attributed to apoptotic responses, it has been shown that the JNK cooperates with other signaling pathways like NF-κB to mediate cell survival. Sustained JNK activation with the absence of a survival pathway may lead to apoptosis (Lamb et al. 2003), while transient JNK activation mediates survival (Liu et al. 1996). Likewise, there are reports indicating the involvement of p38 in paclitaxel-induced activation (Oh et al. 2006; Seidman et al. 2001) as well as inhibition (Yu et al. 2001) of apoptosis. In the present study we observed a transient activation of all the three MAPKs, ERK1/2, JNK, and P38, by paclitaxel and significant down-regulation of the same by curcumin, suggesting that curcumin could be a useful adjunct in therapeutic regimen using paclitaxel. The study also revealed that phosphorylation of MAPKs is completely inhibited when NF-κB is shut down indicating that NF-κB is up-stream of MAPKs in paclitaxel signaling.

AP-1 is a well-known down-stream effector of MAPK pathway. As reported (Amato et al. 1998), we also observed that paclitaxel induces DNA binding of AP-1 and curcumin significantly down-regulated it. Since curcumin inhibited paclitaxel-induced activation of all the three MAPKs that contribute to the increased expression and activation of AP-1, inhibition of AP-1 by curcumin was predictable. Curcumin may also directly inhibit the binding of AP-1 to the DNA response element (Hahm et al. 2002).

Both ERK and JNK signaling pathways have been implicated in NF-κB activation through phosphorylation and subsequent degradation of the inhibitory subunit IκBα (Chen et al. 1999). p38-dependent activation of NF-κB via IKK pathway has also been reported (Chio et al. 2004). Thus, both the transcription factors AP-1 and NF-κB are the targets of MAP kinase signaling cascades (Lee et al. 2002). In our study also, pretreatment with specific inhibitors of MAPKs significantly inhibited nuclear translocation of AP-1, while that of NF-κB was unaffected further confirming that NF-κB is up-stream of MAPKs in paclitaxel signaling. Various studies indicate that NF-κB and AP-1 may modulate the activity of each other. NF-κB transactivation has been found to be elevated by agents that can also activate AP-1 during tumor progression (Li et al. 1997). Besides, NF-κB inhibitors have been found to attenuate AP-1 activity (Li et al. 1998). Further, the response to AP-1 is strikingly enhanced when NF-κB subunits are present and vice versa (Fujioka et al. 2004; Stein et al. 1993).

NF-κB signaling pathway has been considered as a highly attractive target for the development of chemotherapeutic drugs, and several compounds which inhibit this pathway are currently under preclinical or clinical trials. While several of them are general inhibitors of NF-κB activation, some inhibit target-specific steps and others target multiple steps in the NF-κB pathway (Gupta et al. 2010). However, none of them has been approved for human use because most of them lack specificity and thus interfere with the physiological role of NF-κB in maintaining cellular homeostasis. Hence, the most important challenge is to develop NF-κB inhibitors based on their ability to specifically inhibit pathways leading to carcinogenesis, so that the risk of undesired side effects can be avoided. Paclitaxel is a very effective chemotherapeutic drug which acts mainly through induction of tubulin polymerization and cell cycle arrest. However, studies have shown that paclitaxel induces apoptotic cell death via a pathway independent of mitotic arrest (Huang et al. 2000; Lieu et al. 1997). Since lower concentration of paclitaxel leads to the concomitant activation of several survival signals, it fails to induce apoptosis at these concentrations necessitating a higher concentration of the drug for the purpose which in turn becomes the main reason for its toxicity. Hence, compounds like curcumin, which can counteract these survival signals, can be of therapeutic benefit when used in combination with paclitaxel.

Taken together, our results indicate that NF-κB is the central player in the synergism of paclitaxel and curcumin. Though not the only regulator, Akt is a major regulator of NF-κB, which through the phosphorylation of MAPKs regulates a set of survival signals. The study also reveals that NF-κB is the regulator of COX-2, cyclin D1, XIAP, and c-IAP1. While survivin is regulated by Akt, independent of NF-κB, Bcl-2 is operating through a pathway independent of both. However, further studies are required to rule out the role of direct down-stream targets of Akt in the synergistic effect of paclitaxel and curcumin.

Our next attempt was to evaluate the efficacy of the synergism using in vivo tumor models. For this, we used a chemical carcinogen-induced preclinical tumor model and the xenograft cervical cancer model and have shown how a suboptimal dose of the nontoxic dietary phytochemical curcumin circumvents the mechanisms of paclitaxel resistance and sensitizes tumor cells to paclitaxel treatment. The inconsistent findings on curcumin bioavailability in preclinical and clinical studies continue to be a major concern (Anand et al. 2007), and recent evidences suggest that liposomal encapsulation enhances its bioavailability and makes this compound amenable to systemic dosing (Li et al. 2007; Narayanan et al. 2009). In this study we encapsulated curcumin into unilamellar liposomes and injected intraperitoneally in order to improve its bioavailability and to eliminate dosing variability.

The initial gross observations on the percentage of tumor-bearing animals as well as mean tumor volume among different experimental groups provided an early hint about the synergistic anticancer activity of paclitaxel and curcumin against 3-MC-induced carcinogenesis. More interestingly, paclitaxel-curcumin combination therapy afforded significantly better tumor response than standard single-drug treatment. Consistent with previous reports (Chhabra et al. 1995), histopathological analysis of 3-methylcholanthrene-induced cervical tumors derived from our study revealed different stages of squamous cell carcinoma, and such progressive multistage carcinogenesis models better reflect the molecular and cellular complexity of human epithelial tumors.

Consistent with the role of NF-κB in oncogenesis and survival, cumulative experimental and epidemiologic evidence demonstrates the prevalence of aberrant constitutive activation of NF-κB in human tumors of diverse tissue origin and in various cancer cell lines (Aggarwal 2004; Karin et al. 2002). Reports also indicate that inhibition of NF-κB ameliorates the pathogenesis and overcomes therapeutic resistance (Ahn et al. 2007). Moreover, paclitaxel induces NF-κB activation in several cell types, and adjuvants that inhibit NF-κB function can enhance its therapeutic efficiency (Bava et al. 2005; Inoue et al. 2008). To our knowledge this is the first report to reveal the strong association of constitutive NF-κB activity with 3-MC-induced tumorigenesis in mice, and we found that curcumin suppresses the nuclear translocation and DNA-binding activity of NF-κB very effectively in the tumor tissues when given alone or in combination with paclitaxel. The results of the xenograft experiments using HeLa cells also corroborate the central findings of the 3-MC-induced multistage carcinogenesis study, and together they suggest that the administration of curcumin along with paclitaxel can potentially enhance the therapeutic outcome of paclitaxel in vivo.

The transcriptional activation and overexpression of NF-κB target gene products such as the stress response protein COX-2, cell cycle regulatory protein cyclin D1, cell adhesion molecule ICAM-1, proteolytic enzymes such as matrix metalloproteinases 2 and 9, and the angiogenic factor VEGF in human cancers is well documented (Aggarwal et al. 2005). Our data substantiates the ability of curcumin to circumvent the detrimental effects of oncogenic NF-κB, such as induction of proliferation, cell invasion, metastasis, and angiogenesis. The expression patterns of several NF-κB-dependent antiapoptotic genes such as Bcl-2, survivin, XIAP, and c-IAP in the tissue samples showed excellent correlation with the NF-κB activity, and consequently cells with elevated NF-κB activity will be more resistant to paclitaxel-induced cell death. Since these proteins play central roles in the suppression of apoptosis, their inhibition by curcumin can enhance the apoptotic activity of paclitaxel when given together. This notion is confirmed by increased caspase activation observed in the tumor samples treated with the combinatorial regimen.

In many human malignancies, over-expression of the multidrug resistance (MDR-1) gene product P-glycoprotein is a major obstacle to effective chemotherapy, and it functions as an energy-dependent efflux pump for which paclitaxel is a substrate (Bradley and Ling 1994). In addition, MDR-1 gene expression is regulated by NF-κB in different cell types (Bentires-Alj et al. 2003; Zhou and Kuo 1997), and several groups have shown that curcumin down-regulates MDR-1 expression in different cell types either through inhibiting the NF-κB pathway or by direct interaction (Choi et al. 2008; Ganta and Amiji 2009). Our data suggest that the inhibition of MDR-1 expression by curcumin in 3-MC-induced tumor samples can enhance the intracellular accumulation of paclitaxel and contribute at least in part to the synergistic effect of these agents.

Constitutive and drug-induced activation of the serine-threonine kinase Akt and the three major MAPKs – ERK1/2, p38, and JNK – have been widely implicated in cancer cell proliferation, survival, and resistance to apoptotic stimuli (Chang and Karin 2001; Hokeness et al. 2005). Paclitaxel has been reported to activate Akt (Hokeness et al. 2005) and MAPK pathways (Kuo et al. 2006; Yagi et al. 2009) and thereby compromises its apoptotic potential, whereas inhibition of these pathways by curcumin increases susceptibility of cancer cells to chemotherapeutic agents (Aggarwal et al. 2006; Bava et al. 2005; Gagnon et al. 2008). Although activated JNK contributes to some apoptotic responses, the JNK-dependent apoptotic signaling pathways can be blocked by activation of NF-κB and Akt pathways (Xia et al. 1995). Since curcumin remarkably inhibited the activation of MAPKs in 3-MC-induced tumors, it could attenuate the DNA-binding activity of the down-stream transcription factor AP-1. Furthermore, activated Akt can contribute to the induction of NF-κB activity (Kane et al. 1999). Nevertheless, down-regulation of Akt activation, ERK1/2 and JNK pathways, and DNA-binding activity of AP-1 by curcumin are possible mechanisms by which the 3-MC-induced tumors are sensitized to paclitaxel therapy.

Collectively, we have shown that curcumin, the pharmacologically safe chemosensitizer, can significantly augment the anticancer potential of paclitaxel by targeting multiple signaling events using well-defined preclinical models, and these in vivo evidences on the existence of therapeutic synergism between these agents underscore the essential need for validating this combination through clinical trials.

References

Aggarwal BB (2004) Nuclear factor-kappaB: the enemy within. Cancer Cell 6(3):203–208

Aggarwal BB, Shishodia S, Takada Y, Banerjee S, Newman RA, Bueso-Ramos CE, Price JE (2005) Curcumin suppresses the paclitaxel-induced nuclear factor-kappaB pathway in breast cancer cells and inhibits lung metastasis of human breast cancer in nude mice. Clin Cancer Res 11:7490–7498

Aggarwal S, Ichikawa H, Takada Y, Sandur SK, Shishodia S, Aggarwal BB (2006) Curcumin (diferuloylmethane) down-regulates expression of cell proliferation and antiapoptotic and metastatic gene products through suppression of IkappaBalpha kinase and Akt activation. Mol Pharmacol 69:195–206

Ahn KS, Sethi G, Aggarwal BB (2007) Nuclear factor-kappa B: from clone to clinic. Curr Mol Med 7(7): 619–637

Amato SF, Swart JM, Berg M, Wanebo HJ, Mehta SR, Chiles TC (1998) Transient stimulation of the c-Jun-NH2-Terminal Kinase/Activator Protein 1 pathway and inhibition of extracellular signal-regulated kinase are early effects in paclitaxel-mediated apoptosis in human B lymphoblasts. Cancer Res 58:241–247

Anand P, Kunnumakkara AB, Newman RA, Aggarwal BB (2007) Bioavailability of curcumin: problems and promises. Mol Pharm 4(6):807–818

Anto RJ, Maliekal TT, Karunagaran D (2000) L-929 cells harboring ectopically expressed RelA resist curcumin-induced apoptosis. J Biol Chem 275:15601–15604

Anto RJ, Mukhopadhyay A, Denning K, Aggarwal BB (2002) Curcumin (diferuloylmethane) induces apoptosis through activation of caspase-8, BID cleavage and cytochrome c release: its suppression by ectopic expression of Bcl-2 and Bcl-xl. Carcinogenesis 23(1):143–150

Anto RJ, Venkatraman M, Karunagaran D (2003) Inhibition of NF-κB sensitizes A431Cells to EGF-induced apoptosis whereas its activation by ectopic expression of RelA confers resistance. J Biol Chem 278: 25490–25498

Bacus SS, Gudkov AV, Lowe M, Lyass L, Yung Y, Komarov AP (2001) Taxol-induced apoptosis depends on MAP kinase pathways (ERK and p38) and is independent of p53. Oncogene 20:147–155

Banerjee S, Bueso-Ramos C, Aggarwal BB (2002) Suppression of 7,12-dimethylbenz(a)anthracene-induced mammary carcinogenesis in rats by resveratrol: role of nuclear factor-kappaB, cyclooxygenase 2, and matrix metalloprotease 9. Cancer Res 62(17):4945–4954

Bava SV, Puliappadamba VT, Deepti A, Nair A, Karunagaran D, Anto RJ (2005) Sensitization of taxol-induced apoptosis by curcumin involves down-regulation of nuclear factor-kappaB and the serine/threonine kinase Akt and is independent of tubulin polymerization. J Biol Chem 280(8):6301–6308

Bentires-Alj M, Barbu V, Fillet M, Chariot A, Relic B, Jacobs N, Gielen J, Merville MP, Bours V (2003) NF-kappaB transcription factor induces drug resistance through MDR1 expression in cancer cells. Oncogene 22(1):90–97

Bradley G, Ling V (1994) P-glycoprotein, multidrug resistance and tumor progression. Cancer Metastasis Rev 13(2):223–233

Catz SD, Johnson JL (2003) BCL-2 in prostate cancer: a mini review. Apoptosis 8:29–37

Chang L, Karin M (2001) Mammalian MAP kinase signalling cascades. Nature 410(6824):37–40

Chaturvedi MM, Mukhopadhyay A, Aggarwal BB (2000) Assay for redox-sensitive transcription factor. Methods Enzymol 319:585–602

Chen YR, Tan TH (1998) Inhibition of the c-Jun N-terminal kinase (JNK) signalling pathway by curcumin. Oncogene 17:173–178

Chen F, Demers LM, Vallyathan V, Ding M, Lu Y, Castranova V, Shi X (1999) Vanadate induction of NF-kappaB involves IkappaB kinase beta and SAPK/ERK kinase 1 in macrophages. J Biol Chem 274:20307–20312

Chhabra SK, Kaur S, Rao AR (1995) Modulatory influence of the oral contraceptive pill, Ovral, on 3-methylcholanthrene-induced carcinogenesis in the uterus of mouse. Oncology 52(1):32–34

Chio CC, Chang YH, Hsu YW, Chi KH, Lin WW (2004) PKA-dependent activation of PKC, p38 MAPK and IKK in macrophage: implication in the induction of inducible nitric oxide synthase and interleukin-6 by dibutyryl cAMP. Cell Signal 16:565–575

Choi BH, Kim CG, Lim Y, Shin SY, Lee YH (2008) Curcumin down-regulates the multidrug-resistance mdr1b gene by inhibiting the PI3K/Akt/NF kappa B pathway. Cancer Lett 259(1):111–118

Cobb MH (1999) MAP kinase pathways. Prog Biophys Mol Bio 71:479–500

Fujioka S, Niu J, Schmidt C, Sclabas GM, Peng B, Uwagawa T (2004) NF-{kappa}Band AP-1 connection: mechanism of NF-{kappa}B-dependent regulation of AP-1 activity. Mol Cell Biol 24:7806–7819

Gagnon V, Themsche CV, Turner S, Leblanc V, Asselin E (2008) Akt and XIAP regulate the sensitivity of human uterine cancer cells to cisplatin, doxorubicin and taxol. Apoptosis 13:259–271

Ganta S, Amiji M (2009) Coadministration of paclitaxel and curcumin in nanoemulsion formulations to overcome multidrug resistance in tumor cells. Mol Pharm 6(3):928–939

Gupta SC, Sundaram C, Reuter S, Aggarwal BB (2010) Inhibiting NF-kappaB activation by small molecules as a therapeutic strategy. Biochim Biophys Acta 1799:775–787. doi:10.1016/j.bbagrm.2010.05.004

Hahm ER, Cheon G, Lee J, Kim B, Park C, Yang CH (2002) New and known symmetrical curcumin derivatives inhibit the formation of Fos-Jun-DNA complex. Cancer Lett 184:89–96

Hokeness K, Qiu LH, Vezeridis M, Yan BF, Mehta S, Wan YS (2005) IFN-gamma enhances paclitaxel-induced apoptosis that is modulated by activation of caspases 8 and 3 with a concomitant down regulation of the AKT survival pathway in cultured human keratinocytes. Oncol Rep 13(5):965–969

Huang Y, Fan W (2002) IkappaB kinase activation is involved in regulation of paclitaxel-induced apoptosis in human tumor cell lines. Mol Pharmacol 61:105–113

Huang Y, Johnson KR, Norris JS, Fan W (2000) Nuclear factor-kappaB/IkappaB signaling pathway may contribute to the mediation of paclitaxel-induced apoptosis in solid tumor cells. Cancer Res 60:4426–4432

Hussain SP, Rao AR (1991) Chemopreventive action of mace (Myristica fragrans, Houtt) on methylcholanthrene-induced carcinogenesis in the uterine cervix in mice. Cancer Lett 56(3):231–234

Inoue M, Matsumoto S, Saito H, Tsujitani S, Ikeguchi M (2008) Intraperitoneal administration of a small interfering RNA targeting nuclear factor-kappa B with paclitaxel successfully prolongs the survival of xenograft model mice with peritoneal metastasis of gastric cancer. Int J Cancer 123(11):2696–2701

Kane LP, Shapiro VS, Stokoe D, Weiss A (1999) Induction of NF-kappaB by the Akt/PKB kinase. Curr Biol 9(11):601–604

Karin M, Cao Y, Greten FR, Li ZW (2002) NF-kappaB in cancer: from innocent bystander to major culprit. Nat Rev Cancer 2(4):301–310

Kuo HC, Lee HJ, Hu CC, Shun HI, Tseng TH (2006) Enhancement of esculetin on Taxol-induced apoptosis in human hepatoma HepG2 cells. Toxicol Appl Pharmacol 210(1–2):55–62

Kuttan R, Bhanumathy P, Nirmala K, George MC (1985) Potential anticancer activity of turmeric (Curcuma longa). Cancer Lett 29(2):197–202

Lamb JA, Ventura JJ, Hess P, Flavell RA, Davis RJ (2003) JunD mediates survival signaling by the JNK signal transduction pathway. Mol Cell 11:1479–1489

Lee LF, Li G, Templeton DJ, Ting JP (1998) Paclitaxel (Taxol)-induced gene expression and cell death are both mediated by the activation of c-Jun NH2-terminal kinase (JNK/SAPK). J Biol Chem 273:28253–28260

Lee SW, Han SI, Kim HH, Lee ZH (2002) TAK1-dependent activation of AP-1 and c-Jun N-terminal kinase by receptor activator of NF-kappaB. J Biochem Mol Biol 35:371–376

Li JJ, Westergaard C, Ghosh P, Colburn NH (1997) Inhibitors of both nuclear factor kappaB and activator protein-1 activation block the neoplastic transformation response. Cancer Res 57:3569–3576

Li JJ, Rhim JS, Schlegel R, Vousden KH, Colburn NH (1998) Expression of dominant negative Jun inhibits elevated AP-1 and NF-kappaB transactivation and suppresses anchorage independent growth of HPV immortalized human keratinocytes. Oncogene 16:2711–2721

Li L, Ahmed B, Mehta K, Kurzrock R (2007) Liposomal curcumin with and without oxaliplatin: effects on cell growth, apoptosis, and angiogenesis in colorectal cancer. Mol Cancer Therap 6(4):1276–1282

Lieu CH, Chang YN, Lai YK (1997) Dual cytotoxic mechanisms of submicromolar taxol on human leukemia HL-60 cells. Biochem Pharmacol 53:1587–1596

Liu ZG, Hsu H, Goeddel DV, Karin M (1996) Dissection of TNF receptor 1 effector functions: JNK activation is not linked to apoptosis while NF-kappaB activation prevents cell death. Cell 87:565–576

Livak KJ, Schmittgen TD (2001) Analysis of relative gene expression data using real time quantitative PCR and the 2(−Delta Delta C(T)) method. Methods 25(4):402–408

Mabuchi S, Ohmichi M, Nishio Y, Hayasaka T, Kimura A, Ohta T, Kawagoe J, Yada-Hashimoto N, Takahashi K, Seino-Noda H, Sakata M, Motoyama T, Kurachi H, Testa JR, Tasaka K, Murata Y (2004) Inhibition of inhibitor of nuclear factor-kappaB phosphorylation increases the efficacy of paclitaxel in *in vitro* and *in vivo* ovarian cancer models. Clin Cancer Res 10: 7645–7654

Murphy ED (1961) Carcinogenesis of the uterine cervix in mice: effect of diethylstilbestrol after limited application of 3-methylcholanthrene. J Natl Cancer Inst 27:611–653

Narayanan NK, Nargi D, Randolph C, Narayanan BA (2009) Liposome encapsulation of curcumin and resveratrol in combination reduces prostate cancer incidence in PTEN knockout mice. Int J Cancer 125(1):1–8

Oh SY, Song JH, Gil JE, Kim JH, Yeom YI, Moon EY (2006) ERK activation bythymosin-beta-4 (TB4) over expression induces paclitaxel-resistance. Exp Cell Res 312:1651–1657

Seidman R, Gitelman I, Sagi O, Horwitz SB, Wolfson M (2001) The role of ERK ½ and p38 MAP-kinase pathways in Taxol-induced apoptosis in human ovarian carcinoma cells. Exp Cell Res 268:84–92

Stein B, Baldwin AS Jr, Ballard DW, Greene WC, Angel P, Herrlich P (1993) Cross coupling of the NF-kappa B p65 and Fos/Jun transcription factors produces potentiated biological function. EMBO J 12:3879–3891

Xia Z, Dickens M, Raingeaud J, Davis RJ, Greenberg ME (1995) Opposing effects of ERK and JNK-p38 MAP kinases on apoptosis. Science 270(5240):1326–1331

Yagi H, Yotsumoto F, Sonoda K, Kuroki M, Mekada E, Miyamoto S (2009) Synergistic anti-tumor effect of paclitaxel with CRM197, an inhibitor of HB-EGF, in ovarian cancer. Int J Cancer 124(6):1429–1439

Yu C, Wang S, Dent P, Grant S (2001) Sequence-dependent potentiation of paclitaxel mediated apoptosis in human leukemia cells by inhibitors of the mitogen-activated protein kinase kinase/mitogen-activated protein kinase pathway. Mol Pharmacol 60:143–154

Zhao P, Meng Q, Liu LZ, You YP, Liu N, Jiang BH (2010) Regulation of survivin byPI3K/Akt/p70S6K1 pathway. Biochem Biophys Res Commun 395: 219–224

Zhou G, Kuo MT (1997) NF-kappaB-mediated induction of mdr1b expression by insulin in rat hepatoma cells. J Biol Chem 272(24):15174–15183

Zhu N, Gu L, Li F, Zhou M (2008) Inhibition of the Akt/survivin pathway synergizes the antileukemia effect of nutlin-3 in acute lymphoblastic leukemia cells. Mol Cancer Ther 7:1101–1109

Azadirachta indica (Neem) and Neem Limonoids as Anticancer Agents: Molecular Mechanisms and Targets

4

Siddavaram Nagini and Ramamurthi Vidya Priyadarsini

Abstract

Neem (*Azadirachta indica* A. Juss), one of the most versatile medicinal plants that grows ubiquitously in India has attained worldwide prominence owing to its wide range of medicinal properties. The bioactivity of neem has been attributed to its rich content of complex limonoids. Neem extracts and limonoids have been documented to exert antiproliferative effects both in vitro and in vivo. Accumulating evidence indicates that the anticancer effects of neem extracts and neem limonoids are mediated by preventing carcinogen activation; enhancing host antioxidant and detoxification systems; inhibiting cell proliferation, inflammation, invasion and angiogenesis; inducing apoptosis; modulating oncogenic transcription factors and signalling kinases; and influencing the epigenome. Neem and its constituent limonoids that target multiple signalling pathways aberrant in cancer are promising candidates for anticancer drug development.

Keywords

Anticancer • Azadirachtin • Nimbolide • Limonoids • Neem

Abbreviations

Apaf-1	Apoptosis associated factor-1
Bcl-2	B-cell lymphoma-2
B(a)P	Benzo(a)pyrene
CDK	Cyclin-dependent kinases
DR	Death receptor
Dvl	Dishevelled
DMBA	7,12-dimethylbenz(a)anthracene
ECM	Extracellular matrix
ERK	Extracellular signal-regulated kinase
GSK-3β	Glycogen synthase kinase 3 beta
HDAC	Histone deacetylase
HIF-1α	Hypoxia-inducible factor 1α
IAPs	Inhibitors of apoptosis proteins
IκB-α	Inhibitor of kappa B alpha
IKK	IκB kinase
IL	Interleukin
JNK	c-Jun N-terminal kinase
MAPK	Mitogen-activated protein kinase
MMP	Matrix metalloproteinases

S. Nagini (✉) • R. Vidya Priyadarsini
Department of Biochemistry and Biotechnology, Faculty of Science, Annamalai University, Annamalainagar 608 002, Tamil Nadu, India
e-mail: s_nagini@yahoo.com

P.R. Sudhakaran (ed.), *Perspectives in Cancer Prevention – Translational Cancer Research*, DOI 10.1007/978-81-322-1533-2_4, © Springer India 2014

MTMP	Mitochondrial permeability transition pore
NF-κB	Nuclear factor kappa B
NLGP	Neem leaf glycoproteins
PCNA	Proliferating cell nuclear antigen
PARP	Poly(ADP-ribose) polymerase
PI3K	Phosphoinositide 3-kinase
RECK	Reversion-inducing cysteine-rich protein with Kazal motifs
ROS	Reactive oxygen species
Smac/Diablo	Second mitochondria derived activator of caspases/direct IAP binding protein with low pI
TIMP-2	Tissue inhibitor of matrix metalloproteinases-2
TNF	Tumour necrosis factor
TRAIL	TNF-related apoptosis-inducing ligand
Ub	Ubiquitin ligase
VEGF	Vascular endothelial growth factor
XME	Xenobiotic metabolizing enzyme

4.1 Introduction

Azadirachta indica A. Juss (*Meliaceae*), commonly known as neem, is a large, evergreen tree belonging to the *Meliaceae* family ubiquitously present in the Indian subcontinent. Neem is one of the most researched trees globally because of its beneficial effects on the ecosystem and health. Neem is used both as a fertilizer and as a pesticide. The neem tree is recognized to control soil erosion and salinity and improve fertility of the soil. Biopesticides manufactured from neem are effective, eco-friendly, and acceptable to the farmers. Neem products have been shown to possess insecticidal, larvicidal, and mosquito-repellent properties (van der Nat et al. 1991; Udeinya 1993; Brahmachari 2004). Neem seeds are the richest source of pesticidal and insecticidal compounds. In particular, azadirachtin, the most active principle of neem-based insecticides and pesticides extracted from neem seed kernels, has been documented to be effective against approximately 200 insect pests (Mordue and Blackwell 1993; Morgan 2009).

The neem tree has gained worldwide attention in recent years, owing to its wide spectrum of medicinal properties. All parts of the neem tree—leaves, flowers, seeds, fruits, roots, and bark—have been used in traditional systems of medicine including Ayurveda, Siddha, Unani, Roman, and Greek to treat numerous human ailments. In India, the neem tree is considered as '*sarva roga nivarini*' (the panacea for all diseases) and has been hailed as '*heal all*', '*divine tree*', '*village dispensary*', and '*nature's drug store*' (Puri 1999).

The neem is a broad-leaved tree that can grow up to 30 m in height with branches spreading over 20 m and roots that deeply penetrate the soil. The trunk has a moderately thick, furrowed bark. The leaves are broad, alternate, and bitter in taste, and the flowers and fruits are borne in axillary clusters. The drupes are ellipsoidal and greenish yellow in colour and comprise a sweet pulp enclosing the seed composed of shell and kernels. Neem seed oil accounting for about 45 % of the total weight of the seeds is extracted from the kernel that contains secretory cells, which are the sites for the synthesis and storage of neem chemicals (Puri 1999; Biswas et al. 2002; Brahmachari 2004).

4.1.1 Chemistry

Over 300 structurally complex bioactive, organic compounds have been isolated and characterized from various parts of the neem tree (Kumar et al. 1996; Biswas et al. 2002; Tan and Luo 2011). These compounds have been categorized into two major classes: isoprenoids or terpenoids and non-isoprenoids. The isoprenoids include diterpenoids, triterpenoids, vilasinin type of compounds, and C-secomeliacins. Among these, the triterpenoids are the most abundant and occur in all parts of the neem tree especially in seeds and leaves. These are categorized into protolimonoids and mono- to nonanortriterpenoids. The tetranortriterpenoids are also known as limonoids. The non-isoprenoids include polysaccharides, proteins, amino acids, sulphur compounds, hydrocarbons, fatty acids, and their esters, tannins, and polyphenolics such as flavonoids and coumarin (Biswas et al. 2002; Subapriya and Nagini 2005).

Although a large number of compounds have been isolated from neem, only a few pure compounds have been screened for biological activity as shown in Table 4.1. The bioactivity of neem has been largely attributed to the rich content of complex limonoids that constitute about one-third of the phytochemical constituents in neem. Limonoids are highly oxygenated modified triterpenes categorized as tetranorterpenoid. Limonoids with an intact apoeuphol skeleton, a 14,15-β-epoxide, and a reactive site (either 19–28 lactol bridge or a cyclohexane) on the A ring are biologically very active, and absence of these structural features results in reduced activity (Tan and Luo 2011). Activity-guided fractionation of crude ethanolic extract of neem leaf revealed the presence of nimbolide, nimbin, 2′3′-dehydrosalannol, 6-desacetyl nimbinene, nimolinone, and quercetin (Manikandan et al. 2008, 2009; Mahapatra et al. 2012).

4.1.2 Medicinal Properties

Of late, neem has attracted increasing research attention because of the plethora of health benefits that it confers. Although all parts of the neem tree have been successfully used for centuries to treat a variety of disorders, the medicinal utilities have been described especially for leaf and seeds (Biswas et al. 2002; Brahmachari 2004; Subapriya and Nagini 2005). Extracts of neem seeds and leaves were shown to provide protection against various strains of malarial parasite and human fungi including *Candida* (Badam et al. 1987; Khan and Wassilew 1987). The antibacterial effects of neem leaves, seeds, and bark have been demonstrated against Gram-positive and Gram-negative bacteria including *M. tuberculosis* and *Streptomycin* resistant strains, *Vibrio cholerae*, *Klebsiella pneumoniae*, and *M. pyogenes* (Chopra et al. 1952; Satyavati et al. 1976). Neem and neem-based products exhibit antiviral activity against chikungunya, herpes simplex virus-1, dengue virus type-2, and human immunodeficiency virus (HIV) (Udeinya et al. 2004).

Alcoholic neem leaf extracts were found to be effective against chronic skin diseases such as eczema, scabies, and ringworm infection (Singh et al. 1979). Neem has been used in the treatment of gingivitis, periodontitis, oral infections, and inhibition of plaque growth (Patel and Venkatakrishna-Bhatt 1988). A dental gel containing neem leaf extract (25 mg/g) was documented to reduce plaque index and bacterial count (Pai et al. 2004). Herbal chewing sticks of neem were found to be effective against *Streptococcus* spp. involved in causing dental caries (Prashant et al. 2007). Both the aqueous and alcoholic neem leaf extracts are reported to exhibit hepatoprotective effects against liver damage induced by paracetamol and antitubercular drugs (Bhanwra et al. 2000; Chattopadhyay 2003). Neem preparations were demonstrated to be useful in the control of gastric hyperacidity and ulcer by blocking acid secretion through inhibition of H^+–K^+-ATPase and by prevention of oxidative damage and apoptosis (Chattopadhyay et al. 2004). Studies have documented that oral administration of aqueous as well as alcoholic extract of neem leaf decreased blood glucose level in experimentally induced diabetes by releasing endogenous insulin (Khosla et al. 2000).

Neem extracts have been shown to exert potent anticancer effects attributed to the presence of limonoids (Roy and Saraf 2006). Azadirachtin isolated from seed kernels, and nimbolide, abundant in neem leaves and flowers are the most active neem limonoids that display anticancer effects.

4.2 Anticancer Properties

The evidence for the anticancer property of neem extracts and neem limonoids stems from both in vitro and in vivo studies (Biswas et al. 2002; Subapriya and Nagini 2005; Paul et al. 2011).

4.2.1 In Vitro Studies

Several studies have demonstrated the inhibitory effects of neem extracts and limonoids on the

Table 4.1 Structure and biological activity of neem phytochemicals

Neem compound	Structure	Biological activity
Azadirachtin	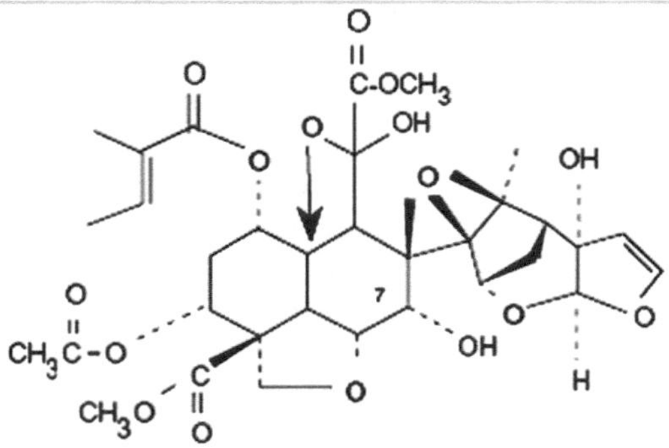	Insecticidal, antimicrobial, antioxidant, antimutagenic, anticancer
Azadirone	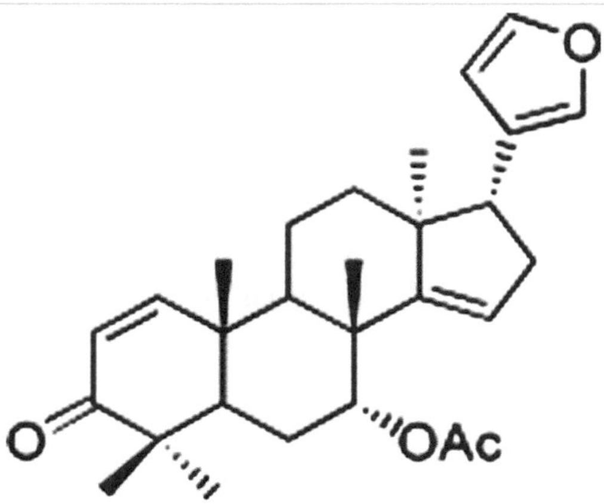	Anticancer
Deacetyl nimbin	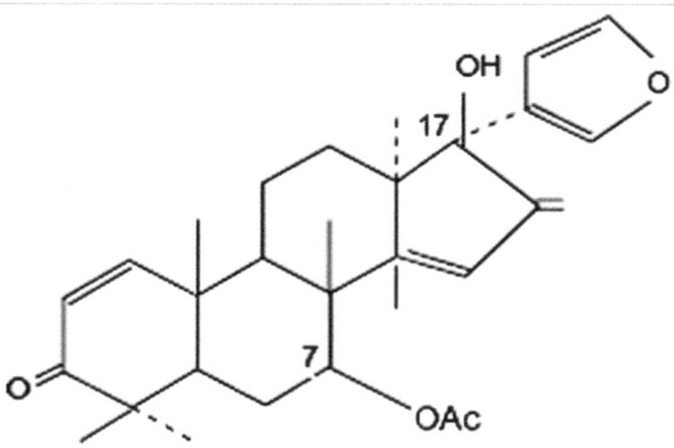	Spermicidal, anticancer
Gedunin	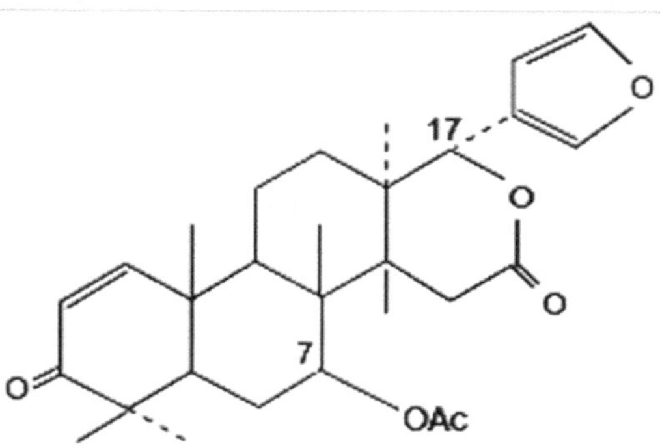	Antimicrobial, diuretic, antiarthritic, antipyretic, spermicidal, anti-inflammatory, anti-ulcerogenic, anticancer

(continued)

Table 4.1 (continued)

Neem compound	Structure	Biological activity
Nimbin	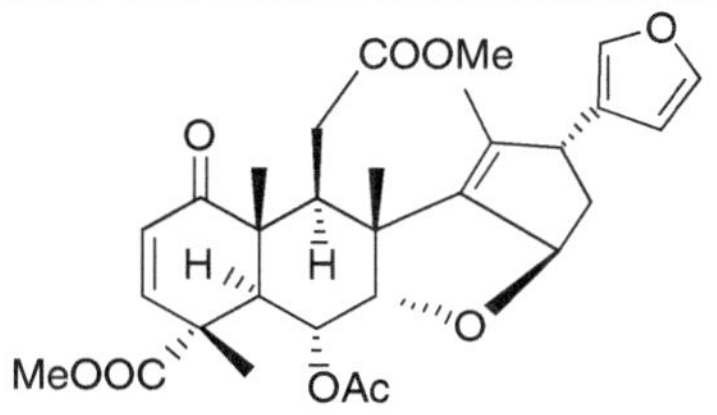	Spermicidal, anticancer
Nimbolide	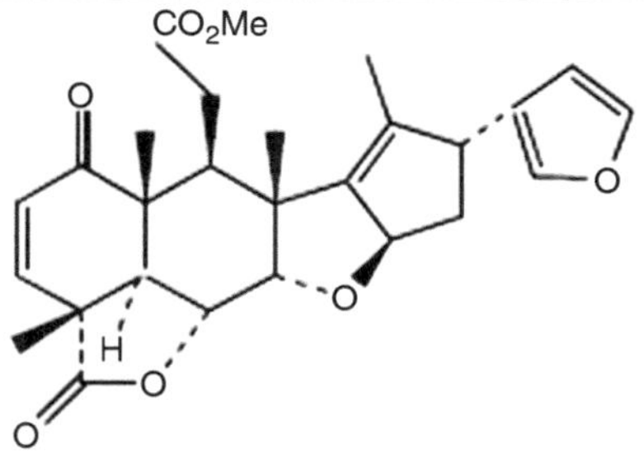	Insecticidal, antimicrobial, cytotoxicity, antioxidant, antimutagenic, anticancer
Salannin	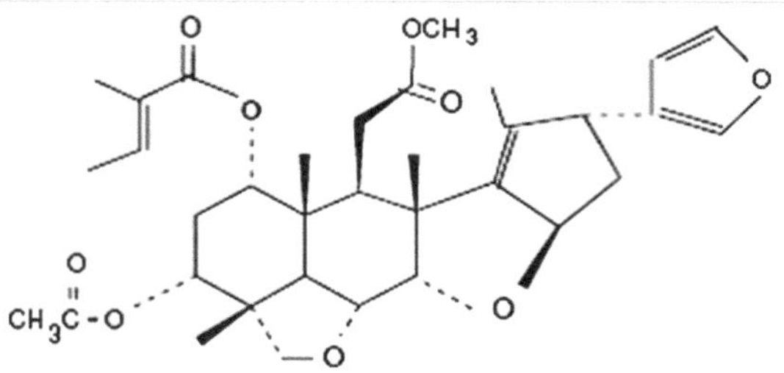	Antigastric ulcer, anticancer
Quercetin	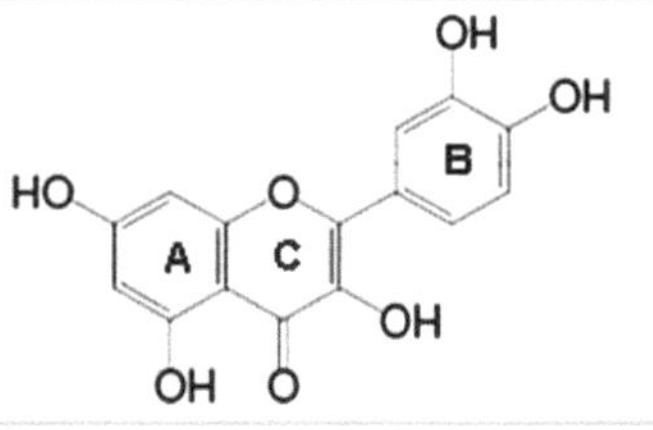	Antioxidant, anticancer

growth of diverse cancer cells in vitro. Neem leaf extracts exerted anticancer effects against human pancreatic carcinoma cell lines Panc-1, BxPC-3, and MIA PaCa-2; prostate cancer cells such as LNCaP, C4-2B, and PC-3; as well as murine Ehrlich's carcinoma (EC) and B16 melanoma cells (Baral and Chattopadhyay 2004; Gunadharini et al. 2011; Mahapatra et al. 2011; Veeraraghavan et al. 2011a, b).

Among the 35 limonoids from *Azadirachta indica* seed extracts evaluated for cytotoxicity against five human cancer cell lines, three limonoids 7-deacetyl-7-benzoylepoxyazadiradione, 7-deacetyl-7-benzoylgeduin, and 28-deoxonimbolide displayed potent cytotoxic effects against HL60 leukaemia cells with IC_{50} values in the range 2.7–3.1 μM. In particular, 7-deacetyl-7-benzoylepoxyazadiradione exhibited selective cytotoxicity to leukaemic cells and only weak cytotoxicity against the normal RPMI 1788 lymphocyte cell line (Kikuchi et al. 2011).

Azadirachtin has been reported to have potent cytotoxic effects against glioblastoma cell lines (G-28, G-112, G-60, G-44, G-62, G-120) by increasing micronuclei formation and decreasing the mitotic index (Akudugu et al. 2011). Azadirachtin was also demonstrated to inhibit the growth of human cervical cancer cells (HeLa),

MCF7 breast cancer cells, 143B.TK- human osteosarcoma, and ovarian cell lines (Cohen et al. 1996a; Priyadarsini et al. 2010). Nanduri et al. (2003) have documented the cytotoxic effect of azadirone against a panel of cancer cell lines.

Gedunin was shown to manifest anticancer activity via inhibition of the 90 kDa heat shock protein 90 (hsp90) folding machinery in MCF-7 and SkBr3 breast cancer cells (Brandt et al. 2008). Kamath et al. (2009) found that gedunin inhibits the proliferation of SKOV3, OVCAR4, and OVCAR8 ovarian cancer cell lines and enhances the antiproliferative effect of cisplatin. 2′-3′-Dehydrosalannol has been reported to inhibit the growth of MDA-MB 231 and MDA-MB 468 triple-negative breast cancer cells (Boopalan et al. 2012).

Studies have revealed that nimbolide is the most potent anticancer agent among the various neem limonoids examined. Nimbolide has been documented to exert significant cytotoxic effects against a panel of human cancer cell lines including 143B TK osteosarcoma, HL-60, U-937 and THP-1 leukaemic, B16 melanoma, SMMC 7721, A-549, MCF-7 breast, HT-29, SW-620, SW-480, HOP-62, A-549, PC-3, and OVCAR-5 cell lines (Cohen et al. 1996b; Sastry et al. 2006; Roy et al. 2007; Chen et al. 2011). Studies from this laboratory as well as by others have shown that nimbolide induces a dose- and time-dependent suppression of the viability of human choriocarcinoma (BeWo), leukaemic (HeLa), and WiDr and HCT-116 colon adenocarcinoma cells (Harish Kumar et al. 2009; Priyadarsini et al. 2010; Babykutty et al. 2012).

4.2.2 In Vivo Studies

Accumulating evidence from experimental animal models have provided convincing evidence to indicate that neem preparations and its constituents are highly effective in affording protection against malignant tumours induced by a variety of chemical carcinogens. Tepsuwan et al. (2002) demonstrated the chemopreventive potential of neem flowers on carcinogen-induced rat mammary and liver carcinogenesis. Extensive investigations from this laboratory provide evidence that neem leaf extracts inhibit the development of experimental oral and gastric carcinogenesis (Subapriya and Nagini 2003; Subapriya et al. 2005, 2006). Dasgupta et al. (2004) reported the chemopreventive potential of neem leaf extract in murine carcinogenesis model systems. Gangar et al. (2006) have demonstrated that *A. indica* exerts chemopreventive effects against benzo(a)pyrene-induced forestomach murine tumours. Oral administration of aqueous neem leaf extract was demonstrated to significantly reduce the incidence of N-nitrosodiethylamine (NDEA)-induced hepatocellular carcinomas and delayed changes in hepatocyte differentiation, metabolism, and morphology (Bharati and Rishi 2012). Neem leaf was found to exhibit short-term chemopreventive effects on preneoplastic lesions in rat colon carcinogenesis (Arakaki et al. 2006). Haque and Baral (2006) have shown that neem leaf preparation induces Ehrlich carcinoma prophylactic growth restriction in Swiss and C57BL mice. Recently, Mahapatra et al. (2011) have demonstrated that ethanolic neem leaf extracts inhibit the growth of C4-2B and PC-3M-luc2 prostate cancer xenografts in nude mice.

Although neem limonoids have been extensively tested for cytotoxicity against a panel of human cancer cell lines, evidence for the in vivo inhibition of tumour growth in animal models is rather scanty. Limonin 17-β-D-glucopyranoside, a neem limonoid, was shown to inhibit DMBA-induced oral carcinogenesis (Miller et al. 1992). Nortriterpenoids, isolated from the seed extract of neem, exhibited marked inhibitory effect on melanogenesis in the B16 melanoma cells. Akihisa et al. (2009) have documented the anti-tumour-initiating activity of azadirachtin B isolated from the seed extract of neem on the two-stage carcinogenesis of mouse skin tumour induced by peroxynitrite (ONOO−; PN) as an initiator and 12-*O*-tetradecanoylphorbol-13-acetate (TPA) as a promoter. Recently, we have demonstrated that administration of both azadirachtin and nimbolide inhibit the development of 7,12-dimethylbenz(a)anthracene

(DMBA)-induced hamster buccal pouch carcinomas by modulating the hallmark capabilities of cancer (Vidya Priyadarsini et al. 2009; Harish Kumar et al. 2010).

4.3 Molecular Mechanisms Underlying Anticancer Effects

4.3.1 Carcinogen Metabolism

A key molecular mechanism responsible for the anticancer effects of neem and its limonoids is the modulation of phase I and II xenobiotic metabolizing enzymes (XME), which play a central role in xenobiotic/drug metabolism. Phase I enzymes, namely, cytochrome P450 monooxygenases and their isoforms, catalyze the biotransformation of procarcinogens to highly reactive electrophilic intermediates that can damage cellular macromolecules. In contrast, the phase II enzymes such as glutathione *S*-transferases (GSTs), uridine diphosphate-glucuronosyl transferases (UGTs), and NADH quinine oxidoreductase (NQO1) catalyze the neutralization of electrophilic intermediates generated in phase I reactions, thereby resulting in reduced chemical reactivity and cellular damage (Iyanagi 2007).

Ethanolic neem leaf extracts, neem leaf fractions, and the limonoids azadirachtin and nimbolide function as *dual-acting agents* offering protection against chemically induced carcinogenesis by constraining the activities of total cytochrome P450 as well as its isoforms CYP1A1, 1A2, 2B and CYP1B1, and cytochrome b_5 and simultaneously enhancing the activities of the phase II detoxification enzymes—GST and DT-diaphorase (Manikandan et al. 2008, 2009; Vidya Priyadarsini et al. 2009). Aqueous extracts of neem leaf were shown to inhibit the formation of benzo(a)pyrene (B(a)P) DNA adducts during B[a]P-induced murine forestomach carcinogenesis via modulating the activities of phase I and II XMEs (Gangar et al. 2006).

4.3.2 Antioxidants

Extensive investigations have provided evidence for the antioxidative properties of neem leaves, fruits, flowers, and stem bark extracts as well as the neem limonoids azadirachtin and nimbolide against various free radicals both in vitro and in vivo (Hanasaki et al. 1994; Sithisarn et al. 2005, 2007; Manikandan et al. 2008, 2009; Vidya Priyadarsini et al. 2009). Farah et al. (2006) reported that ethanolic neem leaf extract exerts significant antimutagenic activity against pentachlorophenol (PCP) and 2,4-dichlorophenoxyacetic acid-induced chromosomal aberrations and incidence of micronuclei in *Channa punctatus*. Studies from this laboratory have unequivocally demonstrated that ethanolic neem leaf extract significantly mitigates carcinogen-induced genotoxicity and oxidative stress by augmenting GSH-dependent antioxidant defence mechanisms (Subapriya et al. 2004, 2005). Activity-guided fractionation identified subfractions that displayed significant protective effects against various free radicals and H_2O_2-induced oxidative damage to erythrocytes and pBR322 DNA (Manikandan et al. 2009). Both azadirachtin and nimbolide exhibited concentration-dependent ROS scavenging activity and reductive potential in vitro and protected against oxidative DNA damage in vivo by upregulation of antioxidants (Vidya Priyadarsini et al. 2009).

4.3.2.1 Cell Proliferation, Cell Cycle Arrest, and DNA Repair

Perturbation of cell cycle control with consequent uncontrolled cell proliferation is a major hallmark of cancer. Sequential activation and deactivation of cyclins and cyclin-dependent kinases (CDKs) regulates progression of the cell cycle through the various phases (Csikasz-Nagy et al. 2011).

Ethanolic extracts of neem leaf have also been reported to inhibit cell proliferation and tumour growth by downregulating a wide array of proteins involved in cellular assembly and organization, DNA replication, recombination, and repair such as HMOX1, AKR1C2, AKR1C3, and AKR1B10 (Mahapatra et al. 2011). Niture et al. (2006) showed that ethanolic and aqueous extracts of neem reduce the expression of O6-alkylguanine lesions in human peripheral blood lymphocytes by increasing the levels of O6-methylguanine-DNA methyltransferase (MGMT) repair protein. Neem limonoids have been documented to induce cell cycle arrest at G1/S or G2/M phase accompanied by p53-dependent accumulation of $p21^{Cip1/waf1}$ and Chk2 associated with downregulation of the cell cycle regulatory proteins cyclin A, cyclin B1, cyclin D1, cyclin E, Cdk2, Rad17, PCNA, and c-myc (Roy et al. 2006; Priyadarsini et al. 2010). 2′3′-Dehydrosalannol has been shown to inhibit the growth of triple-negative breast cancer cells by downregulating phosphorylated protein kinase B (pAKT) and cyclin D1 (Boopalan et al. 2012). Azadirachtin exerts antimitotic effects by interfering with the polymerization of tubules and formation of the mitotic spindle, thereby preventing replication (Salehzadeh et al. 2003). Studies in vitro and in vivo have revealed the regulatory effects of nimbolide on cell cycle progression. Treatment of U937 cells with nimbolide disrupted the cell cycle by decreasing the number of cells in G0/G1 phase (Roy et al. 2007). In colon cancer cells, nimbolide was shown to interfere with cell cycle kinetics and induce S phase arrest by inhibiting cyclin A/cyclin D1 (Babykutty et al. 2012).

4.3.2.2 Induction of Apoptosis

Apoptosis, a form of programmed cell death, plays a crucial role in the maintenance of adult tissue homeostasis. Apoptosis is initiated via complex interactions between the pro- and anti-apoptotic members of the Bc-2 family that dictate the integrity of the mitochondrial membrane. Permeabilization of the outer mitochondrial membrane by pro-apoptotic Bcl-2 family proteins results in the efflux of apoptogenic factors such as cytochrome c, SMAC/DIABLO, and Omi/HtrA2 from the mitochondrial intermembrane space into the cytosol. In the cytosol, cytochrome c engages apoptotic protease activating factor-1 (APAF-1) and pro-caspase-9 to form the apoptosome complex. Formation of the apoptosome complex subsequently activates the downstream caspase cascade and cleavage of vital proteins essential for cell survival (Ulukaya et al. 2011).

Neem leaf extracts induce apoptosis in human neuroblastoma xenografts, Panc-1, BxPC-3, MIA PaCa-2, LNCaP, and PC-3 cancer cells by modulating the expression of Bcl-2 family proteins and upregulating caspases (Gunadharini et al. 2011; Kumar et al. 2006; Baral and Chattopadhyay 2004; Mahapatra et al. 2011; Veeraraghavan et al. 2011a, b).

Neem limonoids have been shown to induce apoptosis in various cancer cells as evidenced by detachment of cells from the substratum, an increase in the number of sub-diploid cells, chromatin condensation, and appearance of annexin-V-positive cells. Studies by us and other workers have revealed that neem limonoids transduce apoptosis by both the death receptor and mitochondrial pathways (Harish Kumar et al. 2009; Priyadarsini et al. 2010). Gupta et al. (2011) reported that nimbolide sensitizes colon cancer cells to tumour necrosis factor-related apoptosis-inducing ligand (TRAIL)-induced apoptosis by enhancing the expression of the death receptors DR5 and DR4 through activation of ERK and p38 MAP kinase and generation of ROS. Recently, Babykutty et al. (2012) also demonstrated that nimbolide induces caspase-mediated apoptosis by inhibiting ERK1/2 and activating p38 and JNK1/2.

Accumulating evidence indicates that neem limonoids induce apoptosis via the mitochondrial pathway. The mechanism involved generation of reactive oxygen species (ROS); decline in the mitochondrial transmembrane potential; downregulation of anti-apoptotic Bcl-2 proteins such as Bcl-2 and Bcl-xL; upregulation of pro-apoptotic Bax, Bak, Bim, Bid, and p53; reduced expression of inhibitor of apoptosis proteins (IAPs), namely, survivin, neuronal apoptosis inhibitory protein (NAIP), IAP-1, IAP-2, I-FLICE, and XIAP; release of cytochrome *c* from the mitochondria; apoptosome complex formation; and activation of initiator and effector caspases and CARD domains, eventually culminating in poly (ADP-ribose) polymerase (PARP) cleavage. Interestingly, azadirachtin and nimbolide enforced nuclear localization of survivin, enabling increased susceptibility to intrinsic apoptosis (Gupta et al. 2010, 2011; Priyadarsini et al. 2010; Boopalan et al. 2012).

4.3.2.3 Inhibition of Tumour Invasion and Angiogenesis

Cancer cell invasion and endothelial transmigration, critical events in tumour progression and metastasis, depend on an intricate balance between proinvasive and proangiogenic factors and their inhibitors. Matrix metalloproteinases (MMPs), a family of zinc-dependent endopeptidases, play a pivotal role in extracellular matrix (ECM) processing during which process several proangiogenic molecules predominantly vascular endothelial growth factor (VEGF) and hypoxia-inducible factor-1α (HIF-1α) are released. MMP activity is tightly regulated by tissue inhibitors of matrix metalloproteinases (TIMPs) and reversion-inducing cysteine-rich protein with Kazal motifs (RECK) (Brew and Nagase 2010; Gialeli et al. 2011; Nagini 2012).

Ethanolic neem leaf extracts are reported to exhibit antiangiogenic effects in human umbilical vein endothelial cells (HUVECs) by attenuating VEGF stimulation (Mahapatra et al. 2012). Studies from this laboratory have provided evidence that the neem limonoids azadirachtin and nimbolide induce a shift of balance from a proinvasive, proangiogenic phenotype by downregulating the expression of MMPs, VEGF, VEGF receptors, and HIF-1α and upregulating TIMP-2 and RECK expression in the hamster buccal pouch carcinogenesis model (Vidya Priyadarsini et al. 2009). In a recent study, nimbolide was demonstrated to block tumour cell invasion, migration, and angiogenesis in colon cancer cells in vitro by downregulating the expression of MMP and VEGF via abrogation of ERK1/2 and NF-κB signalling (Babykutty et al. 2012).

4.3.2.4 Modulation of Oncogenic Transcription Factors

Neem extracts and its constituent limonoids are reported to modulate various transcription factors associated with oncogenesis, chiefly nuclear factor kappa B (NF-κB) and β-catenin. In unstimulated cells, NF-κB exists in the cytosol as an inactive heterodimer of p50 and p65 subunits tightly sequestered to the IκB inhibitory protein. Activation of NF-κB occurs through phosphorylation of IκB at serine-32 and serine-36 residues by IKKβ. This results in proteasomal degradation of IκB and subsequent translocation of free NF-κB heterodimer to the nucleus. In the nucleus, NF-κB binds to the κB enhancer element and transactivates over 500 target genes that are implicated in various processes such as cell proliferation, cell survival, apoptosis evasion, invasion, metastasis, and angiogenesis (Chaturvedi et al. 2011).

Neem extracts and limonoids restrict NF-κB signalling by inhibiting the kinase activity of IKKβ, phosphorylation and proteasomal degradation of IκB, and nuclear translocation of the p50/p65 heterodimer (Manikandan et al. 2008; Priyadarsini et al. 2010; Kavitha et al. 2012). Veeraraghavan et al. (2011a) showed that neem leaf extracts inhibit proliferation of irradiated Panc-1, BxPC-3, and MIA PaCa-2 pancreatic cancer cells through selective abrogation of radiotherapy-induced NF-κB signalling. Gupta et al. (2010) demonstrated that nimbolide inhibits NF-κB activation by modifying cys179 residue in the activation loop of IKKβ, thereby abrogating its kinase activity and subsequent NF-κB signalling. Recent studies from our laboratory have demonstrated that nimbolide inhibits both the constitutive as well as tumour necrosis factor-α (TNF-α)-induced NF-κB activation in NF-κB-responsive luciferase reporter plasmid transfected human hepatocarcinoma (HepG2) cells.

Reciprocal activation of NF-κB and Wnt/β-catenin signalling pathways has been documented in malignant tumours (Du and Geller 2010). Activation of the Wnt/β-catenin pathway involves dissociation of a multiprotein complex containing glycogen synthase kinase 3β

(GSK-3β) that results in cytosolic accumulation and nuclear translocation of β-catenin that interacts with TCF/lymphoid enhancer factor (LEF) to form a functional transcription factor to transactivate various target genes involved in cell proliferation, apoptosis, invasion, and angiogenesis (Sethi and Vidal-Puig 2010). Treatment of HepG2 cells with nimbolide abrogated canonical Wnt/β-catenin signalling by downregulating GSK-3β and impeding the cytosolic accumulation and nuclear translocation of free β-catenin (Kavitha et al. 2012).

4.3.2.5 Modulation of Intracellular Signalling Cascades

The upstream components of the cytoplasmic signalling networks include the protein kinase B/Akt, mitogen-activated protein kinases (MAPKs), protein kinase C, and phosphatidylinositol-3-kinase (PI3K). Inappropriate regulation of these kinases transmit mitogenic signals to transcription factors, coactivators, and co-repressors resulting in transcription of target genes that promote carcinogenesis. Akt, a serine/threonine kinase, plays a pivotal role in various cellular processes particularly cell proliferation and survival. The Akt cascade is activated by receptor tyrosine kinases, integrins, and various other stimuli through the production of phosphatidylinositol 3,4,5 triphosphates. Akt influences cell growth and proliferation through its effects on the mTOR and p70 S6 kinase pathways, cyclin D1, p53, and the CDK inhibitors- p21 and p27. Akt also mediates cell survival through direct inhibition of pro-apoptotic molecules such as Bad and the Forkhead family of transcription factors (Jazirehi et al. 2012). Mitogen-activated protein kinases (MAPK) comprising extracellular signal-regulated kinase (ERK), c-Jun N-terminal kinase (JNK), and p38 kinases are conserved signalling modules that play a key role in oncogenic transformation. Upon activation, these kinases integrate various extracellular and intracellular cues, translocate to the nucleus and induce transcriptional programmes involved in cell growth, apoptosis evasion and matrix invasion (Cargnello and Roux 2011).

Neem extracts and limonoids have been shown to target Akt, phosphoinositide 3-kinase (PI3K), p38, JNK1/2, and ERK signalling pathways and promote apoptosis induction and NF-κB abrogation in diverse malignant cell lines. Gunadharini et al. (2011) reported that ethanolic neem leaf extracts decreased the expression of Akt 1/2 as well as the expression of pAkt and total Akt in PC-3 and LNCaP prostate cancer cells. Babykutty et al. (2012) demonstrated that nimbolide modulates the expression of pERK1/2, pP38, and pJNK1/2 in WiDr colon adenocarcinoma cells. Gupta et al. (2010) found that nimbolide targets ERK and p38 MAPK molecules via generation of reactive oxygen species (ROS) in HCT-116 colon adenocarcinoma cells.

4.3.2.6 Anti-inflammatory Effects

Neem leaf extracts and limonoids have been reported to exert potent anti-inflammatory effects by inhibiting the activation of tumour necrosis factor (TNF)-α, a multifunctional pro-inflammatory cytokine that plays a key role in inflammation through signalling via TNFR1 and TNFR2 and by inhibiting NF-κB activation. Azadirachtin has been shown to exert anti-inflammatory effects via modulating cell surface TNF receptors, thereby blocking TNF-induced inflammatory responses. Inhibition of TNF activation by azadirachtin reduces NF-κB activation and the expression of NF-κB dependent pro-inflammatory mediator COX-2 (Thoh et al. 2010). Epoxyazadiradione is demonstrated to inhibit macrophage migration inhibitory factor (MIF)-mediated pro-inflammation activities in RAW 264.7 cells by inhibiting MIF-induced macrophage chemotactic migration, NF-κB nuclear translocation, and upregulation of inducible nitric oxide synthase and nitric oxide production. Epoxyazadiradione also exhibits anti-inflammatory activity in BALB/c mice by preventing the release of pro-inflammatory cytokines TNF-α and interleukin (IL)-1α, IL-1β, and IL-6 (Alam et al. 2012). The limonoids 1,3-diacetylvilasinin, 28-deoxonimbolide, salannin, 2′,3′-dihydrosalannin, and 3-deacetylsalannin were also found to exhibit potent anti-inflammatory activity against TPA-induced inflammation (Akihisa et al. 2011).

4.3.2.7 Immunomodulatory Effects

Immunosuppression occurring as a result of increased cytokine secretion is a key phenomenon that promotes tumour growth and development. Aqueous extracts of neem were also shown to enhance both humoral immunity and cell-mediated immunity (Ray et al. 1996). Neem leaf glycoproteins (NLGP) and extracts exhibit potential to enhance immunogenicity and block negative immunoregulatory host mechanisms in various tumours. Sarkar et al. (2008, 2010) reported that NLGP induces anti-tumour immunity by enhancing carcinoembryonic antigen (CEA) presentation of dendritic cells to T and B cells. In addition, NLGP inhibits T-regulatory cell (Tregs)-associated murine tumour growth by downregulating the expression of Foxp3, CTLA4, and GITR and facilitating reconditioning of the tumour microenvironment by increasing interferon-γ (IFN-γ) and IL-12 secretion (Chakraborty et al. 2011). Chakraborty et al. (2010) showed that NLGP exhibits anti-tumour activity in patients with head and neck squamous cell carcinoma by activating cytotoxic T lymphocytes and natural killer cells. Neem leaf preparations are also reported to enhance Th1-type immune responses and anti-tumour immunity against breast tumour associated antigen by inhibiting the release of IL-10 and promoting IFN-γ secretion (Mandal-Ghosh et al. 2007).

4.3.2.8 Epigenetic Alterations

Epigenetic modifications such as DNA methylation and histone acetylation play a major role in regulating the dynamics of gene expression. DNA methyltransferases (DNMTs), DNA demethylases, histone acetyltransferases (HATs) and histone deacetylases (HDACs) act as key mediators of the epigenetic processes. While CpG island methylation by DNMTs and histone deacetylation by HDACs result in repression of gene expression, histone hyperacetylation by HATs activates gene expression (Hassler and Egger 2012). The limonoids azadirachtin and nimbolide exhibit the potential to inhibit the expression of HDAC-1 and restrict tumour invasion and angiogenesis during DMBA-induced HBP carcinogenesis (Vidya Priyadarsini et al. 2009). HDAC inhibition by these limonoids is of particular significance in the perspective of the emerging interest in epigenetic reprogramming in cancer and the potential anticancer effects of HDAC inhibitors (Carew et al. 2008). Figure 4.1 summarizes the molecular targets of neem and its constituent phytochemicals.

4.4 Toxicity Studies

Several in vivo studies have demonstrated neem extracts and limonoids to be potentially safe. Aqueous extracts of neem leaf were non-toxic to mice up to oral doses of 1,000 mg/kg body weight (Biswas et al. 2002). Acute toxicity studies in mice have revealed that the LD_{50} value for methanolic neem leaf extract is 13 g/kg body weight (Okpanyi and Ezeukwu 1981). Azadirachtin at daily doses of 15, 0.26 and 0.3 mg/kg body weight was found to be potentially safe for human consumption (Boeke et al. 2004). Technical azadirachtin, a mixture of seven structurally related tetranorterpenoid isomers, is also reported to lack toxicity in rats (Srivastava and Raizada 2007). However, higher doses of azadirachtin ($LD_{50} > 5{,}000$ mg/kg bw) were found to exhibit acute toxicity (Raizada et al. 2001). Pillai and Santhakumari (1984) demonstrated that oral doses of nimbidin up to 100 mg/kg body weight are non-toxic. Intragastric administration of nimbolide was also found to be non-toxic to experimental animals. However, intravenous and intraperitoneal administrations were found to cause death in experimental animals by lowering the arterial blood pressure and inducing dysfunctions in the kidney, small intestine, pancreas, and liver (Glinsukon et al. 1986).

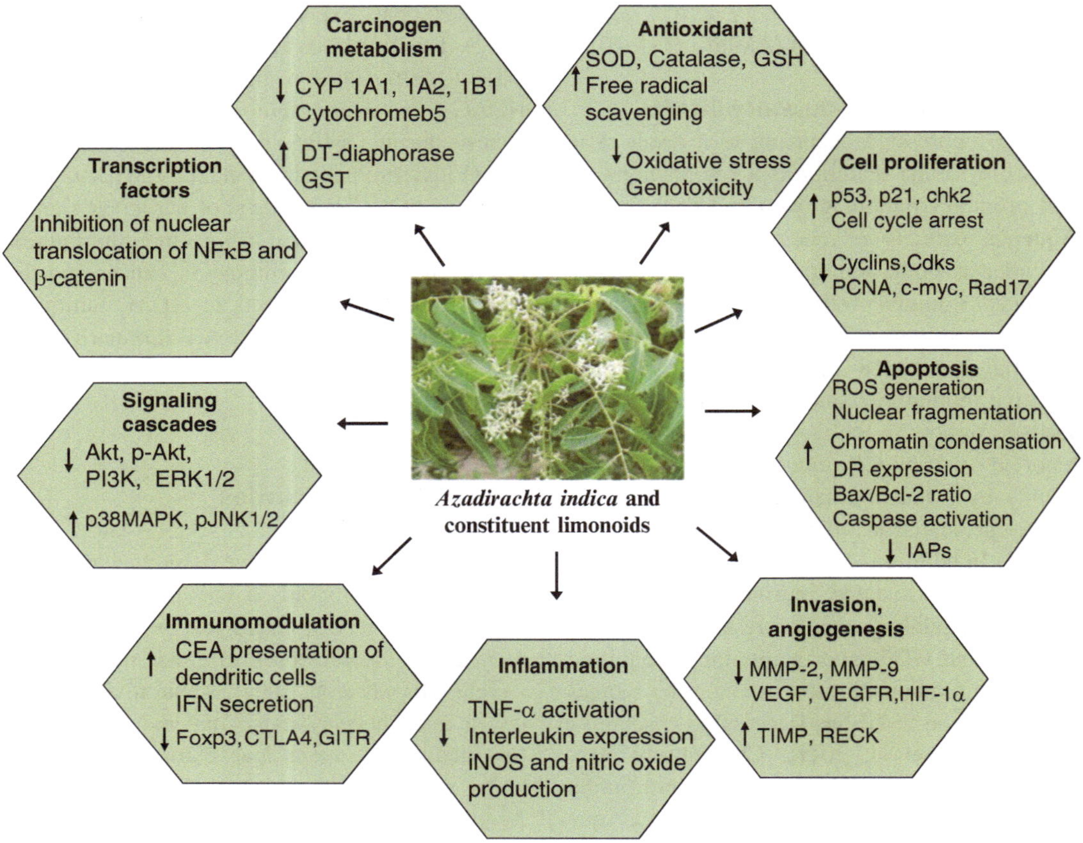

Fig. 4.1 Molecular targets of neem and its constituent phytochemicals

4.5 Conclusions and Future Perspectives

Globally, there is an increasing trend towards the use of natural products for medicinal purposes owing to their chemical diversity, intrinsic biologic activity, affordability, and lack of substantial toxic effects. Neem, a medicinal treasure of the Indian subcontinent with its wide array of phytochemicals is a promising candidate for anticancer drug development. Neem extracts and the constituent limonoids target multiple molecular and cellular pathways that are dysregulated in cancer including xenobiotic metabolism, cell cycle, DNA repair, apoptosis, matrix invasion, angiogenesis, immune surveillance, and intracellular signalling. However, the efficacy of neem extracts and limonoids has been tested only in preclinical models, and the cancer preventive and therapeutic potential in humans are largely unexplored. There is therefore a need for extensive investigations on the metabolism, pharmacokinetics, toxicity, precise molecular mechanism of action, expression profiling using high-throughput microarrays, and epigenetic remodelling in rigorous well-designed clinical trials for translating the beneficial effects of neem from the bench to the bedside.

Acknowledgements The authors gratefully acknowledge financial support from the Department of Science and Technology, Government of India, New Delhi, India.

References

Akihisa T, Noto T, Takahashi A, Fujita Y, Banno N, Tokuda H, Koike K, Suzuki T, Yasukawa K, Kimura Y (2009) Melanogenesis inhibitory, anti-inflammatory, and chemopreventive effects of limonoids from the seeds of Azadirachta indica A. Juss. (neem). J Oleo Sci 58:581–594

Akihisa T, Takahashi A, Kikuchi T, Takagi M, Watanabe K, Fukatsu M, Fujita Y, Banno N, Tokuda H, Yasukawa K (2011) The melanogenesis-inhibitory, anti-inflammatory, and chemopreventive effects of limonoids in n-hexane extract of Azadirachta indica A. Juss. (neem) seeds. J Oleo Sci 60:53–59

Akudugu J, Gade G, Bohm L (2011) Cytotoxicity of azadirachtin A in human glioblastoma cell lines. Life Sci 68:1153–1160

Alam A, Halder S, Thulasiram HV, Kumar R, Goyal M, Iqbal MS, Pal C, Dey S, Bindu S, Sarkar S, Pal U, Maiti NC, Bandyopadhyay U (2012) Novel anti-inflammatory activity of epoxyazadiradione against macrophage migration inhibitory factor: inhibition of tautomerase and pro-inflammatory activities of macrophage migration inhibitory factor. J Biol Chem 287(29):24844–24861

Arakaki J, Suzui M, Morioka T, Kinjo T, Kaneshiro T, Inamine M, Sunagawa N, Nishimaki T, Yoshimi N (2006) Antioxidative and modifying effects of a tropical plant Azadirachta indica (neem) on azoxymethane-induced preneoplastic lesions in the rat colon. Asian Pac J Cancer Prev 7:467–471

Babykutty S, Priya PS, Nandini RJ, Kumar MA, Nair MS, Srinivas P, Gopala S (2012) Nimbolide retards tumor cell migration, invasion, and angiogenesis by downregulating MMP-2/9 expression via inhibiting ERK1/2 and reducing DNA-binding activity of NF-kB in colon cancer cells. Mol Carcinog 51:475–490

Badam L, Deolankar RP, Kulkarni MM, Nagsampgi BA, Wagh UV (1987) In vitro antimalarial activity of neem (Azadirachta indica A. Juss) leaf and seed extract. Indian J Malariol 24:111–117

Baral R, Chattopadhyay U (2004) Neem (Azadirachta indica) leaf mediated immune activation causes prophylactic growth inhibition of murine Ehrlich carcinoma and B16 melanoma. Int Immunopharmacol 4:355–366

Bhanwra S, Singh J, Khosla P (2000) Effect of Azadirachta indica (Neem) leaf aqueous extract on paracetamol-induced liver damage in rats. Indian J Physiol Pharmacol 44:64–68

Bharati S, Rishi P (2012) Azadirachta indica exhibits chemopreventive action against hepatic cancer: studies on associated histopathological and ultrastructural changes. Microsc Res Tech 75:586–595

Biswas K, Chattopadhyay I, Banerjee RK, Bandyopadhyay U (2002) Biological activities and medicinal properties of neem (Azadirachta indica). Curr Sci 82:1336–1345

Boeke SJ, Boersma MG, Alink GM, van Loon JJA, van Huis A, Dicke M, Rietjens IMCM (2004) Safety evaluation of neem (Azadirachta indica) derived pesticides. J Ethnopharmacol 94:25–41

Boopalan T, Arumugam A, Damodaran C, Rajkumar L (2012) The anticancer effect of 2′-3′-dehydrosalannol on triple-negative breast cancer cells. Anticancer Res 32:2801–2806

Brahmachari G (2004) Neem- an omnipotent plant: a retrospection. Chem Biochem 5:408–421

Brandt GE, Schmidt MD, Prisinzano TE, Blagg BS (2008) Gedunin, a novel hsp90 inhibitor: semisynthesis of derivatives and preliminary structure-activity relationships. J Med Chem 51:6495–6502

Brew K, Nagase H (2010) The tissue inhibitors of metalloproteinases (TIMPs): an ancient family with structural and functional diversity. Biochim Biophys Acta 1803:55–71

Carew JS, Giles FJ, Nawrocki ST (2008) Histone deacetylase inhibitors: mechanisms of cell death and promise in combination cancer therapy. Cancer Lett 269:7–17

Cargnello M, Roux PP (2011) Activation and function of the MAPKs and their substrates, the MAPK-activated protein kinases. Microbiol Mol Biol Rev 75:50–83

Chakraborty K, Bose A, Chakraborty T, Sarkar K, Goswami S, Pal S, Baral R (2010) Restoration of dysregulated CC chemokine signaling for monocyte/macrophage chemotaxis in head and neck squamous cell carcinoma patients by neem leaf glycoprotein maximizes tumor cell cytotoxicity. Cell Mol Immunol 7:396–408

Chakraborty T, Bose A, Barik S, Goswami KK, Banerjee S, Goswami S, Ghosh D, Roy S, Chakraborty K, Sarkar K, Baral R (2011) Neem leaf glycoprotein inhibits CD4+CD25+Foxp3+ Tregs to restrict murine tumor growth. Immunotherapy 3:949–969

Chattopadhyay RR (2003) Possible mechanism of hepatoprotective activity of Azadirachta indica leaf extract: part II. J Ethnopharmacol 89:217–219

Chattopadhyay I, Nandi B, Chatterjee R, Biswas K, Bandyopadhyay U, Banerjee RK (2004) Mechanism of antiulcer effect of Neem (Azadirachta indica) leaf extract: effect on H+-K+-ATPase, oxidative damage and apoptosis. Inflammopharmacology 12:153–176

Chaturvedi MM, Sung B, Yadav VR, Kannappan R, Aggarwal BB (2011) NF-kB addiction and its role in cancer: 'one size does not fit all'. Oncogene 30:1615–1630

Chen J, Chen J, Sun Y, Yan Y, Kong L, Li Y, Qiu M (2011) Cytotoxic triterpenoids from Azadirachta indica. Planta Med 77:1844–1847

Chopra IC, Gupta KC, Nazir BN (1952) Preliminary study of antibacterial substances from Melia azadirachta. Indian J Med Res 40:511–515

Cohen E, Quistad GB, Casida JE (1996a) Cytotoxicity of nimbolide, epoxyazadiradione and other limonoids from neem insecticide. Life Sci 58:1075–1081

Cohen E, Quisted GB, Jefferies PR (1996b) Nimbolide is the principle cytotoxic component of neem seed insecticide preparations. Pest Sci 48:135–140

Csikasz-Nagy A, Palmisano A, Zamborszky J (2011) Molecular network dynamics of cell cycle control: transitions to start and finish. Methods Mol Biol 761:277–291

Dasgupta T, Banerjee S, Yadava PK, Rao AR (2004) Chemopreventive potential of Azadirachta indica (neem) leaf extract in murine carcinogenesis model systems. J Ethnopharmacol 92:23–36

Du Q, Geller DA (2010) Cross-regulation between Wnt and NF-κB signaling pathways. For Immunopathol Dis Therap 1:155–181

Farah MA, Ateeq B, Ahmad W (2006) Antimutagenic effect of neem leaves extract in freshwater fish, Channa punctatus evaluated by cytogenetic tests. Sci Total Environ 364:200–214

Gangar SC, Sandhir R, Rai DV, Koul A (2006) Modulatory effects of Azadirachta indica on benzo(a)pyrene-induced forestomach tumorigenesis in mice. World J Gastroenterol 12:2749–2755

Gialeli C, Theocharis AD, Karamanos NK (2011) Roles of matrix metalloproteinases in cancer progression and their pharmacological targeting. FEBS J 278:16–27

Glinsukon T, Somjaree R, Piyachaturawat P, Thebtaranonth Y (1986) Acute toxicity of nimbolide and nimbic acid in mice, rats and hamsters. Toxicol Lett 30:159–166

Gunadharini DN, Elumalai P, Arunkumar R, Senthilkumar K, Arunakaran J (2011) Induction of apoptosis and inhibition of PI3K/Akt pathway in PC-3 and LNCaP prostate cancer cells by ethanolic neem leaf extract. J Ethnopharmacol 134:644–650

Gupta SC, Prasad S, Reuter S, Kannappan R, Yadav VR, Ravindran J, Hema PS, Chaturvedi MM, Nair M, Aggarwal BB (2010) Modification of cysteine 179 of IkappaBalpha kinase by nimbolide leads to down-regulation of NF-kappa B-regulated cell survival and proliferative proteins and sensitization of tumor cells to chemotherapeutic agents. J Biol Chem 285:35406–35417

Gupta SC, Reuter S, Phromnoi K, Park B, Hema PS, Nair M, Aggarwal BB (2011) Nimbolide sensitizes human colon cancer cells to TRAIL through reactive oxygen species- and ERK-dependent up-regulation of death receptors, p53, and Bax. J Biol Chem 286:1134–1146

Hanasaki Y, Ogawa S, Fukui S (1994) The correlation between active oxygens scavenging and antioxidative effects of flavonoids. Free Radic Biol Med 16:845–850

Haque E, Baral R (2006) Neem (Azadirachta indica) leaf preparation induces prophylactic growth inhibition of murine Ehrlich carcinoma in Swiss and C57BL/6 mice by activation of NK cells and NK-T cells. Immunobiology 211:721–731

Harish Kumar G, Chandra Mohan KVP, Rao AJ, Nagini S (2009) Nimbolide a limonoid from Azadirachta indica inhibits proliferation and induces apoptosis of human choriocarcinoma (BeWo) cells. Invest New Drugs 27:246–252

Harish Kumar G, Vidya Priyadarsini R, Vinothini G, Vidjaya Letchoumy P, Nagini S (2010) The neem limonoids azadirachtin and nimbolide inhibit cell proliferation and induce apoptosis in an animal model of oral oncogenesis. Invest New Drugs 28:392–401

Hassler MR, Egger G (2012) Epigenomics of cancer—emerging new concepts. Biochimie 94(11):2219–2230

Iyanagi T (2007) Molecular mechanism of phase I and phase II drug-metabolizing enzymes: implications for detoxification. Int Rev Cytol 260:35–112

Jazirehi AR, Wenn PB, Damavand M (2012) Therapeutic implications of targeting the PI3Kinase/AKT/mTOR signaling module in melanoma therapy. Am J Cancer Res 2:178–191

Kamath SG, Chen N, Xiong Y, Wenham R, Apte S, Humphrey M, Cragun J, Lancaster JM (2009) Gedunin, a novel natural substance, inhibits ovarian cancer cell proliferation. Int J Gynecol Cancer 19:1564–1569

Kavitha K, Vidya Priyadarsini R, Anitha P, Ramalingam K, Sakthivel R, Purushothaman G, Singh AK, Karunagaran D, Nagini S (2012) Nimbolide, a neem limonoid abrogates canonical NF-κB and Wnt signaling to induce caspase dependent apoptosis in human hepatocarcinoma HepG2 cells. Eur J Pharmacol 681:6–14

Khan M, Wassilew SW (1987) The effect of raw material from the neem tree, neem oil and neem extracts on fungi pathogenic to humans. In: Schmutterer H, Asher KRS (eds) Natural pesticides from the neem tree and other tropical plants. GTZ, Eschborn, pp 645–650

Khosla P, Bhanwra S, Singh J, Seth S, Srivastava RK (2000) A study of hypoglycaemic effects of Azadirachta indica (neem) in normal and alloxan diabetic rabbits. Indian J Physiol Pharmacol 44:69–74

Kikuchi T, Ishii K, Noto T, Takahashi A, Tabata K, Takashi Suzuki T, Akihisa T (2011) Cytotoxic and apoptosis-inducing activities of limonoids from the seeds of Azadirachta indica (Neem). J Nat Prod 74:866–870

Kumar SR, Srinivas M, Yakkundi S (1996) Limonoids from the seeds of Azadirachta indica. Phytochemistry 43:451–455

Kumar S, Suresh PK, Vijayababu MR, Arunkumar A, Arunakaran J (2006) Anticancer effects of ethanolic neem leaf extract on prostate cancer cell line (PC-3). J Ethnopharmacol 105:246–250

Mahapatra S, Karnes RJ, Holmes MW, Young CY, Cheville JC, Kohli M, Klee EW, Tindall DJ, Donkena KV (2011) Novel molecular targets of Azadirachta indica associated with inhibition of tumor growth in prostate cancer. AAPS J 13:365–377

Mahapatra S, Young CY, Kohli M, Karnes RJ, Klee EW, Holmes MW, Tindall DJ, Donkena KV (2012) Antiangiogenic effects and therapeutic targets of azadirachta indica leaf extract in endothelial cells. Evid Based Complement Alternat Med 2012:303019

Mandal-Ghosh I, Chattopadhyay U, Baral R (2007) Neem leaf preparation enhances Th1 type immune response and anti-tumor immunity against breast tumor associated antigen. Cancer Immun 7:8

Manikandan P, Vidjaya Letchoumy P, Gopalakrishnan M, Nagini S (2008) Evaluation of Azadirachta indica leaf fractions for in vitro antioxidant potential and in vivo modulation of biomarkers of chemoprevention in the hamster buccal pouch carcinogenesis model. Food Chem Toxicol 46:2332–2343

Manikandan P, Anandan R, Nagini S (2009) Evaluation of Azadirachta indica leaf fractions for in vitro antioxidant potential and protective effects against H_2O_2-induced oxidative damage on pBR322 DNA and RBCs. J Agric Food Chem 57:6990–6996

Miller EG, Gonzales-Sanders AP, Couvillon AM, Wright JM, Hasegawa S, Lam LK (1992) Inhibition of hamster buccal pouch carcinogenesis by limonin 17-beta-D-glucopyranoside. Nutr Cancer 17:1–7

Mordue AJ, Blackwell A (1993) Azadirachtin: an update. J Insect Physiol 39:903–924

Morgan DE (2009) Azadirachtin, a scientific gold mine. Bioorg Med Chem 17:4096–4105

Nagini S (2012) RECKing MMP: relevance of reversion-inducing cysteine-rich protein with kazal motifs as a prognostic marker and therapeutic target for cancer (a review). Anticancer Agents Med Chem 12(7):718–725

Nanduri S, Thunuguntla SS, Nyavanandi VK, Kasu S, Kumar PM, Ram PS, Rajagopal S, Kumar RA, Deevi DS, Rajagopalan R, Venkateswarlu A (2003) Biological investigation and structure-activity relationship studies on azadirone from Azadirachta indica A. Juss. Bioorg Med Chem Lett 13:4111–4115

Niture SK, Rao US, Srivenugopal KS (2006) Chemopreventative strategies targeting the MGMT repair protein: augmented expression in human lymphocytes and tumor cells by ethanolic and aqueous extracts of several Indian medicinal plants. Int J Oncol 29:1269–1278

Okpanyi SN, Ezeukwu GC (1981) Anti-inflammatory and antipyretic activities of Azadirachta indica. Planta Med 41:34–39

Pai MR, Acharya LD, Udupa N (2004) Evaluation of antiplaque activity of Azadirachta indica leaf extract gel-a 6-week clinical study. J Ethnopharmacol 90:99–103

Patel VK, Venkatakrishna-Bhatt H (1988) Folklore therapeutic indigenous plants in periodontal disorders in India (review, experimental and clinical approach). Int J Clin Pharmacol Ther Toxicol 26:176–184

Paul R, Prasad M, Sah NK (2011) Anticancer biology of Azadirachta indica L (Neem): a mini review. Cancer Biol Ther Cancer Biol Ther 12:467–476

Pillai NR, Santhakumari G (1984) Toxicity studies on nimbidin, a potential antiulcer drug. Planta Med 50:146–148

Prashant GM, Chandu GN, Muralikrishna KS, Shafiulla MD (2007) The effect of mango and neem extract on four organisms causing dental caries: Streptococcus mutans, Streptococcus salivavius, Streptococcus mitis and Streptococcus sangui: an in vitro study. Indian J Dent Res 18:148–151

Priyadarsini RV, Murugan RS, Sripriya P, Karunagaran D, Nagini S (2010) The neem limonoids azadirachtin and nimbolide induce cell cycle arrest and mitochondria-mediated apoptosis in human cervical cancer (HeLa) cells. Free Radic Res 44:624–634

Puri HS (1999) Plant sources. In: Hardman R (ed) Neem. The divine tree. Azadirachta indica. Harwood Academic Publishers, Singapore, pp 9–21

Raizada RB, Srivastava MK, Kaushal RA, Singh RP (2001) Azadirachtin, a neem biopesticide: subchronic toxicity assessment in rats. Food Chem Toxicol 39:477–483

Ray A, Banerjee BD, Sen P (1996) Modulation of humoral and cell-mediated immune responses by Azadirachta indica (neem) in mice. Indian J Exp Biol 34:698–701

Roy A, Saraf S (2006) Limonoids: overview of significant bioactive triterpenes distributed in plant kingdom. Biol Pharm Bull 29:191–201

Roy MK, Kobori M, Takenaka M, Nakahara K, Shinmoto H, Tsushida T (2006) Inhibition of colon cancer (HT-29) cell proliferation by a triterpenoid isolated from Azadirachta indica is accompanied by cell cycle arrest and upregulation of p21. Planta Med 72:917–923

Roy MK, Kobori M, Takenaka M, Nakahara K, Shinmoto H, Isobe S, Tsushida T (2007) Antiproliferative effect on human cancer cell lines after treatment with nimbolide extracted from an edible part of the neem tree (Azadirachta indica). Phytother Res 21:245–250

Salehzadeh A, Akhkha A, Cushley W, Adams RLP, Kusel JR, Strang RHC (2003) Antimitotic effects of the neem terpenoid azadirachtin on cultured insect cells. Insect Biochem Mol Biol 33:681–689

Sarkar K, Bose A, Chakraborty K, Haque E, Ghosh D, Goswami S, Chakraborty T, Laskar S, Baral R (2008) Neem leaf glycoprotein helps to generate carcinoembryonic antigen specific anti-tumor immune responses utilizing macrophage-mediated antigen presentation. Vaccine 26:4352–4362

Sarkar K, Goswami S, Roy S, Mallick A, Chakraborty K, Bose A, Baral R (2010) Neem leaf glycoprotein enhances carcinoembryonic antigen presentation of dendritic cells to T and B cells for induction of anti-tumor immunity by allowing generation of immune effector/memory response. Int Immunopharmacol 10:865–874

Sastry BS, Suresh Babu K, Hari Babu T, Chandrasekhar S, Srinivas PV, Saxena AK, Madhusudana Rao J (2006) Synthesis and biological activity of amide derivatives of nimbolide. Bioorg Med Chem Lett 16:4391–4394

Satyavati GV, Raina MK, Sharma M (1976) Medicinal plants of India 1976, vol I. Indian Council of Medical Research, New Delhi, pp 112–117

Sethi JK, Vidal-Puig A (2010) Wnt signalling and the control of cellular metabolism. Biochem J 427:1–17

Singh N, Misra N, Singh SP, Kohli RP (1979) Melia azadirachta in some common skin disorders- a clinical evaluation. Antiseptic 76:677–679

Sithisarn P, Supabphol R, Gritsanapan W (2005) Antioxidant activity of Siamese neem tree (VP1209). J Ethnopharmacol 99:109–112

Sithisarn P, Carlsen CU, Andersen ML, Gritsanapan W, Skibsted LH (2007) Antioxidative effects of leaves from Azadirachta species of different provenience. Food Chem 104:1539–1549

Srivastava MK, Raizada RB (2007) Lack of toxic effect of technical azadirachtin during postnatal development of rats. Food Chem Toxicol 45:465–471

Subapriya R, Nagini S (2003) Ethanolic neem leaf extract protects against N-methyl -N′-nitro-N-nitrosoguanidine-induced gastric carcinogenesis in Wistar rats. Asian Pac J Cancer Prev 4:215–223

Subapriya R, Nagini S (2005) Medicinal properties of neem leaves: a review. Curr Med Chem Anticancer Agents 5:149–156

Subapriya R, Kumaraguruparan R, Abraham SK, Nagini S (2004) Protective effects of ethanolic neem leaf extract on N-methyl-N′-nitro-N-nitrosoguanidine-induced genotoxicity and oxidative stress in mice. Drug Chem Toxicol 27:15–26

Subapriya R, Bhuvaneswari V, Ramesh V, Nagini S (2005) Ethanolic leaf extract of neem (Azadirachta indica) inhibits buccal pouch carcinogenesis in hamsters. Cell Biochem Funct 23:229–238

Subapriya R, Kumaraguruparan R, Nagini S (2006) Expression of PCNA, cytokeratin, Bcl-2 and p53 during chemoprevention of hamster buccal pouch carcinogenesis by ethanolic neem (Azadirachta indica) leaf extract. Clin Biochem 39:1080–1087

Tan QG, Luo XD (2011) Meliaceous limonoids: chemistry and biological activities. Chem Rev 111:7437–7522

Tepsuwan A, Kupradinun P, Kusamran WR (2002) Chemopreventive potential of neem flowers on carcinogen-induced rat mammary and liver carcinogenesis. Asian Pac J Cancer Prev 3:231–238

Thoh M, Kumar P, Nagarajaram HA, Manna SK (2010) Azadirachtin interacts with the tumor necrosis factor (TNF) binding domain of its receptors and inhibits TNF-induced biological responses. J Biol Chem 285:5888–5895

Udeinya IJ (1993) Antimalarial activity of Nigerian neem leaves. Trans R Soc Trop Ned Hyg 87:471

Udeinya IJ, Mbah AU, Chijioke CP, Shu EN (2004) An antimalarial extract from neem leaves is antiretroviral. Trans R Soc Trop Med Hyg 98:435–447

Ulukaya E, Acilan C, Yilmaz Y (2011) Apoptosis: why and how does it occur in biology? Cell Biochem Funct 29:468–480

Van der Nat JM, Van der Sluis WG, De Silva KTD, Labadie RP (1991) Ethnopharmacognostical survey of Azadirachta indica A. Juss (Meliaceae). J Ethnopharmacol 35:1–24

Veeraraghavan J, Aravindan S, Natarajan M, Awasthi V, Herman TS, Aravindan N (2011a) Neem leaf extract induces radiosensitization in human neuroblastoma xenograft through modulation of apoptotic pathway. Anticancer Res 31:161–170

Veeraraghavan J, Natarajan M, Lagisetty P, Awasthi V, Herman TS, Aravindan N (2011b) Impact of curcumin, raspberry extract, and neem leaf extract on rel protein-regulated cell death/radiosensitization in pancreatic cancer cells. Pancreas 40:1107–1119

Vidya Priyadarsini R, Manikandan P, Kumar GH, Nagini S (2009) The neem limonoids azadirachtin and nimbolide inhibit hamster cheek pouch carcinogenesis by modulating xenobiotic-metabolizing enzymes, DNA damage, antioxidants, invasion and angiogenesis. Free Radic Res 43:492–504

In Vitro Studies on the Antioxidant/Antigenotoxic Potential of Aqueous Fraction from *Anthocephalus cadamba* Bark

5

Madhu Chandel, Upendra Sharma, Neeraj Kumar, Bikram Singh, and Satwinderjeet Kaur

Abstract

Cancer is a major public health problem in all parts of the world. With the increasing number of cancer cases worldwide, considerable attention is now being given to natural products for their possible cancer-preventing properties. Increasing evidence suggests that oxidative stress-mediated cardiovascular diseases and cancer-causing oxidation of the DNA molecule can be counteracted by natural antioxidants. The present study was conducted to evaluate the antioxidant/antigenotoxic potential of aqueous fraction from the bark of *Anthocephalus cadamba*, an important Ayurvedic medicinal plant. The antioxidant activity was assessed by in vitro assays, namely, DPPH (2,2-diphenyl-2-picrylhydrazyl), ABTS 2,2-azino-bis-(3-ethylbenzthiazoline-6-sulphonic acid) assay, reducing power assay, superoxide anion radical scavenging assay and plasmid DNA nicking assay. The antigenotoxicity was studied against 4NQO-induced DNA damage in *E. coli* PQ37 tester strain using SOS chromotest. The fraction exhibited potent antioxidant activity in all the antioxidant assays. The fraction exhibited 90.77 % activity in DPPH and 97.46 % in ABTS assay at highest tested concentration (200 μg/ml). The fraction showed 67.13 % reduction potential and percent inhibition of 81.00 % in superoxide anion radical scavenging assay at 1,000 μg/ml. The fraction at a concentration of 1,000 μg/ml decreased the SOS-inducing potency

M. Chandel • S. Kaur (✉)
Department of Botanical and Environmental Sciences,
Guru Nanak Dev University, Amritsar 143 005, India
e-mail: sjkaur@rediffmail.com; sjkaur2001@yahoo.co.in

U. Sharma • N. Kumar • B. Singh
Natural Plant Products Division, CSIR-Institute of
Himalayan Bioresource Technology, Palampur,
HP 176 061, India

P.R. Sudhakaran (ed.), *Perspectives in Cancer Prevention – Translational Cancer Research*, DOI 10.1007/978-81-322-1533-2_5, © Springer India 2014

(SOSIP) of 4NQO (20 μg/ml) by 21.86 %. Phytochemical analysis of aqueous fraction (AQAB) by UPLC-ESI-QTOF-MS revealed the fraction to be rich in alkaloids.

Keywords
Anthocephalus cadamba • Antioxidant activity • Antigenotoxicity

5.1 Introduction

Chronic diseases such as arteriosclerosis and cancer, which are the leading causes of death in the western world, are likely to be mediated by free radical and lipid peroxidation mechanisms (Halliwell and Gutteridge 1990). Cancer is expected to claim nine million deaths worldwide by the year 2015. Oxidative stress has been generating much interest primarily because of its accepted role as a major contributor to the aetiology of both normal senescence and severe pathologies with serious public health implications such as obesity, diabetes, atherosclerosis, metabolic syndrome and cancer. Antioxidants play a crucial role to protect human body against oxidative damage caused by reactive oxygen species. Reactive oxygen species (ROS) are by-products of biological metabolism with important roles in cell signalling, inflammation and immune defence (Valko et al. 2007). Under physiological conditions, the balance between oxidation and antioxidation is maintained by enzymatic systems and chemical scavengers; all of them are able to remove free radicals formed in cells and thus protect against oxidative damage (Bouayed and Bohn 2010). However, excessive formation of ROS and/or inadequate antioxidant defence may be a primary cause of oxidative damage (Valko et al. 2004). Antioxidants are those compounds that inhibit or delay the oxidation of other molecules by inhibiting the initiation or propagation of oxidising chain reactions (Velioglu et al. 1998). They are effective in protecting living organisms against oxidative damages caused by ROS. Several synthetic antioxidants, such as butylated hydroxyanisole (BHA), butylated hydroxytoluene (BHT) and tert-butylhydroquinone (TBHQ), are commercially available, but their applications are restricted for use in foods because of their toxicity (Ito et al. 1986; Peters et al. 1996; Li et al. 2002). In recent times, there has been an increasing interest in antimutagenic and antioxidant activity of compounds from plants. Natural plant products are efficient chemopreventive agents (Surh and Ferguson 2003). Moreover, several studies have reported a positive correlation of the increased dietary intake of natural antioxidants with reduced coronary heart disease, reduced cancer mortality and longer life expectancy (Halliwell 2007; Rios et al. 2009). *Anthocephalus cadamba* (Roxb.) Miq. (*Rubiaceae*) is an Ayurvedic medicinal plant, used in treating various ailments. It is used as a folk medicine in the treatment of fever and anaemia, as antidiuretic and for improvement of semen quality. The present study was undertaken to evaluate the water fraction (AQAB) from bark of this plant for its antioxidant/antigenotoxic potential in various in vitro assays.

5.2 Materials and Methods

5.2.1 Bacterial Strain and Chemicals

Escherichia coli PQ37 strain was purchased from Institut Pasteur, France. 2,2-Diphenyl-1-picrylhydrazyl (DPPH), Ferric chloride, L-Ascorbic acid, NADH (nicotinamide adenine dinucleotide), PMS (phenazine methosulphate), NBT (nitroblue tetrazolium chloride), Ortho-nitrophenyl β-D-galactopyranoside (ONPG) and para-nitrophenylphosphate (PNPP) were obtained from HiMedia Pvt. Limited Mumbai, India. Potassium persulphate, ABTS [2,2-azinobis (3-ethylbenzothiazoline-6-sulphonic acid) diammonium salt] and rutin were from Sigma (St. Louis, MO, USA). Plasmid pBR322 was purchased from Genei Pvt. Ltd., Bangalore. All other reagents used were of analytical grade (AR).

5.2.2 Collection of Plant Material

The bark of *Anthocephalus cadamba* was collected from the trees growing in the campus of Guru Nanak Dev University, Amritsar.

5.2.3 Extraction and Fractionation

The bark was washed with running water to remove any dust impurities and dried at 40 °C. The material was finely powdered and extracted with 80 % MeOH. The methanol extract was concentrated under reduced pressure using rotary evaporator. It was then made aqueous with distilled water in a separating funnel and further fractionated with organic solvents in order of increasing polarity, namely, *n*-hexane, chloroform, ethyl acetate and *n*-butanol. The remaining fraction was the aqueous fraction (AQAB) which was subjected to various in vitro assays in the present study.

5.2.4 Antioxidant Activity

5.2.4.1 DPPH Radical Scavenging Assay

DPPH radical scavenging assay was carried out by the method of Blois (1958) with some modifications. Different concentrations (20–200 μg/ml) of AQAB fraction from *Anthocephalus cadamba* bark were dissolved in methanol and taken in test tubes in triplicates. Then, 2 ml of 0.1 mM methanol solution of DPPH was added to each of the test tubes and were shaken vigorously. After 30 min, absorbance was taken at 517 nm using UV-VIS spectrophotometer.

$$\% \text{ Radical scavengingactivity } (\%) = [\text{Abs (control)} - \text{Abs (sample)} / \text{Abs (control)}] \times 100$$

where

Abs (control) is the absorbance of DPPH radical + solvent alone and

Abs (sample) is the absorbance of DPPH radical + AQAB fraction.

5.2.4.2 ABTS Radical Scavenging Assay

The spectrophotometric analysis of $ABTS^{+\bullet}$ scavenging activity was determined according to the protocol given by Re et al. (1999). ABTS radical cations were produced by reacting ABTS solution (7 mM) and potassium persulphate (2.45 mM) solution in the ratio of 1: 0.5 and allowing the mixture to stand in the dark at room temperature for 12–16 h before use. The ABTS radical cation solution was diluted with ethanol to an absorbance of 0.70 (±0.02) at 734 nm. 300 μl of different concentrations (20–200 μg/ml) of AQAB fraction were added to the diluted ABTS radical cation solution and absorbance was taken up to 5 min.

$$\text{Radical scavenging activity } \% = A_0 - A_1/A_0 \times 100$$

where

A_0 is the absorbance of ABTS solution and

A_1 is the absorbance of reaction mixture (containing test sample & ABTS solution).

5.2.4.3 Reducing Power Assay

Reducing potential of the AQAB fraction was determined using the method of Oyaizu (1986). Different concentrations (200–1,000 μg/ml) of AQAB fraction from *Anthocephalus cadamba* bark were dissolved in methanol and taken in test tubes in triplicates. To the test tubes, 2.5 ml of phosphate buffer (pH 6.6, 0.2 M) and 2.5 ml of 1 % potassium ferricyanide solution was added. These contents were mixed well and were incubated at 50 °C for 20 min. After incubation, 10 % TCA (trichloroacetic acid) was added. 2.5 ml of supernatant was taken and mixed with double distilled water (2.5 ml) and ferric chloride (0.1 %). The OD (absorbance) was measured spectrophotometrically at 700 nm. Increase in absorbance of reaction mixture was interpreted as increase in reducing ability of the sample, and ascorbic acid and rutin were used as standard.

5.2.4.4 Superoxide Anion Radical Scavenging Assay

The measurement of superoxide anion scavenging activity of AQAB fraction was performed according to the method of Nishikimi et al. (1972) with slight modifications. About 1 ml of nitroblue tetrazolium (NBT) solution (156 μM prepared in phosphate buffer, pH 7.4), 1 ml of NADH solution (468 μM prepared in phosphate buffer pH 7.4) and 1 ml of various concentrations of the AQAB fraction (100, 200, 400, 600, 800 and 1,000 μg/ml) and the reference compound ascorbic acid and rutin were mixed, and the reaction was started by adding 100 μl of phenazine methosulphate (PMS) solution (60 μM in phosphate buffer, pH 7.4). The reaction mixture was incubated at 25 °C for 5 min and the absorbance was measured at 560 nm. The percentage inhibition was calculated by formula:

$$[(\text{Abs. of control}) - (\text{Abs. of sample})/(\text{Abs. of control})] \times 100.$$

5.2.4.5 Plasmid DNA Protection Assay

To measure the hydroxyl radical scavenging effect of AQAB fraction, DNA nicking experiment was performed according to the protocol of Lee et al. (2002). Plasmid DNA was incubated with Fenton's reagent containing different concentrations of AQAB fraction, and finally the volume of the mixture was raised up to 20 μl. The mixture was then incubated for 30 min at 37 °C followed by addition of loading dye. Electrophoresis was carried out in TAE (tris-acetic acid-EDTA) buffer and DNA was analysed followed by ethidium bromide staining.

5.2.5 Genotoxic/Antigenotoxic Activity

5.2.5.1 SOS Chromotest

The SOS chromotest is an SOS transcriptional-fusion-based assay to estimate primary DNA damage produced by chemicals and physical agents by measuring the expression of a reporter gene (β-galactosidase) that becomes coloured in the presence of a substrate. It was carried out with the method of Quillardet and Hofnung (1985). Exponential-phase culture of *E. coli* PQ37 was grown at 37 °C in Luria broth medium (1 % bactotryptone, 0.5 % yeast extract and 1 % NaCl) plus 20 μg/ml ampicillin and diluted 1:9 into fresh medium; 100 μl aliquots were distributed into glass test tube containing 20 μl of genotoxicant [4NQO (20 μg/ml)] and 20 μl of AQAB fraction of different concentrations (10–1,000 μg/ml) each and made final volume 0.6 ml with L medium. Positive control was prepared by exposure of bacteria to 4NQO. After incubation for 2 h at 37 °C, 300 μl samples were used for assay of β-galactosidase and alkaline phosphatase activities, respectively. The activity of the constitutive enzyme alkaline phosphatase was used as a measure of protein synthesis and toxicity. In order to determine the β-galactosidase activity, 2.7 ml of B-buffer (adjusted to pH 7.5) was added, and after 10 min, 600 μl of 0.4 % 4-nitrophenyl-β-galactopyranoside (ONPG) solution was added to each of the test tubes of one set. To determine the constitutive alkaline phosphatase activity, P-buffer (adjusted to pH 8.8) was added, and after 10 min, 600 μl of 0.4 % 4-nitrophenyl phosphate (PNPP) solution was added to another set of tubes. All mixtures were incubated at 37 °C and observed for the colour development. After 30 min, the conversion of ONPG was stopped with 2 ml of 1 M sodium carbonate and that of PNPP with 1 ml of 2.5 M HCl and after 5 min added 1 ml of 2 M tris (hydroxymethyl) amino-methane. The absorption was measured at 420 nm using a reference solution in which culture is replaced by L medium.

The enzyme activities were calculated according to the simplified method:

$$\text{Enzyme units } (U) = A_{420} \times 1{,}000/t$$

(A_{420} = optical density at 420 nm; t = substrate conversion time in minutes).

$$\text{Induction factor (IF)} = \text{Rc}/\text{Ro}$$

Rc = β-galactosidase activity/alkaline phosphatase activity determined for the test compound at concentration c,

Ro = β-galactosidase activity/alkaline phosphatase activity in the absence of the test compound.

Anti-genotoxicity was expressed as percentage inhibition of genotoxicity according to the formula:

$$\text{Inhibition }(\%) = 100 - (\text{IF}_1 - \text{IF}_0/\text{IF}_2 - \text{IF}_0) \times 100$$

where

IF_1 is the induction factor of the test compound,
IF_2 is the induction factor of positive control (4NQO) and
IF_0 the induction factor of the blank (without any test compound).

5.2.6 UPLC-Electrospray Ionisation-Quadrupole Time-of-Flight Mass Spectrometry

5.2.6.1 Sample Preparation

For UPLC-ESI-QTOF-MS analysis, samples were prepared in a mixture of acetonitrile/water (80/20; v/v) and filtered through a 0.22 μ MILLEX GV syringe filter (Millipore, MA, USA) prior to inject into the UPLC system.

5.2.6.2 UPLC Instruments and Chromatographic Conditions

All analysis were performed on Waters ACQUITY UPLC system (Waters, MA, USA), including binary solvent manager, sample manager, column comportment and photo diode array (PDA) detector, connected with Waters Mass Lynx software. An ACQUITY UPLC BEH C_{18} column (100 mm × 2.1 mm i.d, 1.7 μm) also from Waters was used. The column temperature was maintained at 30 °C. Samples were separated using a gradient mobile phase consisting of 0.05 % formic acid in water (A) and acetonitrile (B). The gradient elution is 0–0.2 min, 82 %A; 0.2–1.4 min, 75 % A; 1.4–2.0 min, 65 % A; 2.2–3.5 min, 65 % A, and finally reconditioning the column with 82 % A for 1 min. The flow rate was set 0.28 ml min^{-1} and the injection volume was 1 μl.

5.2.7 Statistical Analysis

The results are presented as the mean ± standard error. Regression analysis was carried out by best-fit method and IC_{50} values were calculated using regression equation.

5.3 Results

5.3.1 DPPH Radical Scavenging Assay

The scavenging of DPPH radicals increased with increasing concentrations (20–200 μg/ml) of the fraction. The percent of DPPH radical scavenging was 21.59, 43.26, 66.75, 87.78 and 90.77 % at concentrations of 20, 60, 100, 140 and 200 μg/ml, respectively (Fig. 5.1). The IC_{50} was found to be 58.26 μg/ml. The results were compared with ascorbic acid (IC_{50} 13.74 μg/ml) and rutin (IC_{50} 54.05 μg/ml).

5.3.2 ABTS Radical Scavenging Assay

The inhibitory effect on $ABTS^{+\bullet}$ radicals of different concentrations of the AQAB fraction was assayed at various concentrations ranging from 20 to 200 μg/ml. The absorption was taken upto 5 min and there was decrease in the absorption with time. The inhibitory activity of 97.46 % was observed at highest tested concentration of 200 μg/ml (Fig. 5.2). The IC_{50} of the fraction was found to be 51.42 μg/ml compared with standard compounds rutin and BHT which showed IC_{50} value of 24.78 and 42.75 μg/ml, respectively.

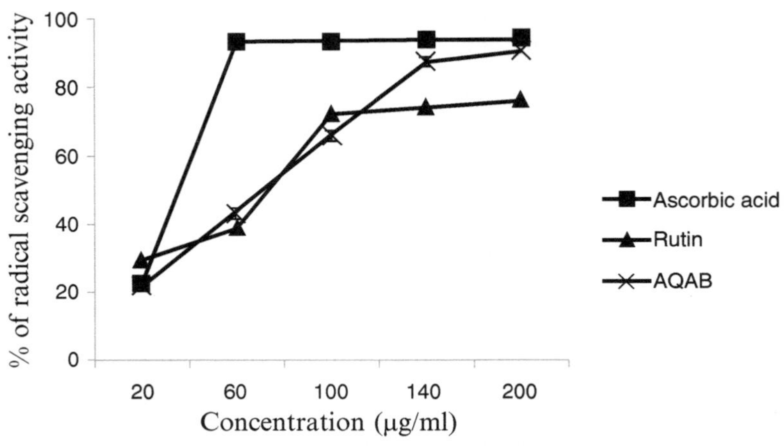

Fig. 5.1 Scavenging effect on DPPH radicals of AQAB fraction from bark of *Anthocephalus cadamba*

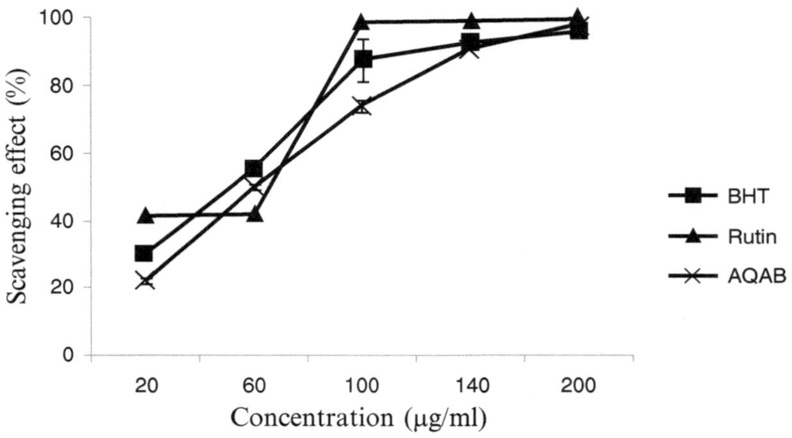

Fig. 5.2 ABTS radical scavenging activity of AQAB fraction from bark of *Anthocephalus cadamba*

5.3.3 Reducing Power Assay

The increased absorbance of the reaction mixture indicates increased reducing power. The reducing power of AQAB fraction from *A. cadamba* bark is presented in Fig. 5.3. As described in Fig. 5.3, the AQAB fraction was found to have strong and increased reducing ability at concentrations of 200–1,000 μg/ml. The reducing power of AQAB fraction increased with increasing concentration and was compared with standard ascorbic acid and rutin. It showed reducing power of 61.93 and 67.13 % when compared with ascorbic acid and rutin and the IC_{50} values were 764.98 and 708.24 μg/ml, respectively.

5.3.4 Superoxide Scavenging Assay

AQAB fraction showed superoxide scavenging activity which was dose dependent (Fig. 5.4). The highest tested concentration of 1,000 μg/ml showed the scavenging activity of 81.00 %. IC_{50} value of AQAB fraction on superoxide radical scavenging activity was found to be 51.42 μg/ml, whereas IC_{50} value of ascorbic acid and rutin was found to be 13.96 and 58.75 μg/ml, respectively.

5.3.5 Plasmid DNA Nicking Assay

DNA protective activity was assessed by measuring the degree of protection on DNA scission

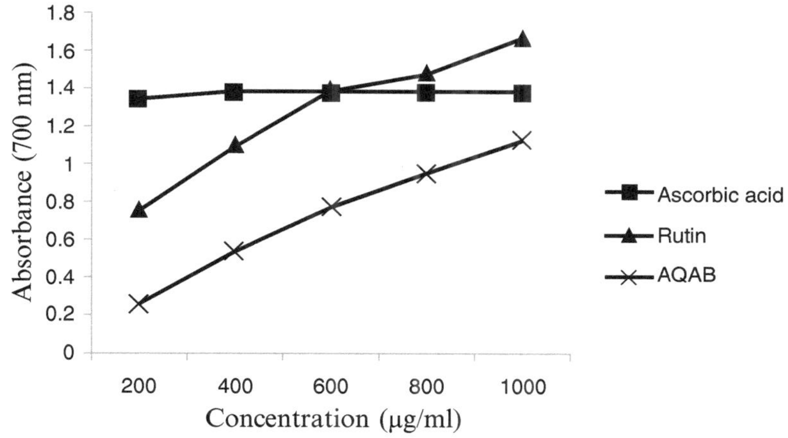

Fig. 5.3 Reducing power of AQAB fraction from bark of *Anthocephalus cadamba*

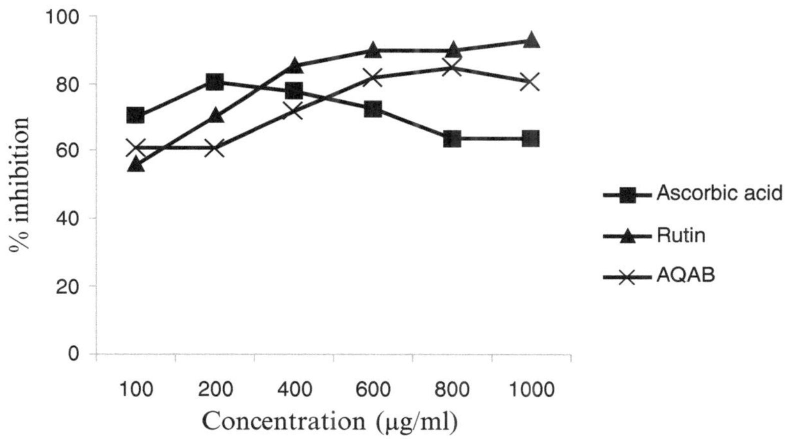

Fig. 5.4 Superoxide anion radical scavenging activity of AQAB fraction from bark of *Anthocephalus cadamba*

that was induced by the attack of hydroxyl radicals, which was shown by the agarose gel electrophoresis pattern. It is clear from the results that the AQAB fraction scavenged the hydroxyl radicals and protected the pBR322 plasmid DNA quite effectively (Fig. 5.5).

5.3.6 Genotoxic/Antigenotoxic Activity

In the SOS chromotest, it was ascertained that different concentrations of AQAB fraction of *A. cadamba* added to the indicator bacteria were not genotoxic as the induction factor induced by the tested doses was below 1.5. The AQAB fraction reduced the genotoxicity of 4NQO by 21.86 % at a concentration of 1,000 μg/ml. The induction factor induced by 4NQO was 16.01 ± 0.82 which was reduced to 12.73 ± 0.90 at 1,000 μg/ml concentration of AQAB fraction (Table 5.1).

5.3.7 Identification of Bioactive Compounds by UPLC

UPLC chromatogram of AQAB fraction is shown in Fig. 5.6. The retention times (t_R), *m/z* and λ_{max} are listed in Table 5.2. Tentative identification of compounds was based on comparison of mass and λ_{max} from literature. UPLC-ESI-QTOF-MS study of AQAB fraction from bark of *A. cadamba* showing peaks at t_R 1.70, 2.03, 2.51 which correspond

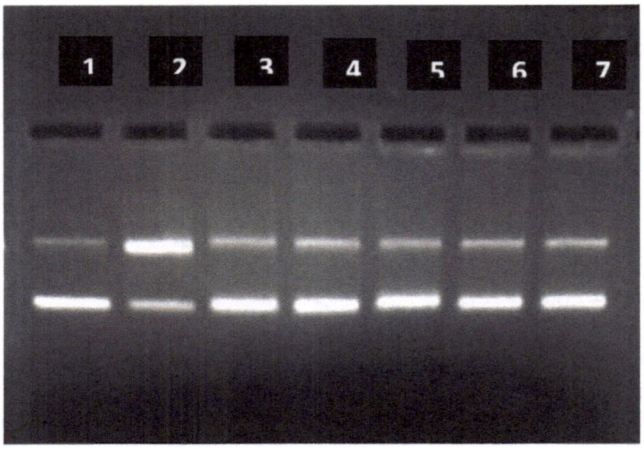

Fig. 5.5 *Effect of AQAB fraction from bark of A. cadamba in plasmid DNA nicking assay. Lane 1*: Negative Control (DW + pBR322 plasmid DNA). *Lane 2*: pBR322 DNA + Fenton's reagent (FR). *Lane 3*: pBR322 plasmid DNA + FR + AQAB (100 μg/ml). *Lane 4*: pBR322 plasmid DNA + FR + AQAB (200 μg/ml). *Lane 5*: pBR322 plasmid DNA + FR + AQAB (300 μg/ml). *Lane 6*: pBR322 plasmid DNA + FR + AQAB (400 μg/ml). *Lane 7*: pBR322 plasmid DNA + FR + AQAB (500 μg/ml)

Table 5.1 Genotoxic/antigenotoxic effect of AQAB fraction from bark of *Anthocephalus cadamba* in SOS chromotest using *E. coli* PQ37 tester strain

		β-Galactosidase units	Alkaline phosphatase units		Percent
Treatment	Dose (μg/ml)	Mean ± SD	Mean ± SD	Induction factor	inhibition
Control		4.83 ± 0.32	14.62 ± 1.20		
Positive control					–
4NQO	20 μg/ml	65.84 ± 1.71	12.93 ± 1.00	16.01 ± 0.82	
Negative control	10	2.31 ± 1.01	13.36 ± 0.67	0.73 ± 0.19	–
	30	3.29 ± 0.47	12.63 ± 1.09	0.79 ± 0.17	–
	100	2.32 ± 0.59	13.30 ± 0.75	0.53 ± 0.14	–
	300	2.97 ± 1.00	14.12 ± 0.48	0.63 ± 0.22	–
	1,000	3.33 ± 0.46	13.36 ± 0.46	0.72 ± 0.07	–
4NQO + AQAB	10	54.42 ± 2.09	11.89 ± 1.29	14.29 ± 2.27	11.50 %
	30	52.36 ± 1.10	11.53 ± 0.65	13.79 ± 0.68	14.79 %
	100	51.99 ± 3.45	11.32 ± 0.68	13.95 ± 1.30	13.72 %
	300	51.28 ± 3.27	11.57 ± 1.43	13.61 ± 0.89	15.99 %
	1,000	49.98 ± 3.69	11.87 ± 0.57	12.73 ± 0.90	21.86 %

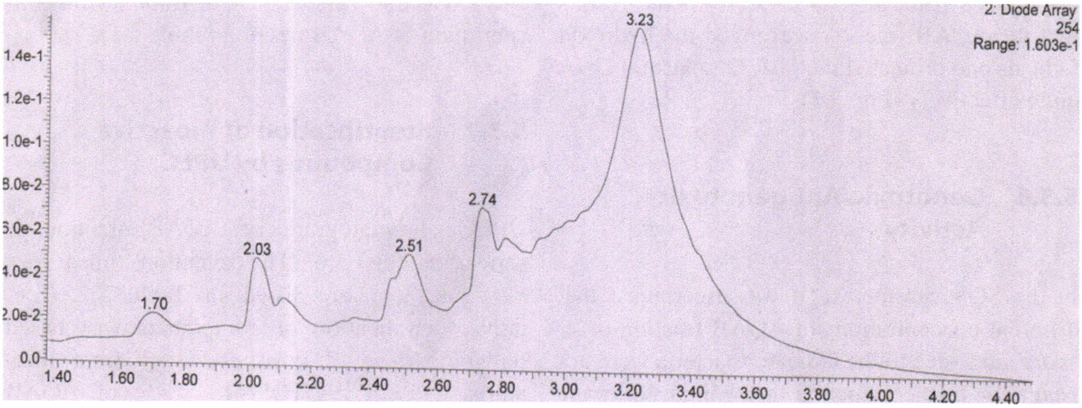

Fig. 5.6 UPLC chromatogram of AQAB fraction from bark of *A. cadamba*

Table 5.2 Tentative identification of compounds in AQAB fraction from bark of *A. cadamba* by UPLC

Sl. No.	t_R	m/z $[M+H]^+$	UV λ_{max}	Tentative identification
1	1.70	563	268, 366	3β-isodihydrocadambine- 4oxide [Glycosidic monoterpenoid indole alkaloid]
2	2.03	543	233, 308	3′-*O*-caffeoylsweroside [iridoid glucoside]
3	2.51	545	220, 360	Cadambine [indole alkaloid glucoside]
4	2.74	547	221, 280	3β-dihydrocadambine [indole alkaloid]
5	3.23	547	278	3β-isodihydrocadambine

to glycosidic monoterpenoid indole alkaloid ($m/z = 563$; $\lambda_{max} = 268$, 366) (Zhou et al. 2008), iridoid glucoside ($m/z = 543$; $\lambda_{max} = 233$, 308) (Kitagawa et al. 1996) and Cadambine, indole alkaloid glucoside ($m/z = 545$; $\lambda_{max} = 220$, 360) (Handa et al. 1984), respectively. The occurrence of peaks at t_R 2.74 ($\lambda_{max} = 221$, 280) and 3.23 ($\lambda_{max} = 278$) having m/z 547 are identified as dihydrocadambine and/or isodihydrocadambine (Zhou et al. 2008; on the basis of m/z only).

5.4 Discussion

Radical scavenging activities are very important due to the deleterious role of free radicals in foods and in biological systems. DPPH$^{\bullet}$ and ABTS$^{+\bullet}$ radical scavenging methods are spectrophotometric procedures for evaluating the antioxidant potential of various plant extracts/bioactive phytoconstituents (Bretan et al. 2011; Liu et al. 2011; Tai et al. 2011; Suh et al. 2011; Pan et al. 2007; Mathew and Abraham 2006). These chromogens (the violet DPPH radical and the blue green ABTS radical cation) are easy to use, have a high sensitivity and allow the rapid analysis of the antioxidant activity of large number of samples. DPPH is a stable free radical at room temperature and accepts an electron to become a stable diamagnetic molecule. The reduction capability of DPPH was determined by the decrease in its absorbance (517 nm) in the presence of antioxidant. In the present study, the AQAB fraction showed dose-response relationship in DPPH radical scavenging assay. The IC_{50} of AQAB fraction was comparable to that of rutin. The AQAB fraction also showed potent antioxidant potential in ABTS radical cation scavenging method. Fragoso et al. (2008) reported the antioxidant and antigenotoxic activity of psychollatine, a monoterpene indole alkaloid from *Psychotria umbellata*. The antimutagenic activity was assayed using *Saccharomyces cerevisiae* N123 strain in the presence of H_2O_2, and the antioxidant capacity of the extract and indole alkaloid was investigated using the hypoxanthine/xanthine oxidase assay. Psychollatine and the crude foliar extract of *P. umbellata* showed protective effect against oxidative stress in yeast, acting both as antioxidant and antimutagenic agents. Iridoid glucosides were isolated from the methanolic stem-bark extract of *Fagraea blumei* which were reported to show scavenging properties towards the 2,2-diphenyl-1-picryl-hydrazyl (DPPH) radical in TLC autographic and spectrophotometric assays (Cuendet et al. 1997). The high free radical scavenging activity of AQAB fraction in DPPH and ABTS assay may be attributed to the presence of free hydroxyl groups present in iridoid glucoside (3′-*O*-caffeoylsweroside) and indole alkaloid glucosides (3β-isodihydrocadambine 4-oxide, 3β-dihydrocadambine, cadambine and 3β-isodihydrocadambine) (Fig. 5.7) analysed by UPLC. The DPPH radical scavenging activity of three alkaloids isolated from *Mahonia aquifolium* –berberine, jatrorrhizine and magnoflorine – were studied by Rackova et al. (2004), and it was observed that alkaloids bearing free phenolic groups – jatrorrhizine and magnoflorine – showed better activities than berberine not bearing any readily abstractable hydrogen on its skeleton. In a report by Shirwaikar et al. (2006), the ABTS$^{+\bullet}$ radicals were scavenged by berberine (benzyl tetra isoquinoline alkaloid) in a concentration dependent manner with the maximum scavenging activity observed at 512 µg/ml and the minimum scavenging activity found at 2 µg/ml and IC_{50} was found to

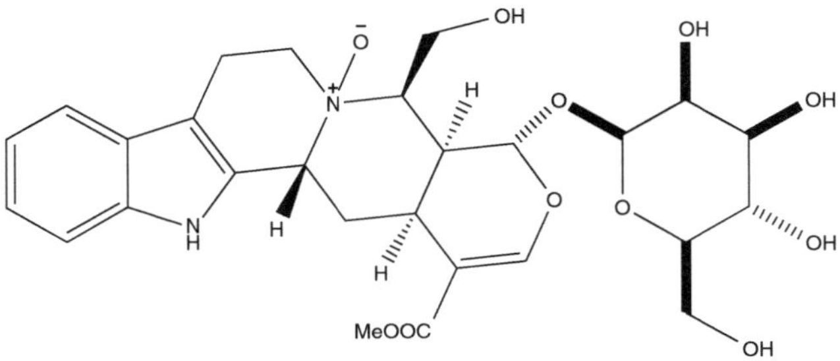

3β-isodihydrocadambine 4-oxide

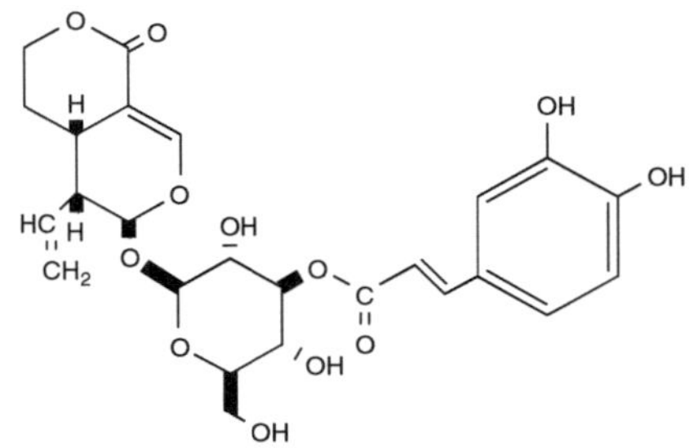

3' -O-caffeoylsweroside

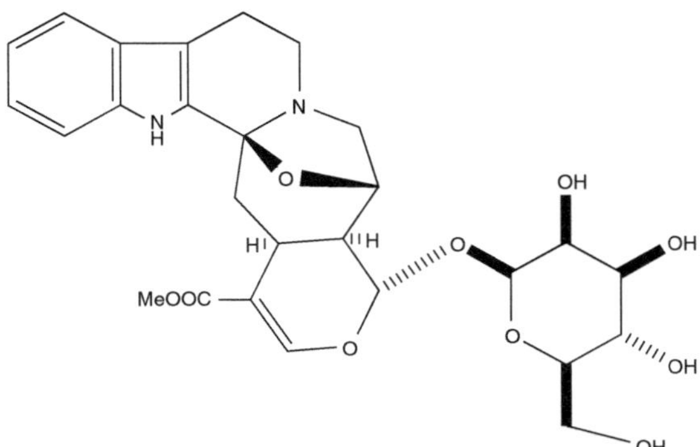

Cadambine

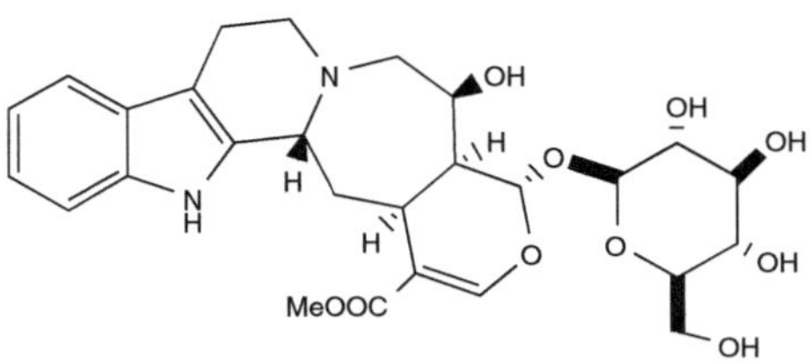

3β-dihydrocadambine

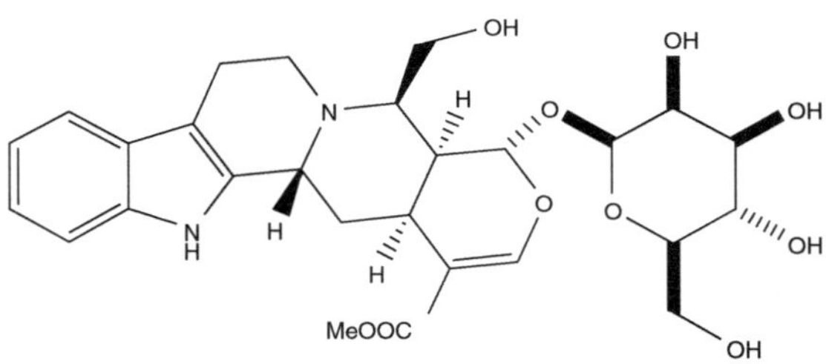

3β-isodihydrocadambine

Fig. 5.7 Structures of compounds identified from AQAB fraction from *A. cadamba* bark

be 38.7 μg/ml. The reducing power can serve as a significant reflection of the antioxidant activity. AQAB fraction showed potent reducing power in a dose-dependent manner. In this assay, the yellow colour of the test solution changes to various shades of green and blue, depending on the reducing power of test compound. The presence of reducers (i.e. antioxidants) causes the reduction of the Fe^{3+}/ferricyanide complex to the ferrous form. Superoxide radical is biologically quite toxic and is formed in almost all aerobic cells, one important source being the 'respiratory burst' of phagocytic cells when they contact foreign particles and immune complexes (Halliwell and Gutteridge 1984). The biological toxicity of superoxide is due to its capacity to inactivate iron-sulphur cluster containing enzymes, which are critical in wide variety of metabolic pathways, thereby liberating free iron in the cell, which can undergo Fenton chemistry and generate the secondary ROS such as hydrogen peroxide and hydroxyl radical (Valko et al. 2006). In superoxide scavenging assay, the fraction showed IC_{50} value of 51.42 μg/ml which was comparable to standard rutin ($IC_{50} = 58.75$ μg/ml). The AQAB fraction was tested in SOS chromotest for its genotoxic and antigenotoxic potential. It was found to be non-genotoxic as the IF was less than 1.5. The compounds are classified as non-genotoxic if the IF (induction factor) remains <1.5, as marginally genotoxic if the IF ranges between 1.5 and 2 and as genotoxic if the IF exceeds 2 (Kevekordes et al. 1999). AQAB fraction showed weak antigenotoxic activity against the genotoxic effect of 4NQO. However, AQAB fraction when studied for its protective activity against the DNA damage caused by hydroxyl radicals generated by Fenton's reagent in plasmid DNA nicking assay showed that it possessed the potential to protect the DNA from the damage caused by hydroxyl radicals. Hydroxyl radical is the most reactive free radical and its formation causes the oxidation of lipids, proteins and nucleic acids. Damage to DNA may cause strand breaks, base modifications and DNA cross links (Cadet et al. 1999). Nascimento et al. (2007) showed that brachycerine (monoterpene indole alkaloid) and the crude foliar extract of *Psychotria brachyceras* have antioxidant and antimutagenic effects in yeast, and probably this action is mainly due to the scavenging of $OH^{\bullet}$ radicals. The potent antioxidant activity of AQAB fraction in various in vitro assays and its potential to prevent DNA damage caused by hydroxyl radicals may be attributed to the presence of iridoid glucoside and alkaloid glucosides which can be exploited for cancer chemoprevention.

Acknowledgements The authors are thankful to UGC (DRS-SAP), New Delhi, for providing financial assistance. Director of CSIR-IHBT, Palampur, is gratefully acknowledged for providing the lab facility. Upendra Sharma is grateful to CSIR for SRF. We also thank Shiv Kumar for the UPLC analysis.

References

Blois MS (1958) Antioxidant determinations by the use of a stable free radical. Nature 29:1199–1200

Bouayed J, Bohn T (2010) Exogenous antioxidants-double-edged swords in cellular redox state. Oxid Med Cell Longev 3:228–237

Bretan F, Cerantola S, Gall EA (2011) Distribution and radical scavenging activity of phenols in *Ascophyllum nodosum* (Phaeophyceae). J Exp Mar Biol Ecol 399:167–172

Cadet J, Delatour T, Douki T, Gasparutto D, Pouget J-P, Ravanat J-L, Sauvaigo S (1999) Hydroxyl radicals and DNA base damage. Mutat Res 424:9–21

Cuendet M, Hostettmann K, Potterat O, Dyatmiko W (1997) Iridoid glucosides with free radical scavenging properties from *Fagraea blumei*. Helv Chim Acta 80:1144–1152

Fragoso V, Nascimento NC, Moura DJ, Silva ACR, Richter MF, Saffi J, Fett-Neto AG (2008) Antioxidant and antimutagenic properties of the monoterpeneindolealkaloid psychollatine and the crude foliar extract of *Psychotria umbellata* Vell. Toxicol In Vitro 22:559–566

Halliwell B (2007) Dietary polyphenols: good, bad, or indifferent for your health? Cardiovasc Res 73: 341–347

Halliwell B, Gutteridge JMC (1984) Oxygen toxicity, oxygen radicals, transition metals and disease. Biochem J 219:1–14

Halliwell B, Gutteridge JM (1990) Role of free radicals and catalytic metal ions in human disease: an overview. Methods Enzymol 186:1–85

Handa SS, Gupta SK, Vasisht K, Keene AT, Phillipson JD (1984) Quinoline alkaloids from *Anthocephalus chinensis*. Planta Med 50:358

Ito N, Hirose M, Fukishima S, Tsuda H, Shirai T, Tatematsu M (1986) Studies on antioxidants: their anticarcinogenic and modifying effects on chemical carcinogenesis. Food Chem Toxicol 24: 1099–1102

Kevekordes S, Mersch-Sundermann V, Burghaus CM, Spielberger J, Schmeiser HH, Arlt VM, Dunkelberg H (1999) SOS induction of selected naturally occurring substances in *Escherichia coli* (SOS chromotest). Mutat Res 15:81–91

Kitagawa I, Wei H, Nagao S, Mahmud T, Hori K, Kobayashi M, Uji T, Shibuya H (1996) Characterization of 3′-O-caffeoylsweroside, a new secoiridoid glucoside, and kelampayosides A and B, two new phenolic apioglucosides, from the bark of *Anthocephalus chinensis* (Rubiaceae). Chem Pharm Bull 44:1162–1167

Lee JC, Kim HR, Kim J, Jang YS (2002) Antioxidant activity of ethanol extract of the stem of *Opuntia ficus*-indica var. saboten. J Agric Food Chem 50:6490–6496

Li Y, Seacat A, Kuppusamy P, Zweier JL, Yager JD, Trush MA (2002) Copper redox-dependent activation of 2-*tert*-butyl(1,4)hydroquinone: formation of reactive oxygen species and induction of oxidative DNA damage in isolated DNA and cultured rat hepatocytes. Mutat Res 518:123–133

Liu J, Wang C, Wang Z, Zhang C, Lu S, Liu J (2011) The antioxidant and free-radical scavenging activities of extract and fractions from corn silk (*Zea mays* L.) and related flavone glycosides. Food Chem 126: 261–269

Mathew S, Abraham TE (2006) Studies on the antioxidant activities of cinnamon (*Cinnamomum verum*) bark extracts, through various *in vitro* models. Food Chem 94:520–528

Nascimento NC, Fragoso V, Moura DJ, Silva ACR, Fett-Neto AG, Saffi J (2007) Antioxidant and antimutagenic effects of the crude foliar extract and the alkaloid brachycerine of *Psychotria brachyceras*. Environ Mol Mutagen 48:728–734

Nishikimi M, Rao NA, Yagi K (1972) The occurrence of superoxide anion in the reaction of reduced phenazine methosulphate and molecular oxygen. Biochem Biophys Res Commun 46:849–853

Oyaizu M (1986) Studies on product of browning reaction prepared from glucose amine. Jpn J Nutr 44:307–315

Pan Y, Zhu J, Wang H, Zhang X, Zhang Y, He C, Ji X, Li H (2007) Antioxidant activity of ethanolic extract of *Cortex fraxini* and use in peanut oil. Food Chem 103:913–918

Peters MMCG, Rivera MI, Jones TW, Monks TJ, Lau SS (1996) Glutathione conjugates of tert-butyl-hydroquinone, a metabolite of the urinary tract tumor promoter 3-tert-butyl-hyroxyanisole, are toxic to kidney and bladder. Cancer Res 56:1006–1011

Quillardet P, Hofnung M (1985) The SOS Chromotest, a colorimetric bacterial assay for genotoxins: procedures. Mutat Res 147:65–78

Rackova L, Majekova M, Kostalova D, Stefek M (2004) Antiradical and antioxidant activities of alkaloids isolated from *Mahonia aquifolium*. Structural aspects. Bioorg Med Chem 12:4709–4715

Re R, Pellegrini N, Proreggente A, Pannala A, Yang M, Rice-Evans C (1999) Antioxidant activity applying an improved ABTS radical cation decolourization assay. Free Radic Biol Med 26:1231–1237

Rios ADO, Antunes LMG, Bianchi MDLP (2009) Bixin and lycopene modulation of free radical generation induced by cisplatin–DNA interaction. Food Chem 113:1113–1118

Shirwaikar A, Shirwaikar A, Rajendran K, Punitha ISR (2006) *In vitro* antioxidant studies on the benzyl tetra isoquinoline alkaloid berberine. Biol Pharm Bull 29:1906–1910

Suh H-J, Kim S-R, Hwang J-S, Kim MJ, Kim I (2011) Antioxidant activity of aqueous methanol extracts from the lucanid beetle, *Serrognathus platymelus castanicolor* Motschulsky (Coleoptera: Lucanidae). J Asia Pac Entomol 14:95–98

Surh Y, Ferguson LR (2003) Dietary and medicinal antimutagens and anticarcinogens: molecular mechanisms and chemopreventive potential highlights of a symposium. Mutat Res 9485:1–8

Tai Z, Cai L, Dai L, Dong L, Wang M, Yang Y, Cao Q, Ding Z (2011) Antioxidant activity and chemical constituents of edible flower of *Sophora viciifolia*. Food Chem 126:1648–1654

Valko M, Izakovic M, Mazur M, Rhodes CJ, Telser J (2004) Role of oxygen radicals in DNA damage and cancer incidence. Mol Cell Biochem 266:37–56

Valko M, Rhodes CJ, Moncol J, Izakovic M, Mazur M (2006) Free radicals, metals and antioxidants in oxidative stress-induced cancer. Chem Biol Interact 160:1–40

Valko M, Leibfritz D, Moncola J, Cronin MTD, Mazura M, Telser J (2007) Free radicals and antioxidants in normal physiological functions and human disease. Int J Biochem Cell Biol 39:44–84

Velioglu YS, Mazza G, Gao L, Oomah BD (1998) Antioxidant activity and total phenolics in selected fruits, vegetables and grain products. J Agric Food Chem 46:4113

Zhou Z, He H-P, Kong N-C, Wang T-J, Hao X-J (2008) Indole alkaloids from the leaves of *Anthocephalus chinensis*. Helv Chim Acta 91:2148–2152

Possible Involvement of Signal Transducer and Activator of Transcription-3 (STAT3) Signaling Pathway in the Initiation and Progression of Hepatocellular Carcinoma

6

Aruljothi Subramaniam, Muthu K. Shanmugam, Ekambaram Perumal, Feng Li, Alamelu Nachiyappan, Alan P. Kumar, Benny K.H. Tan, and Gautam Sethi

Abstract

Hepatocellular carcinoma (HCC) is the most common type of liver cancer and the third leading cause of cancer death worldwide, with 75 % of cases occurring in Southeast Asian countries like China, Hong Kong, Taiwan, Singapore, Korea, and Japan. The etiology of HCC is likely to involve interactions between multiple risk factors. The most commonly reported risk factors are nonspecific cirrhosis (21 %), followed by alcohol-induced liver disease (16 %), HCV infection (10 %), and HBV infection (5 %). In addition, obesity and type II diabetes are also suspected to increase the risk of acquiring liver cancer. Persistent activation of signal transducers and activators of transcription-3 (STAT3) is frequently observed several human cancers and transformed cell lines including HCC. The significance of constitutively STAT3 in HCC is due to its induction of several tumorigenic genes that substantially contribute to the initiation and progression of the malignancy. These include antiapoptotic proteins like Bcl-2, Bcl-xL,

A. Subramaniam
Department of Pharmacology, Yong Loo Lin School of Medicine, National University of Singapore, Singapore 117597, Singapore

Molecular Toxicology Lab, Department of Biotechnology, Bharathiar University, Coimbatore 641046, Tamil Nadu, India

M.K. Shanmugam • F. Li • A. Nachiyappan • B.K.H. Tan
Department of Pharmacology, Yong Loo Lin School of Medicine, National University of Singapore, Singapore 117597, Singapore

E. Perumal
Molecular Toxicology Lab, Department of Biotechnology, Bharathiar University, Coimbatore 641046, Tamil Nadu, India

A.P. Kumar • G. Sethi (✉)
Department of Pharmacology, Yong Loo Lin School of Medicine, National University of Singapore, Singapore 117597, Singapore

Cancer Science Institute of Singapore, National University of Singapore, Centre for Translational Medicine, 14 Medical Drive, #11-01M, Singapore 117599, Singapore
e-mail: phcgs@nus.edu.sg

P.R. Sudhakaran (ed.), *Perspectives in Cancer Prevention – Translational Cancer Research*, DOI 10.1007/978-81-322-1533-2_6, © Springer India 2014

Mcl-1, XIAP, and survivin. Examples of other STAT3-regulated oncogenic genes include c-Myc and cyclin D1, which regulates cell proliferation; matrix metalloproteinase-9 which mediates cellular invasion; and vascular endothelial growth factor, which controls angiogenesis. Thus, novel agents that can suppress constitutive and/or inducible activation of STAT3 have the potential for HCC therapy. In this chapter, we discuss in detail the potential role of STAT3 signaling cascade both in HCC initiation and progression and also various therapeutic strategies employed to block aberrant activation of this proinflammatory transcription factor in HCC.

Keywords
HCC • STAT3 • Proliferation • Apoptosis • Angiogenesis

Abbreviations

Bad	Bcl2 associated death promoter protein
Bax	Bcl-2-associated X protein
Bcl2	B-cell lymphoma 2
Bcl-xL	B-cell lymphoma extra large
Bid	BH3 interacting-domain death agonist
c-myc	Myelocytomatosis cellular oncogene
CSF-1R	Colony-stimulating factor-1R
EGF	Epidermal growth factor
G-CSF	Granulocyte colony-stimulating factor
HBV	Hepatitis B virus
HCV	Hepatitis C virus
HGF	Hepatocyte growth factor
IGF	Insulin-like growth factor
IL	Interleukin
IFN-γ	Interferon-gamma
JAK	Janus kinase
MMPs	Matrix metalloproteases
NAFLD	Nonalcoholic fatty liver disease
NASH	Nonalcoholic steatohepatitis
NF-κB	Nuclear factor kappa B
PDGF	Platelet-derived growth factor
PTPase	Protein tyrosine phosphatase
ROS	Reactive oxygen species
SOCS	Suppressor of cytokine signaling
STAT3	Signal transducer and activator of transcription 3
TGF	Transforming growth factor
VEGF	Vascular endothelial growth factor

6.1 Introduction: Risk Factors Associated with Initiation and Development of HCC

Hepatocellular carcinoma (HCC) is the fifth most prevalent cancer worldwide (Ferlay et al. 2010) and possibly the most common malignant tumor found among men (Dominguez-Malagon and Gaytan-Graham 2001; Subramaniam et al. 2013). Due to its late presentation, aggressiveness, and limited response to therapy, HCC has become the third most deadly cancer and causes approximately one million deaths annually (Ferlay et al. 2010; Carr et al. 2010). While considered a rare form of cancer in many western countries, HCC is endemic in East and Southeast Asia where over three-quarters of liver cancer-caused deaths occur (Ferlay et al. 2010). Infections with chronic hepatitis B (HBV)/hepatitis C virus (HCV) and associated liver cirrhosis/hepatitis have been attributed to more than 80 % of the cases of HCC (Lau and Lai 2008). For example, chronic hepatitis caused by HBV/HCV can cause significant damage to hepatocytes and adversely affect their normal functioning (Subramaniam et al. 2013; Nakamoto and Kaneko 2003) (Fig. 6.1).

In addition, various environmental risk factors also including aflatoxin B1 exposure, alcohol over-abuse, and cigarette smoking have been reported to contribute to the development of HCC (Subramaniam et al. 2013; Abdel-Hamid 2009). For example, an increased risk of mortality in

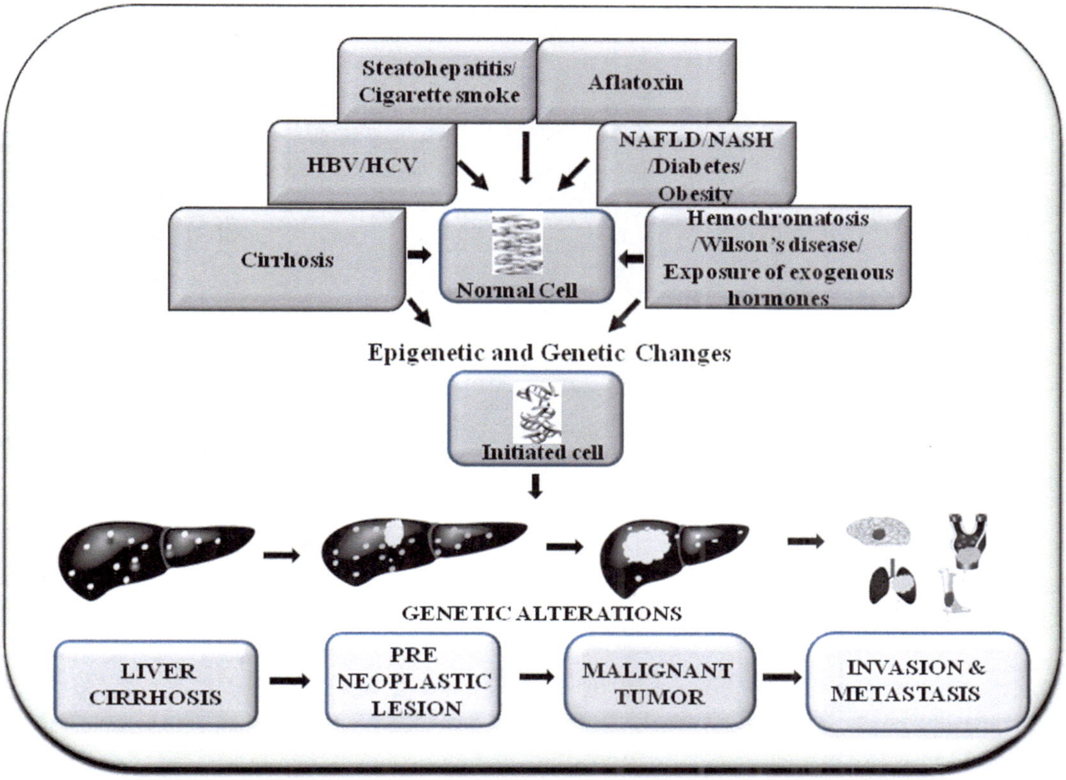

Fig. 6.1 A multi step cascade for HCC initiation and development

HCC patients has been closely associated with obesity. It has been found that obesity can induce an inflammatory response, which in turn may increase levels of proinflammatory cytokines [interleukin-6 (IL-6) and tumor necrosis factor-alpha (TNF-α) expression] in adipose tissue and Kupffer cells (Subramaniam et al. 2013; Toffanin et al. 2010).

6.2 Role of STAT3 Signaling Pathway in the Initiation of HCC

Signal transducer and activator of transcription (STATs) were initially discovered in 1993 by James Darnell and can be activated by diverse stimuli to activate gene transcription (Shuai et al. 1993). STAT proteins have been in particular shown to play a critical role in cytokine signaling cascades that regulate various cell growth and differentiation signal transduction (Subramaniam et al. 2013). The STAT family consists of seven members; these are STAT1, STAT2, STAT3, STAT4, STAT5a, STAT5b, and STAT6 that can be further classified into two groups, according to their biological functions. The first group comprising of STAT2, STAT4, and STAT6 is reported to actively participate interferon-gamma (IFN-γ) signaling and T cell maturation. On the other hand, the second group consisting of STAT1, STAT3, and STAT5 is involved in development of mammary glands, embryogenesis, as well as oncogenesis (Subramaniam et al. 2013; He and Karin 2011).

Among various STAT family proteins, STAT3 has gained significant attention as it has been found to be an important regulator of distinct signal transduction pathways involved in liver damage and repair mechanisms (Subramaniam et al.

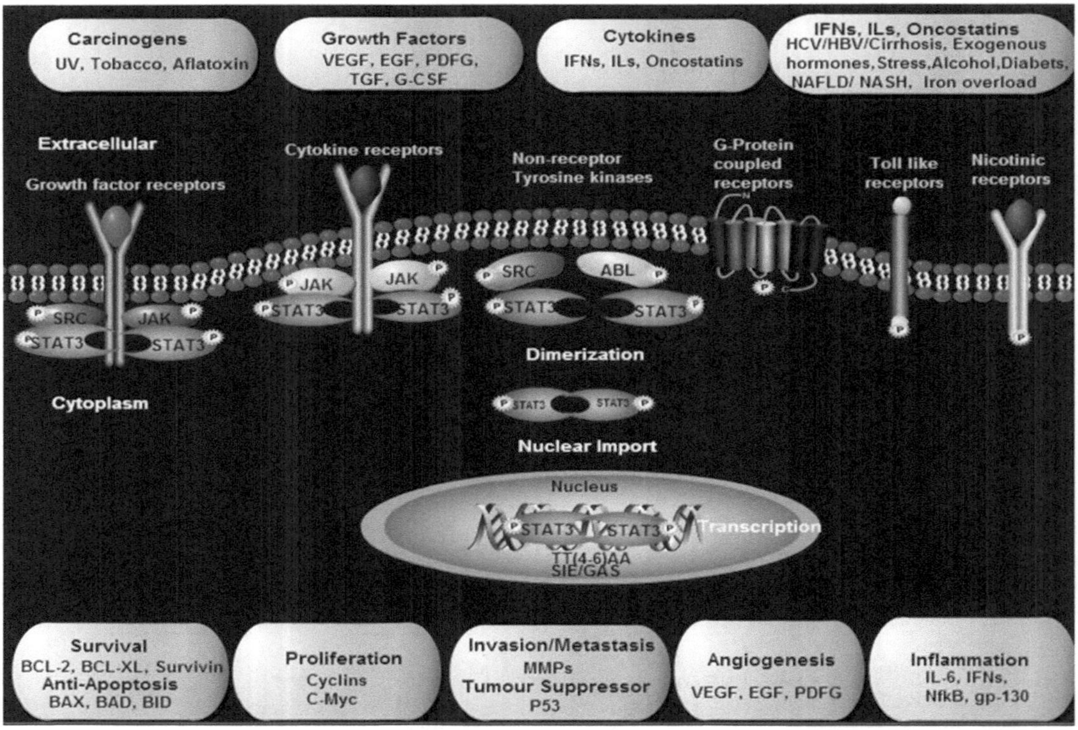

Fig. 6.2 STAT3 activation cascade involved in HCC progression

2013; Strain 1998; Taub 2003). STAT3 was initially demonstrated to be an acute-phase response factor that can bind to the IL-6 responsive element (Wegenka et al. 1993) and subsequently as a DNA-binding protein in response to epidermal growth factor stimulation (Zhong et al. 1994). STAT3 can be induced by various cytokines such as IL-6, leukemia inhibitory factor (LIF), oncostatin M, and ciliary neurotrophic factor (CNTF) that transmit their signals through the gp130 protein (Akira et al. 1994; Hibi et al. 1990; Hirano et al. 1997). Interestingly, the expression of IL-6 is elevated in various liver ailments and HCC (Subramaniam et al. 2013; Trikha et al. 2003; Naugler et al. 2007), and even IL-22-induced STAT3 phosphorylation on Ser727 residue can induce acute-phase genes in the liver (Dumoutier et al. 2000). In addition, STAT proteins can also be substantially stimulated by receptor tyrosine kinases such as epidermal growth factor receptor (EGFR), platelet-derived growth factor (PDGF-R), transforming growth factor (TGF), and colony stimulating factor-1R (CSF-1R) and seven-transmembrane G-protein-coupled receptors such as angiotensin II receptors (Karras et al. 1997). In fact, EGF, TGF-β, and PDGF receptors can even directly activate STAT3 proteins leading to enhanced proliferation and transformation (Subramaniam et al. 2013; Levy and Darnell 2002) (Fig. 6.2). The possible role of STAT3 in different aspects of liver tumorigenesis including transformation, inflammation, antiapoptosis, angiogenesis, cell cycle progression, and cellular invasion is discussed in detail below.

6.2.1 Oncogenic Transformation

Persistent activation of STAT3 is involved in several critical biological processes including growth, survival, invasion, and angiogenesis, all of which promote HCC initiation and progression (Turkson et al. 1998; Subramaniam et al. 2013). The first evidence related to the involvement of STAT3 in transformation came to light initially after studies showed that STAT3 is constitutively activated during transformation induced by oncogene v-Src. Several subsequent studies also reemphasized the important finding that STAT3 signaling is indeed required for oncogenic transformation by v-Src (Cao et al. 1996; Chaturvedi et al. 1997; Bromberg et al. 1998). Deregulated STAT3 activation has been consistently observed in HCC clinical samples and cell lines but not in non-transformed liver cells (Subramaniam et al. 2013; Yoshikawa et al. 2001; Niwa et al. 2005; Li et al. 2006). On the contrary, in a recent study, Schneller and colleagues elucidated the role of STAT3 in Ras-dependent HCC progression in the presence and absence of p19 (ARF)/p14 (ARF). They found that constitutive active STAT3 is tumor suppressive in Ras-transformed p19 (ARF−/−) hepatocytes, whereas the expression of STAT3 lacking Tyr (705) phosphorylation (U-Stat3) can enhance tumor formation. Accordingly, Ras-transformed STAT3 (Δhc)/p19 (ARF−/−) hepatocytes showed increased tumor growth, compared to those expressing STAT3, demonstrating a tumor-suppressor activity of STAT3 in cells lacking p19 (ARF) (Schneller et al. 2011). Moreover, Wu et al. found in another study that phosphorylated STAT3 expression in monocyte was significantly correlated to advanced clinical stage of HCC and a poor prognosis. They also noticed that pharmacological STAT3 inhibitor, NSC 74859, significantly suppressed tumor growth in mice with diethylnitrosamine (DEN)-induced HCC. Interestingly, NSC 74859 treatment also attenuated cancer-associated inflammation in DEN-induced HCC model (Wu et al. 2011). Moreover, Chen and coworkers evaluated the efficacy of combination therapy using cetuximab and NSC 74859 (a novel STAT3 inhibitor) in EGFR and STAT3 overexpressing hepatoma cells and found that NSC 74859 potentiated the antiproliferative effect of cetuximab in all three cell lines. siRNA knockdown of STAT3 increased the sensitivity of these cell lines to cetuximab, whereas STAT3 overexpression antagonized these effects (Chen et al. 2012a). Also, it has been reported that even multitargeted tyrosine kinase inhibitor sorafenib can inhibit growth and metastasis of HCC in part by blocking the MEK/ERK/STAT3 and PI3K/Akt/STAT3 signaling pathways, but independent of JAK2 and phosphatase shatterproof 2 (SHP2) activation (Pfitzner et al. 2004). All these above-cited reports and also the findings of our recently published review article (Subramaniam et al. 2013) clearly establish that the aberrant activation of STAT3 indeed plays a pivotal role in both HCC initiation and development. This is further supported by the fact that various novel STAT3 inhibitors have been identified in recent years that can suppress proliferation and induce apoptosis in various HCC cell lines and mouse models (Table 6.1).

6.2.2 Inflammation

Several reports indicate the potential role of HCC as a proinflammatory transcription factor in HCC and other liver diseases (Subramaniam et al. 2013; Pfitzner et al. 2004). STAT3 was initially discovered as an acute-phase response protein, thus suggesting its possible connection to inflammation (Wegenka et al. 1993). IL-6 is one of the key regulators of inflammation and predominantly exerts its biological effects through the activation of the STAT3 pathway (Zhong et al. 1994). Liang et al. recently tested the effect of IL-6 family cytokines Golgi phosphoprotein (GP73) mRNA and/or protein levels in human hepatoblastoma HepG2 cells. They found that levels of GP73 mRNA and protein were upregulated in HepG2 cells following treatment with either proinflammatory cytokine IL-6 or the related cytokine oncostatin M (OSM). Induction required the shared receptor subunit gp130 and correlated with increased tyrosine phosphorylation of STAT3. ELISA measurement of GP73 and IL-6 levels in the sera of patients with premalignant liver disease revealed a significant correlation between circulating levels of the two proteins. OSM levels were also elevated six- to sevenfold in sera from patients

Table 6.1 Reported STAT3 blockers in HCC cell lines and mouse models

Natural/synthetic inhibitors	Mechanism of inhibition	*Cell lines/mouse models*	References
Celecoxib	Inhibited JAK2 phosphorylation	Hep3B, HepG2, Huh-7, SNU-387, and SNU-449	Liu et al. (2011a)
Parthenolide along with TRAIL	Suppressed activation of JAK proteins	HepG2, Hep3B, and SK-Hep1	Carlisi et al. (2011)
Galiellalactone – a fungal metabolite from the ascomycete *Galiella rufa*	Exerted STAT3 inhibitory effect by covalently modifying a cysteine residue in the STAT3 DNA-binding domain	HepG2	Lavecchia et al. (2011)
XZH-5 small molecule	Reduced constitutive STAT3 phosphorylation at Tyr705 and the expression of STAT3- regulated genes	Hep3B, HepG2, Huh-7, SNU-387, and SNU-449	Liu et al. (2011b)
Sorafenib SC-1-synthetic molecule	Caused SHP-1-dependent STAT3 inactivation	HCC cell lines (PLC5, Huh-7, Hep3B, and Sk-Hep1)/nude mice with Huh xenografts	Tai et al. (2011)
Sorafenib with TRAIL	Upregulated SHP-1 activity	PLC5, Huh-7, Hep3B, and Sk-Hep1/nude mice with PLC5 xenografts	Chen et al. (2010)
3-[3,4-Dihydroxy-phenyl]-acrylic acid 2-[3,4-dihydroxy-phenyl]-ethyl ester (CADPE)	Inhibited both IL-6-mediated STAT3 activation and recruitment of STAT3 to the cyclin D1 promoter	Huh-7	Won et al. (2010)
FLLL32	JAK/STAT inhibitor suppressed STAT3 phosphorylation, STAT3 DNA-binding activity, and STAT3-regulated gene products	SNU-449, SNU-398, HEP3B, and SNU387	Lin et al. (2010) and Liu et al. (2010b)
LLL12	Inhibited IL-6-induced STAT3 phosphorylation	Hep3B, SNU-387, SNU-398, SNU-449	Liu et al. (2010a)
NSC-74859	Abrogated STAT3 activation	HepG2, PLC/PRF/5, Huh-7, SNU-398, SNU-449, SNU-182 and SNU-475, Huh-7 in nude mice	Lin et al. (2009)
ENMD-1198	Inhibited STAT3 phosphorylation	Huh-7 and HepG2	Moser et al. (2008)
Decoy ODN	Caused abrogation of STAT3-mediated cell cycle and antiapoptotic genes	HepG2, H7402, and PLC/PRF/5	Sun et al. (2008)
AG490	Janus kinase 2-specificinhibitor	Huh-1, Huh-7, HepG2 and Hep3B cells, Huh-7 tumors in athymic mice	Kusaba et al. (2007)

(continued)

Table 6.1 (continued)

Natural/synthetic inhibitors	Mechanism of inhibition	*Cell lines/mouse models*	References
IL-6 receptor fusion protein (IL-6-RFP)	A high-affinity cytokine-binding protein	HepG2	Metz et al. (2007)
YC-1	Inhibited STAT3 activity by enhancing the polyubiquitination of p-STAT3 (705) induced by cisplatin	HepG2, Hep3, and PLC	Lau et al. (2007)
Atiprimod	Suppressed STAT3 mediated through the inhibition of activation of upstream kinases c-Src, JAK1, and JAK2	Huh-7, HepG2, HepG2.2.15, and HepG2	Choudhari et al. (2007)
2′-*O*-methoxyethylribose-modified phosphorothioate antisense oligonucleotide (ASO)	Caused suppression of phosphorylated STAT3 and reduced its DNA-binding activity	HCCLM3, SNU423, Huh7, HCCLM3 nude mouse model	Li et al. (2006)
Stattic (non-peptide small molecule)	Inhibited SH2 domain, STAT3 dimerization, and DNA binding	HepG2	Schust et al. (2006)
Statins	Reduced IL-6-induced serine phosphorylation of transcription factorSTAT3	Hep3B	Arnaud et al. (2005)
SOCS-1 (peptide inhibitor)	(SOCS-1; also known as JAB and SSI-1) switched cytokine signaling "off" by means of its direct interaction with JAK	Human HCC lines SNU-182, SNU-423, SNU-387, SNU-398, SNU-449, SNU-475, and PLC/PRF/5	Yoshikawa et al. (2001)
Cyclopentenones, 2-(1-chloropropenyl)-4,5-dihydroxycyclopent-2-enone (CPDHC)	Suppressed IL-6and IL-6-dependent pathway by inhibiting the tyrosine phosphorylation of the STAT3 and STAT1 as well as the serine phosphorylation of the STAT3 by direct inhibition of JAK	HepG2	Weidler et al. (2000)
Celastrol	Abrogated JAK/STAT pathway and induced apoptosis of HCC cells in vitro and in vivo	C3A, HepG2, Hep3B, PLC/PRF5, and Huh-7	Rajendran et al. (2012)
β-Escin	Inhibited activation of upstream kinases c-Src, JAK1, and JAK2	HepG2, Huh-7, PLC/PRF5, wild, and STAT3 KO mice fibroblasts	Tan et al. (2010)
γ-Tocotrienol	Increased the expression of SHP-1 in HCC cells	HepG2, Huh-7 xenografts in nude mice	Rajendran et al. (2011a)
Butein	Inhibited activation of upstream kinases c-Src and JAK2 induced the expression of SHP-1	HepG2, SNU-387, HCCLM3, and PLC/PRF5/HCCLM3 nude mouse models	Rajendran et al. (2011b)

(continued)

Table 6.1 (continued)

Natural/synthetic inhibitors	Mechanism of inhibition	*Cell lines/mouse models*	References
Diosgenin	Induced the expression of Src homology 2 phosphatase 2 (SH-PTP2) that correlated with downregulation of constitutive STAT3 activation	HepG2, C3A	Li et al. (2010)
Luteolin	Accelerated ubiquitin-dependent degradation in the Tyr705-phosphorylated STAT3	HepG2, HLF, and HAK-1B	Selvendiran et al. (2006)
Cucurbitacin B	Inhibited STAT3 phosphorylation	HepG2 cells and mouse model	Zhang et al. (2009)
17-Hydroxy-jolkinolide B (HJB)	Reacted with cysteine residues of JAKs to form covalent bonds that inactivate JAKs	HepG2	Wang et al. (2009)

with either cirrhosis or HCC relative to controls without liver disease. Although there was an association between levels of GP73 and OSM in serum from people with liver cirrhosis, there was not a statistically significant correlation in HCC, thereby suggesting that the role of the proinflammatory cytokines in determining circulating levels may be complex (Liang et al. 2012). Furthermore, in various tumors, STAT3 can directly interact with nuclear factor NF-κB family member RELA (p65), keeping it localized in the nucleus and thereby contributing to constitutive NF-κB activation in cancer (Lee et al. 2009). Also, in a recent study, Mano and coworkers examined STAT3 activation, cytokine expression, and infiltration of tumor-associated macrophages in resected HCCs as well as the alteration of cell growth and migration by cytokine stimulation in HCC cell lines. They observed that in HCC specimens, the pSTAT3-positive group showed high levels of α-fetoprotein, large tumor size, frequent intrahepatic metastasis, high Ki-67 and Bcl-xL, poor prognosis, and high recurrence rate (Mano et al. 2013). Overall, their findings clearly indicate that STAT3 activation was correlated with aggressive behavior of HCC and may be mediated via tumor-associated macrophage.

6.2.3 Regulation of Apoptosis

STAT3 hyperactivation can also lead to increased transcription of various STAT3-regulated cell survival genes, e.g., Bcl-2, Bcl-xL, and survivin, Mcl-1, and XIAP, and thereby inhibiting pro-apoptotic proteins such as Bax, Bad, and Bid (Subramaniam et al. 2013; Al Zaid Siddiquee and Turkson 2008; Germain and Frank 2007). For example, Chen and coworkers reported that sorafenib can augment the antitumor effect of recombinant tumor necrosis factor-related apoptosis-inducing ligand (TRAIL) in resistant HCC. They found that STAT3 played a significant role in mediating TRAIL sensitization and showed that sorafenib downregulated phospho-STAT3 (pSTAT3) and subsequently reduced the expression levels of STAT3-related proteins (Mcl-1, survivin, and cyclin D1) in a dose- and time-dependent manner in TRAIL-treated HCC cells. Knockdown of STAT3 by RNA interference overcame apoptotic resistance to TRAIL in HCC cells, and ectopic expression of STAT3 in HCC cells abolished the TRAIL-sensitizing effect of sorafenib (Chen et al. 2010). Moreover, Liu et al. reported that IL-6 promoted survival of human liver cancer cells through activating STAT3 in response to doxorubicin treatment. Neutralizing IL-6 with anti-IL-6 antibody decreased survival of SNU-449 cells in response to doxorubicin. Also, targeting STAT3 with STAT3 siRNA reduced the protection of IL-6 against doxorubicin-induced apoptosis, indicating that STAT3 signaling contributed to the antiapoptotic effect of IL-6. They also observed that LLL12, a STAT3 small molecule inhibitor, can block IL-6-induced STAT3 phosphorylation, resulting in the attenuation of the antiapoptotic activity of IL-6. Overall, these results demonstrated that targeting STAT3 signaling could interrupt the antiapoptotic function of IL-6 in HCC cells (Liu et al. 2010a). Furthermore, Peroukides and colleagues studied by immunohistochemistry the protein expression of survivin in relation to cyclin D1, p-STAT3, beta-catenin, E-cadherin, and p-Akt in 69 cases of HCC and adjacent liver cirrhosis. Survivin was expressed in 63/69 (91.3 %) cases of HCC and in 40/47 (85.1 %) cases of liver cirrhosis. Survivin localization in HCC was exclusively nuclear, while intense cytoplasmic and low nuclear expression of survivin was observed in cases of cirrhosis. Survivin expression in HCC correlated significantly with low-grade tumors and expression of cyclin D1 and p-STAT3. Expression of survivin in liver cirrhosis correlated with downregulation of E-cadherin expression. Overall, they noticed a clear association of nuclear survivin with well-differentiated HCC, as well as with the expression of the cell cycle regulator cyclin D1 (Peroukides et al. 2010). Interestingly, Chen and coworkers recently reported that a novel obatoclax derivative, SC-2001, can induce apoptosis through SHP-1-dependent STAT3 inactivation in HCC cells (Chen et al. 2012b).

6.2.4 Cell Cycle Progression

It has been documented that the expression of cyclin D1, which can associate with cdk4 or cdk6 and controls progression from G1 to S phase, is elevated in STAT3-C expressing cells (Bromberg et al. 1999). Also, several studies have shown that dysregulated expression of cell cycle-related proteins, such as cyclin D1, cyclin-dependent kinase 4 (Cdk4), cyclin E, cyclin A, p16, and p27, may significantly contribute to both HCC initiation and progression (Subramaniam et al. 2013; Matsuda and Ichida 2006). Guo and coworkers recently showed that $p27^{-/-}$ mice display increased proliferation and decreased apoptosis of tumor cells, accompanied by an increase in the serum inflammatory cytokines IL-6 and TNF-α. Furthermore, they observed that the increased number and STAT3 phosphorylation status of infiltrated inflammatory cells was accompanied by increased IL-6 and TNF-α mRNA levels in tumor and normal liver tissue in the $p27^{-/-}$ mice. Overall, their data demonstrated that the loss of p27 promotes carcinogen-induced HCC genesis and progression via the elevation of inflammatory cytokines and the augmented activation of STAT3 signaling in tumor cells and infiltrated inflammatory cells (Guo et al. 2013). On the contrary, Hu et al. found that low doses of NSC 78459 (a novel STAT3 inhibitor) had little effect on HCC cell proliferation but efficiently inhibited STAT3 activation. Huh-7, Hep3B, and HepG2 cells, with epithelial phenotypes, displayed significantly enhanced doxorubicin cytotoxicity following co-treatment with NSC 74859, whereas mesenchymal SNU-449 cells did not show significant enhancement. NSC 74859 inhibited STAT3 activity and suppressed doxorubicin-induced epithelial-mesenchymal transition (EMT) in epithelial HCC cells. siRNA-mediated STAT3 knockdown resulted in EMT inhibition, which led to attenuation of NSC 74859-mediated chemosensitivity. Collectively, their data indicated that STAT3 deactivation and associated EMT attenuation contribute to the synergistic antitumor effects of combined NSC 74859/doxorubicin therapy (Hu et al. 2012).

6.2.5 Angiogenesis

A large number of studies have implicated the critical role of STAT3 in the process of angiogenesis that facilitates formation of new blood vessels from existing ones to supply nutrients to tumor cells (Subramaniam et al. 2013; Folkman 1990). Ji and colleagues found that angiotensin II (Ang II) can upregulate angiogenic factors production such as vascular endothelial growth factor (VEGF), angiopoietin-2 (Ang-2), and Tie-2 in HCC (MHCC97H) cells in a time- and concentration-dependent manner. Moreover, Ang II-induced JAK2 and STAT3 phosphorylation was significantly suppressed by losartan but not PD123319. Further, STAT3 phosphorylation and SOCS3 expression induced by Ang II were evidently impaired by AG490. More importantly, SOCS3 siRNA remarkably reinforced Ang II-induced VEGF, Ang-2, and Tie-2 generation in MHCC97H cells (Ji et al. 2012). Additionally, it has been also noticed that the cross-talk pathway between AngII and the EGFR mediated by EGF-like ligands cleaved by a disintegrin and metalloprotease is involved in the proliferation and invasion activities of several HCC cell lines (Itabashi et al. 2008). Moreover, aberrant VEGF expression is considered to be an important clinical feature in HCC and may correlate with HCC tumor invasion and metastasis (Subramaniam et al. 2013; El-Assal et al. 1998). In another recent study, Jia et al. tested the effect of a combination therapy consisting of endostatin (a powerful angiogenesis inhibitor) and STAT3-specific small interfering RNA, using a DNA vector delivered by attenuated *S. typhimurium*, on an orthotopic HCC model in C57BL/6 mice. Although antitumor effects were observed with either single therapeutic treatment, the combination therapy provided superior antitumor effects. Correlated with this finding, the combination treatment resulted in significant alteration of STAT3 and endostatin levels and that of the downstream gene VEGF, decreased cell proliferation, induced cell apoptosis, and inhibited angiogenesis (Jia et al. 2012). Also, silencing of STAT3 expression by RNA interference has been reported to significantly inhibit expression of STAT3 mRNA and protein and suppress the growth of human HCC in tumor-bearing nude mice through the downregulation of survivin, VEGF, and c-myc and upregulation of p53 and caspase-3 expression (Li et al. 2009). Interestingly, Lang and coworkers also found that the dual inhibition of Raf and VEGFR2 reduces growth and vascularization of HCC in a subcutaneous tumor model (Lang et al. 2008).

6.2.6 Cellular Invasion

Several studies have shown that STAT3 is intimately linked to the process of tumor invasion in HCC (Subramaniam et al. 2013). STAT3 activation can modulate the expression of matrix metalloproteinases MMP-1, MMP-2, and MMP-9 which in turn can mediate tumor migration and invasion (Subramaniam et al. 2013; Xie et al. 2006). Yan and colleagues recently identified the presence of mesenchymal stem cells (MSCs) in HCC tissues. They demonstrated that liver cancer-associated MSCs (LC-MSCs) significantly enhanced tumor growth in vivo and promoted tumor sphere formation in vitro. LC-MSCs also promoted HCC metastasis in an orthotopic liver transplantation model. cDNA microarray analysis showed that S100A4 expression was significantly higher in LC-MSCs compared with liver normal MSCs (LN-MSCs) from adjacent cancer-free tissues and that S100A4 secreted from LC-MSCs can promote HCC cell proliferation and invasion. They also noticed that S100A4 promoted the expression of miR-155, which mediates the downregulation of suppressor of cytokine signaling 1 (SOCS1), leading to the subsequent activation of STAT3 signaling. This promoted the expression of MMP9, which resulted in increased tumor invasiveness (Yan et al. 2013). Lin et al. noticed significantly greater STAT3 and tyrosine-phosphorylated STAT3 in human HCC tissues than in human normal liver. Further, in HCC cells with loss of response to TGF-beta, NSC 74859, a STAT3-specific inhibitor, markedly suppresses growth. In contrast, CD133 (+) status did not affect the response to STAT3 inhibition: both CD133 (+) Huh-7 cells and CD133 (−) Huh-7 cells are equally sensitive to NSC 74859 treatment and STAT3 inhibition. Thus, the TGF-beta/beta2 spectrin (beta2SP) pathway may reflect a more functional "stem/progenitor" state than CD133. Overall, their findings indicate that inhibiting interleukin 6 (IL6)/STAT3 in HCCs with inactivation of the TGF-beta/beta2SP pathway may be an effective approach in management of HCCs (Lin et al. 2009).

6.3 Link Between Oxidative Stress and STAT3 Activation

Several reports in literature also indicate a critical link between oxidative stress and STAT3 activation in various human malignancies, including HCC (Wang et al. 2011; Toyokuni et al. 1995). For example, a study by Kamata and coworkers showed that inactivation of IKK-β in HCC cells or hepatocytes favors the accumulation of ROS which oxidize the catalytic cysteine of various protein tyrosine phosphatases (PTPs) (Kamata et al. 2005), including SHP1 and SHP2 [the phosphatases that dephosphorylate STAT3 and JAK2] (Valentino and Pierre 2006). Oxidation of SHP1 and SHP2 results in loss of their catalytic activity and accumulation of phosphorylated and activated JAK2 and STAT3, which stimulate the proliferation and tumorigenic growth of NF-κB-deficient HCC (He et al. 2010). Sustained oxidative stress is continuously maintained in tumor cells (Toyokuni et al. 1995). Interestingly, many HCC risk factors, including HCV infection and hepatosteatosis, cause oxidative stress (El-Serag and Rudolph 2007; Parekh and Anania 2007; Wang and Weinman 2006), and just like JNK, STAT3 can also be activated in response to ROS accumulation (He et al. 2010). STAT3 was required for the activation of several immediate-early genes at the gene expression level, including c-*fos* and *jun*B. These two genes are the most strongly affected immediate-early genes in IL-6/livers, and their expression is likely to be directly regulated by STAT3 because their full transactivation requires the STAT-binding elements in their promoters (Wagner et al. 1990; Coffer et al. 1995). In addition, a positive correlation between c-jun and STAT3 was observed in the HCC progression (Zhang et al. 1999), c-jun being the first discovered nuclear proto-oncogene (Maki et al. 1987). The c-Jun interaction does not occur with STAT1. Furthermore, there are a number of enhancer elements that contain c-Jun and STAT3 sites. The transcription factor c-Jun was found to interact with activated STAT3, and STAT3 supplemented the transcriptional activation capacity of c-Jun in a transfection assay (Schaefer et al. 1995). These results suggest that STAT3/JAKs signaling cascade may also contribute to malignant transformation of hepatocytes besides Ras/Raf/ MAPK signaling pathway in HCC (Feng et al. 2001). Also, Machida et al. reported that HCV infection can cause production of ROS and lead to the reduction of mitochondrial transmembrane potential (Delta Psi(m)) in HCV-infected cell cultures. Furthermore, an inhibitor of ROS production, antioxidant *N*-acetyl-L-cysteine (NAC), or an inhibitor of nitric oxide (NO) prevented the alterations Delta Psi(m). The HCV-induced DSB was also abolished by a combination of NO and ROS inhibitors. These findings indicated that the mitochondrial damage and DSBs in HCV-infected cells were mediated by both NO and ROS (Machida et al. 2006).

6.4 Conclusion and Perspectives

This chapter clearly indicates that STAT3 activation plays a major role in both HCC initiation and development, and thereby the abrogation of STAT3 activation using novel pharmacological inhibitors can form the basis of future HCC therapy. Interestingly, a number of strategies, including the use of antisense oligonucleotide targeting STAT3, synthetic drugs (including AG490, YC-1, ENMD-1198, LLL12, NSC-74859, XZH-5, sorafenib, and celecoxib), small molecules derived from natural sources (diosgenin, β-escin, butein, celastrol, γ-tocotrienol, garcinol, honokiol, emodin, ursolic acid, capsaicin, resveratrol, curcumin), and gene therapy techniques have been reported to suppress STAT3 signaling cascade in different HCC cell lines and mouse models. An important issue related to the safety of these blockers still remains to be addressed as inhibition of STAT3 in normal tissues may have detrimental effects. Hence, to further develop STAT3 pharmacological blockers for potential clinical application, complete toxicological and pharmacokinetics analysis in HCC mouse models should be carried out in future studies.

Acknowledgments This work was supported by grants from NUS Academic Research Fund [Grants R-184-207-112] to GS. APK was supported by grants from Singapore Ministry of Education Tier 2 [MOE2012-T2-2-139],

Academic Research Fund Tier 1 [R-184-000-228-112], and Cancer Science Institute of Singapore, Experimental Therapeutics I Program [Grant R-713-001-011-271].

Conflict of Interest The authors declare that they have no conflict of interest.

References

Abdel-Hamid NM (2009) Recent insights on risk factors of hepatocellular carcinoma. World J Hepatol 1: 3–7

Akira S, Nishio Y, Inoue M, Wang XJ, Wei S, Matsusaka T, Yoshida K, Sudo T, Naruto M, Kishimoto T (1994) Molecular cloning of APRF, a novel IFN-stimulated gene factor 3 p91-related transcription factor involved in the gp130-mediated signaling pathway. Cell 77: 63–71

Al Zaid Siddiquee K, Turkson J (2008) STAT3 as a target for inducing apoptosis in solid and hematological tumors. Cell Res 18:254–267

Arnaud C, Burger F, Steffens S, Veillard NR, Nguyen TH, Trono D, Mach F (2005) Statins reduce interleukin-6-induced C-reactive protein in human hepatocytes: new evidence for direct antiinflammatory effects of statins. Arterioscler Thromb Vasc Biol 25:1231–1236

Bromberg JF, Horvath CM, Besser D, Lathem WW, Darnell JE Jr (1998) Stat3 activation is required for cellular transformation by v-src. Mol Cell Biol 18: 2553–2558

Bromberg JF, Wrzeszczynska MH, Devgan G, Zhao Y, Pestell RG, Albanese C, Darnell JE Jr (1999) Stat3 as an oncogene. Cell 98:295–303

Cao X, Tay A, Guy GR, Tan YH (1996) Activation and association of Stat3 with Src in v-Src-transformed cell lines. Mol Cell Biol 16:1595–1603

Carlisi D, D'Anneo A, Angileri L, Lauricella M, Emanuele S, Santulli A, Vento R, Tesoriere G (2011) Parthenolide sensitizes hepatocellular carcinoma cells to TRAIL by inducing the expression of death receptors through inhibition of STAT3 activation. J Cell Physiol 226:1632–1641

Carr BI, Pancoska P, Branch RA (2010) Tumor and liver determinants of prognosis in unresectable hepatocellular carcinoma: a large case cohort study. Hepatol Int 4:396–405

Chaturvedi P, Sharma S, Reddy EP (1997) Abrogation of interleukin-3 dependence of myeloid cells by the v-src oncogene requires SH2 and SH3 domains which specify activation of STATs. Mol Cell Biol 17: 3295–3304

Chen KF, Tai WT, Liu TH, Huang HP, Lin YC, Shiau CW, Li PK, Chen PJ, Cheng AL (2010) Sorafenib overcomes TRAIL resistance of hepatocellular carcinoma cells through the inhibition of STAT3. Clin Cancer Res 16:5189–5199

Chen W, Shen X, Xia X, Xu G, Ma T, Bai X, Liang T (2012a) NSC 74859-mediated inhibition of STAT3 enhances the anti-proliferative activity of cetuximab in hepatocellular carcinoma. Liver Int 32:70–77

Chen KF, Su JC, Liu CY, Huang JW, Chen KC, Chen WL, Tai WT, Shiau CW (2012b) A novel obatoclax derivative, SC-2001, induces apoptosis in hepatocellular carcinoma cells through SHP-1-dependent STAT3 inactivation. Cancer Lett 321:27–35

Choudhari SR, Khan MA, Harris G, Picker D, Jacob GS, Block T, Shailubhai K (2007) Deactivation of Akt and STAT3 signaling promotes apoptosis, inhibits proliferation, and enhances the sensitivity of hepatocellular carcinoma cells to an anticancer agent, Atiprimod. Mol Cancer Ther 6:112–121

Coffer P, Lutticken C, van Puijenbroek A, Klop-de Jonge M, Horn F, Kruijer W (1995) Transcriptional regulation of the junB promoter: analysis of STAT-mediated signal transduction. Oncogene 10:985–994

Dominguez-Malagon H, Gaytan-Graham S (2001) Hepatocellular carcinoma: an update. Ultrastruct Pathol 25:497–516

Dumoutier L, Van Roost E, Colau D, Renauld JC (2000) Human interleukin-10-related T cell-derived inducible factor: molecular cloning and functional characterization as an hepatocyte-stimulating factor. Proc Natl Acad Sci U S A 97:10144–10149

El-Assal ON, Yamanoi A, Soda Y, Yamaguchi M, Igarashi M, Yamamoto A, Nabika T, Nagasue N (1998) Clinical significance of microvessel density and vascular endothelial growth factor expression in hepatocellular carcinoma and surrounding liver: possible involvement of vascular endothelial growth factor in the angiogenesis of cirrhotic liver. Hepatology 27:1554–1562

El-Serag HB, Rudolph KL (2007) Hepatocellular carcinoma: epidemiology and molecular carcinogenesis. Gastroenterology 132:2557–2576

Feng DY, Zheng H, Tan Y, Cheng RX (2001) Effect of phosphorylation of MAPK and Stat3 and expression of c-fos and c-jun proteins on hepatocarcinogenesis and their clinical significance. World J Gastroenterol 7: 33–36

Ferlay J, Shin HR, Bray F, Forman D, Mathers C, Parkin DM (2010) Estimates of worldwide burden of cancer in 2008: GLOBOCAN 2008. Int J Cancer 127: 2893–2917

Folkman J (1990) What is the evidence that tumors are angiogenesis dependent? J Natl Cancer Inst 82: 4–6

Germain D, Frank DA (2007) Targeting the cytoplasmic and nuclear functions of signal transducers and activators of transcription 3 for cancer therapy. Clin Cancer Res 13:5665–5669

Guo J, Ma Q, Zhou X, Shan T, Fan P, Miao D (2013) Inactivation of p27 promotes carcinogens induced liver hepatocarcinogenesis through enhancing inflammatory cytokine secretion and STAT3 signaling activation. J Cell Physiol 228:1967–1976

He G, Karin M (2011) NF-kappaB and STAT3 – key players in liver inflammation and cancer. Cell Res 21:159–168

He G, Yu GY, Temkin V, Ogata H, Kuntzen C, Sakurai T, Sieghart W, Peck-Radosavljevic M, Leffert HL, Karin M (2010) Hepatocyte IKKbeta/NF-kappaB inhibits tumor promotion and progression by preventing oxidative stress-driven STAT3 activation. Cancer Cell 17:286–297

Hibi M, Murakami M, Saito M, Hirano T, Taga T, Kishimoto T (1990) Molecular cloning and expression of an IL-6 signal transducer, gp130. Cell 63:1149–1157

Hirano T, Nakajima K, Hibi M (1997) Signaling mechanisms through gp130: a model of the cytokine system. Cytokine Growth Factor Rev 8:241–252

Hu QD, Chen W, Yan TL, Ma T, Chen CL, Liang C, Zhang Q, Xia XF, Liu H, Zhi X, Zheng XX, Bai XL, Yu XZ, Liang TB (2012) NSC 74859 enhances doxorubicin cytotoxicity via inhibition of epithelial-mesenchymal transition in hepatocellular carcinoma cells. Cancer Lett 325:207–213

Itabashi H, Maesawa C, Oikawa H, Kotani K, Sakurai E, Kato K, Komatsu H, Nitta H, Kawamura H, Wakabayashi G, Masuda T (2008) Angiotensin II and epidermal growth factor receptor cross-talk mediated by a disintegrin and metalloprotease accelerates tumor cell proliferation of hepatocellular carcinoma cell lines. Hepatol ResOff J Jap Soc Hepatol 38:601–613

Ji Y, Wang Z, Li Z, Li K, Le X, Zhang T (2012) Angiotensin II induces angiogenic factors production partly via AT1/JAK2/STAT3/SOCS3 signaling pathway in MHCC97H cells. Cell Physiol Biochem Int J Exp Cell Physiol Biochem Pharmacol 29: 863–874

Jia H, Li Y, Zhao T, Li X, Hu J, Yin D, Guo B, Kopecko DJ, Zhao X, Zhang L, de Xu Q (2012) Antitumor effects of Stat3-siRNA and endostatin combined therapies, delivered by attenuated Salmonella, on orthotopically implanted hepatocarcinoma. Cancer Immunol Immunother CII 61:1977–1987

Kamata H, Honda S, Maeda S, Chang L, Hirata H, Karin M (2005) Reactive oxygen species promote TNFalpha-induced death and sustained JNK activation by inhibiting MAP kinase phosphatases. Cell 120:649–661

Karras JG, Wang Z, Huo L, Frank DA, Rothstein TL (1997) Induction of STAT protein signaling through the CD40 receptor in B lymphocytes: distinct STAT activation following surface Ig and CD40 receptor engagement. J Immunol 159:4350–4355

Kusaba M, Nakao K, Goto T, Nishimura D, Kawashimo H, Shibata H, Motoyoshi Y, Taura N, Ichikawa T, Hamasaki K, Eguchi K (2007) Abrogation of constitutive STAT3 activity sensitizes human hepatoma cells to TRAIL-mediated apoptosis. J Hepatol 47: 546–555

Lang SA, Brecht I, Moser C, Obed A, Batt D, Schlitt HJ, Geissler EK, Stoeltzing O (2008) Dual inhibition of Raf and VEGFR2 reduces growth and vascularization of hepatocellular carcinoma in an experimental model. Langenbeck's Arch Surg/Deutsche Gesellschaft fur Chirurgie 393:333–341

Lau WY, Lai EC (2008) Hepatocellular carcinoma: current management and recent advances. Hepatobiliary Pancreat Dis Int 7:237–257

Lau CK, Yang ZF, Lam SP, Lam CT, Ngai P, Tam KH, Poon RT, Fan ST (2007) Inhibition of Stat3 activity by YC-1 enhances chemo-sensitivity in hepatocellular carcinoma. Cancer Biol Ther 6:1900–1907

Lavecchia A, Di Giovanni C, Novellino E (2011) STAT-3 inhibitors: state of the art and new horizons for cancer treatment. Curr Med Chem 18:2359–2375

Lee H, Herrmann A, Deng JH, Kujawski M, Niu G, Li Z, Forman S, Jove R, Pardoll DM, Yu H (2009) Persistently activated Stat3 maintains constitutive NF-kappaB activity in tumors. Cancer Cell 15:283–293

Levy DE, Darnell JE Jr (2002) Stats: transcriptional control and biological impact. Nat Rev Mol Cell Biol 3:651–662

Li WC, Ye SL, Sun RX, Liu YK, Tang ZY, Kim Y, Karras JG, Zhang H (2006) Inhibition of growth and metastasis of human hepatocellular carcinoma by antisense oligonucleotide targeting signal transducer and activator of transcription 3. Clin Cancer Res 12: 7140–7148

Li J, Piao YF, Jiang Z, Chen L, Sun HB (2009) Silencing of signal transducer and activator of transcription 3 expression by RNA interference suppresses growth of human hepatocellular carcinoma in tumor-bearing nude mice. World J Gastroenterol 15: 2602–2608

Li F, Fernandez PP, Rajendran P, Hui KM, Sethi G (2010) Diosgenin, a steroidal saponin, inhibits STAT3 signaling pathway leading to suppression of proliferation and chemosensitization of human hepatocellular carcinoma cells. Cancer Lett 292:197–207

Liang H, Block TM, Wang M, Nefsky B, Long R, Hafner J, Mehta AS, Marrero J, Gish R, Norton PA (2012) Interleukin-6 and oncostatin M are elevated in liver disease in conjunction with candidate hepatocellular carcinoma biomarker GP73. Cancer biomarkers: section A of Disease markers 11:161–171

Lin L, Amin R, Gallicano GI, Glasgow E, Jogunoori W, Jessup JM, Zasloff M, Marshall JL, Shetty K, Johnson L, Mishra L, He AR (2009) The STAT3 inhibitor NSC 74859 is effective in hepatocellular cancers with disrupted TGF-beta signaling. Oncogene 28:961–972

Lin L, Deangelis S, Foust E, Fuchs J, Li C, Li PK, Schwartz EB, Lesinski GB, Benson D, Lu J, Hoyt D, Lin J (2010) A novel small molecule inhibits STAT3 phosphorylation and DNA binding activity and exhibits potent growth suppressive activity in human cancer cells. Mol Cancer 9:217

Liu Y, Li PK, Li C, Lin J (2010a) Inhibition of STAT3 signaling blocks the anti-apoptotic activity of IL-6 in human liver cancer cells. J Biol Chem 285: 27429–27439

Liu Y, Fuchs J, Li C, Lin J (2010b) IL-6, a risk factor for hepatocellular carcinoma: FLLL32 inhibits IL-6-

induced STAT3 phosphorylation in human hepatocellular cancer cells. Cell Cycle 9:3423–3427

Liu Y, Liu A, Li H, Li C, Lin J (2011a) Celecoxib inhibits interleukin-6/interleukin-6 receptor-induced JAK2/STAT3 phosphorylation in human hepatocellular carcinoma cells. Cancer Prev Res (Phila) 4: 1296–1305

Liu Y, Liu A, Xu Z, Yu W, Wang H, Li C, Lin J (2011b) XZH-5 inhibits STAT3 phosphorylation and causes apoptosis in human hepatocellular carcinoma cells. Apoptosis 16:502–510

Machida K, Cheng KT, Lai CK, Jeng KS, Sung VM, Lai MM (2006) Hepatitis C virus triggers mitochondrial permeability transition with production of reactive oxygen species, leading to DNA damage and STAT3 activation. J Virol 80:7199–7207

Maki Y, Bos TJ, Davis C, Starbuck M, Vogt PK (1987) Avian sarcoma virus 17 carries the jun oncogene. Proc Natl Acad Sci U S A 84:2848–2852

Mano Y, Aishima S, Fujita N, Tanaka Y, Kubo Y, Motomura T, Taketomi A, Shirabe K, Maehara Y, Oda Y (2013) Tumor-associated macrophage promotes tumor progression via STAT3 signaling in hepatocellular carcinoma. Pathobiol J Immunopathol Mol Cell Biol 80:146–154

Matsuda Y, Ichida T (2006) p16 and p27 are functionally correlated during the progress of hepatocarcinogenesis. Med Mol Morphol 39:169–175

Metz S, Wiesinger M, Vogt M, Lauks H, Schmalzing G, Heinrich PC, Muller-Newen G (2007) Characterization of the Interleukin (IL)-6 Inhibitor IL-6-RFP: fused receptor domains act as high affinity cytokine-binding proteins. J Biol Chem 282:1238–1248

Moser C, Lang SA, Mori A, Hellerbrand C, Schlitt HJ, Geissler EK, Fogler WE, Stoeltzing O (2008) ENMD-1198, a novel tubulin-binding agent reduces HIF-1alpha and STAT3 activity in human hepatocellular carcinoma (HCC) cells, and inhibits growth and vascularization in vivo. BMC Cancer 8:206

Nakamoto Y, Kaneko S (2003) Mechanisms of viral hepatitis induced liver injury. Curr Mol Med 3: 537–544

Naugler WE, Sakurai T, Kim S, Maeda S, Kim K, Elsharkawy AM, Karin M (2007) Gender disparity in liver cancer due to sex differences in MyD88-dependent IL-6 production. Science 317:121–124

Niwa Y, Kanda H, Shikauchi Y, Saiura A, Matsubara K, Kitagawa T, Yamamoto J, Kubo T, Yoshikawa H (2005) Methylation silencing of SOCS-3 promotes cell growth and migration by enhancing JAK/STAT and FAK signalings in human hepatocellular carcinoma. Oncogene 24:6406–6417

Parekh S, Anania FA (2007) Abnormal lipid and glucose metabolism in obesity: implications for non-alcoholic fatty liver disease. Gastroenterology 132: 2191–2207

Peroukides S, Bravou V, Alexopoulos A, Varakis J, Kalofonos H, Papadaki H (2010) Survivin overexpression in HCC and liver cirrhosis differentially correlates with p-STAT3 and E-cadherin. Histol Histopathol 25:299–307

Pfitzner E, Kliem S, Baus D, Litterst CM (2004) The role of STATs in inflammation and inflammatory diseases. Curr Pharm Des 10:2839–2850

Rajendran P, Li F, Manu KA, Shanmugam MK, Loo SY, Kumar AP, Sethi G (2011a) gamma-Tocotrienol is a novel inhibitor of constitutive and inducible STAT3 signalling pathway in human hepatocellular carcinoma: potential role as an antiproliferative, pro-apoptotic and chemosensitizing agent. Br J Pharmacol 163:283–298

Rajendran P, Ong TH, Chen L, Li F, Shanmugam MK, Vali S, Abbasi T, Kapoor S, Sharma A, Kumar AP, Hui KM, Sethi G (2011b) Suppression of signal transducer and activator of transcription 3 activation by butein inhibits growth of human hepatocellular carcinoma in vivo. Clin Cancer Res 17:1425–1439

Rajendran P, Li F, Shanmugam MK, Kannaiyan R, Goh JN, Wong KF, Wang W, Khin E, Tergaonkar V, Kumar AP, Luk JM, Sethi G (2012) Celastrol suppresses growth and induces apoptosis of human hepatocellular carcinoma through the modulation of STAT3/JAK2 signaling cascade in vitro and in vivo. Cancer Prev Res (Phila) 5:631–643

Schaefer TS, Sanders LK, Nathans D (1995) Cooperative transcriptional activity of Jun and Stat3 beta, a short form of Stat3. Proc Natl Acad Sci U S A 92: 9097–9101

Schneller D, Machat G, Sousek A, Proell V, van Zijl F, Zulehner G, Huber H, Mair M, Muellner MK, Nijman SM, Eferl R, Moriggl R, Mikulits W (2011) p19(ARF) /p14(ARF) controls oncogenic functions of signal transducer and activator of transcription 3 in hepatocellular carcinoma. Hepatology 54: 164–172

Schust J, Sperl B, Hollis A, Mayer TU, Berg T (2006) Stattic: a small-molecule inhibitor of STAT3 activation and dimerization. Chem Biol 13:1235–1242

Selvendiran K, Koga H, Ueno T, Yoshida T, Maeyama M, Torimura T, Yano H, Kojiro M, Sata M (2006) Luteolin promotes degradation in signal transducer and activator of transcription 3 in human hepatoma cells: an implication for the antitumor potential of flavonoids. Cancer Res 66:4826–4834

Shuai K, Stark GR, Kerr IM, Darnell JE Jr (1993) A single phosphotyrosine residue of Stat91 required for gene activation by interferon-gamma. Science 261: 1744–1746

Strain A (1998) Liver growth and repair. Chapman & Hall, London

Subramaniam A, Shanmugam MK, Perumal E, Li F, Nachiyappan A, Dai X, Swamy SN, Ahn KS, Kumar AP, Tan BK, Hui KM, Sethi G (2013) Potential role of signal transducer and activator of transcription (STAT)3 signaling pathway in inflammation, survival, proliferation and invasion of hepatocellular carcinoma. Biochim Biophys Acta 1835: 46–60

Sun X, Zhang J, Wang L, Tian Z (2008) Growth inhibition of human hepatocellular carcinoma cells by blocking STAT3 activation with decoy-ODN. Cancer Lett 262:201–213

Tai WT, Cheng AL, Shiau CW, Huang HP, Huang JW, Chen PJ, Chen KF (2011) Signal transducer and activator of transcription 3 is a major kinase-independent target of sorafenib in hepatocellular carcinoma. J Hepatol 55:1041–1048

Tan SM, Li F, Rajendran P, Kumar AP, Hui KM, Sethi G (2010) Identification of beta-escin as a novel inhibitor of signal transducer and activator of transcription 3/Janus-activated kinase 2 signaling pathway that suppresses proliferation and induces apoptosis in human hepatocellular carcinoma cells. J Pharmacol Exp Ther 334:285–293

Taub R (2003) Hepatoprotection via the IL-6/Stat3 pathway. J Clin Invest 112:978–980

Toffanin S, Friedman SL, Llovet JM (2010) Obesity, inflammatory signaling, and hepatocellular carcinoma-an enlarging link. Cancer Cell 17:115–117

Toyokuni S, Okamoto K, Yodoi J, Hiai H (1995) Persistent oxidative stress in cancer. FEBS Lett 358:1–3

Trikha M, Corringham R, Klein B, Rossi JF (2003) Targeted anti-interleukin-6 monoclonal antibody therapy for cancer: a review of the rationale and clinical evidence. Clin Cancer Res 9:4653–4665

Turkson J, Bowman T, Garcia R, Caldenhoven E, De Groot RP, Jove R (1998) Stat3 activation by Src induces specific gene regulation and is required for cell transformation. Mol Cell Biol 18:2545–2552

Valentino L, Pierre J (2006) JAK/STAT signal transduction: regulators and implication in hematological malignancies. Biochem Pharmacol 71:713–721

Wagner BJ, Hayes TE, Hoban CJ, Cochran BH (1990) The SIF binding element confers sis/PDGF inducibility onto the c-fos promoter. EMBO J 9:4477–4484

Wang T, Weinman SA (2006) Causes and consequences of mitochondrial reactive oxygen species generation in hepatitis C. J Gastroenterol Hepatol 21(Suppl 3): S34–S37

Wang Y, Ma X, Yan S, Shen S, Zhu H, Gu Y, Wang H, Qin G, Yu Q (2009) 17-hydroxy-jolkinolide B inhibits signal transducers and activators of transcription 3 signaling by covalently cross-linking Janus kinases and induces apoptosis of human cancer cells. Cancer Res 69:7302–7310

Wang H, Lafdil F, Wang L, Park O, Yin S, Niu J, Miller AM, Sun Z, Gao B (2011) Hepatoprotective versus oncogenic functions of STAT3 in liver tumorigenesis. Am J Pathol 179:714–724

Wegenka UM, Buschmann J, Lutticken C, Heinrich PC, Horn F (1993) Acute-phase response factor, a nuclear factor binding to acute-phase response elements, is rapidly activated by interleukin-6 at the posttranslational level. Mol Cell Biol 13:276–288

Weidler M, Rether J, Anke T, Erkel G (2000) Inhibition of interleukin-6 signaling and Stat3 activation by a new class of bioactive cyclopentenone derivatives. Biochem Biophys Res Commun 276:447–453

Won C, Lee CS, Lee JK, Kim TJ, Lee KH, Yang YM, Kim YN, Ye SK, Chung MH (2010) CADPE suppresses cyclin D1 expression in hepatocellular carcinoma by blocking IL-6-induced STAT3 activation. Anticancer Res 30:481–488

Wu WY, Li J, Wu ZS, Zhang CL, Meng XL (2011) STAT3 activation in monocytes accelerates liver cancer progression. BMC Cancer 11:506

Xie TX, Huang FJ, Aldape KD, Kang SH, Liu M, Gershenwald JE, Xie K, Sawaya R, Huang S (2006) Activation of stat3 in human melanoma promotes brain metastasis. Cancer Res 66:3188–3196

Yan XL, Jia YL, Chen L, Zeng Q, Zhou JN, Fu CJ, Chen HX, Yuan HF, Li ZW, Shi L, Xu YC, Wang JX, Zhang XM, He LJ, Zhai C, Yue W, Pei XT (2013) Hepatocellular carcinoma-associated mesenchymal stem cells promote hepatocarcinoma progression: role of the S100A4-miR155-SOCS1-MMP9 axis. Hepatology 57:2274–2286

Yoshikawa H, Matsubara K, Qian GS, Jackson P, Groopman JD, Manning JE, Harris CC, Herman JG (2001) SOCS-1, a negative regulator of the JAK/STAT pathway, is silenced by methylation in human hepatocellular carcinoma and shows growth-suppression activity. Nat Genet 28:29–35

Zhang X, Wrzeszczynska MH, Horvath CM, Darnell JE Jr (1999) Interacting regions in Stat3 and c-Jun that participate in cooperative transcriptional activation. Mol Cell Biol 19:7138–7146

Zhang M, Zhang H, Sun C, Shan X, Yang X, Li-Ling J, Deng Y (2009) Targeted constitutive activation of signal transducer and activator of transcription 3 in human hepatocellular carcinoma cells by cucurbitacin B. Cancer Chemother Pharmacol 63:635–642

Zhong Z, Wen Z, Darnell JE Jr (1994) Stat3: a STAT family member activated by tyrosine phosphorylation in response to epidermal growth factor and interleukin-6. Science 264:95–98

7 Simple Sequence Repeats in 5′ and 3′ Flanking Sequences of Cell Cycle Genes

Seema Trivedi

Abstract

Simple sequence repeats (SSRs) are hypermutable, and this instability leads to many disorders. Perhaps it is because of this reason SSRs are relatively rare in coding sequences. The present study was undertaken to explore SSRs in 5′ and 3′ flanking sequences (FS) of cell cycle genes (checkpoint; regulation; replication, repair, and recombination (RRR); and transition) in humans and eight mammalian orthologues. The present study shows more SSRs in FS of regulation genes compared to other gene groups. However, differences in repeat numbers between different groups of cell cycle genes are not significant. Trinucleotide repeats are generally more in 3′ FS of human cell cycle genes but not in other mammals (with some exceptions). On the other hand, in 5′ FS of cell cycle genes (except human genes), trinucleotide repeats are more in number compared to other repeat types in almost all mammals (with some exceptions). Repeat numbers do not differ significantly from other mammals except human and cow genes. Many repeats in FS of human genes are conserved, including rare repeats like CG/GC. CG motifs are conserved only in 5′ and 3′ FS of regulation genes but GC motifs are conserved in RRR genes. This paper presents characteristics of SSRs occurring in 5′ and 3′ FS of cell cycle genes, which may be potential mutational hotspots that could be used for further exploration of their potential roles in gene regulation or medical investigations.

Keywords

Cell cycle • Checkpoint • Microsatellites • Replication • Repair • Recombination • Simple sequence repeats (SSRs) • Transition • Flanking sequences

Abbreviations

Di Dinucleotide
FS Flanking sequence(s)

S. Trivedi (✉)
Department of Zoology, JN Vyas University, Jodhpur, Rajasthan 342011, India
e-mail: svtrived@hotmail.com

P.R. Sudhakaran (ed.), *Perspectives in Cancer Prevention – Translational Cancer Research*, DOI 10.1007/978-81-322-1533-2_7, © Springer India 2014

Penta Penta-nucleotide
SSRs Simple sequence repeats
Tetra Tetranucleotide
Tri Trinucleotide

7.1 Introduction

Arrays of DNA motifs of 1–8 base pairs repeated in tandem are known as simple sequence repeats (SSRs, or microsatellites) with density and length variations in different species or even chromosomes of the same species (Chambers and MacAvoy 2000; Toth et al. 2000; Trivedi 2006, 2010). Several factors affect SSR frequency and length in different organisms that include differences in nucleotide content (CG richness) of genome or repeat, repair machinery, mutational pressures, and distance of repeats from replication origin (Jacob and Eckert 2007; Eckert and Hile 2009; Choudhary and Trivedi 2010; Tian et al. 2011). Despite these differences, most organisms have higher SSR density in intergenic regions compared to coding sequences (Chambers and MacAvoy 2000; Toth et al. 2000) with exceptions in Archaea (Trivedi 2006). Moreover, in general trinucleotide and hexanucleotide repeats are more common in coding sequences compared to other repeat types. This may be due to risk of mutations in other repeat types that could lead to nonsense mutation and possible loss of gene expression (Metzgar et al. 2000).

SSRs mutations are mainly due to polymerase strand slippage (Levinson and Gutman 1987) and, to some extent, due to unequal recombination (Li et al. 2002), which may result in expansion or contraction of repeat length. SSR instability can increase by mutations affecting post-replication mismatch mutation repair (MMR) (Strand et al. 1993), or some other mechanism as some prokaryotes do not have MMR (Eisen and Hanawalt 1999).

SSRs may have functional roles (Kashi and King 2006; Lukusa and Fryns 2008; Bacolla and Wells 2009; Eckert and Hile 2009) and may repress transcription (Regelson et al. 2006) or affect efficiency of the cell cycle. For example, AT-rich repeats can affect replication initiation, nucleosome assembly, and DNA supercoiling (Bacolla and Wells 2009). DNA replication time during S-phase can be affected by repeats like (CA)*n* and (ACTG)*n* that are present in the regions flanking later replicating genes and (CATA)n repeats near earlier replicating genes. S-phase checkpoint proteins can influence SSR length mutations especially on SSRs present near the origin of replication or present on lagging strand (Dere et al. 2004).

Since SSRs may affect gene regulation, it might be expected that there would be fewer repeats in 5′ and 3′ flanking sequences (FS) of genes specially cell cycle genes as these regions may also have regulatory elements that may be important for gene expression and may affect cell cyle. Nonetheless, SSRs are present in many genes involved in DNA repair (Chang et al. 2001; Trivedi 2003, 2010). Repeats are also present in genes involved in FS of cell cycle checkpoint, like (CT)19/(CA)16 are present in G0S2 (member of G0S genes actively involved in G0/G1 switch). Mutations in some of these repeats are known to cause tumor or cancer in humans. For example, tumorigenesis is seen due to mutations in the mononucleotide repeat A(9) present in the CtIP gene that plays a role in DNA-damage-induced cell cycle checkpoint control at the G2/M transition and G1/S transition (Russell and Forsdyke 1991).

Though repeats in cell cycle genes have been reported, analysis of SSRs in 5′ and 3′ FS of all cell cycle genes has not been undertaken. The aim of present study is to analyze the distribution of repeats in 5′ and 3′ FS of human cell cycle genes (checkpoint; regulation; replication, repair, and recombination (RRR); and transition) and compare with orthologues in eight mammals. This may help in identification of candidate cell cycle genes that could be vulnerable to mutations in their FS and hence affect cell cycle regulation.

7.2 Material and Methods

7.2.1 Cell Cycle Gene Sequences

Gene Ontology (GO) annotation IDs for *Homo sapiens* cell cycle genes were obtained from AmiGO (Biological Process, all data source, evidence code all, search terms: cell cycle/cell division) (The Gene Ontology Consortium 2000). These GO IDs were used for obtaining *H. sapiens* gene IDs from the Ensembl Genome Browser version 55 (http://www.ensembl.org/biomart/martview/). Human orthologue IDs of chimpanzee (*Pan troglodytes*), orangutan (*Pongo pygmaeus*), macaque (*Macaca mulatta*), horse (*Equus caballus*), cow (*Bos taurus*), dog (*Canis familiaris*), mouse (*Mus musculus*), and rat (*Rattus norvegicus*) were also obtained from Ensembl by using human cell cycle genes' Ensembl gene IDs. Unspliced genes with 50 nucleotides (nts) upstream and downstream flanks from Ensembl were obtained by using these Ensembl gene IDs.

Note: Only GO IDs for genes that have a direct role in the cell cycle were used for further analysis. Further, IDs for genes not directly associated with cell cycle but associated with signaling pathways that affect cell cycle regulation were not included.

7.2.2 Grouping/Classification of Genes

Classification of human cell cycle-related genes was done on the basis of reported function/expression in the cell cycle as per GO "biological process" names (The Gene Ontology Consortium 2000), cell cycle base (Gauthier et al. 2008), reactome (Joshi-Tope et al. 2003; Matthews et al. 2007, 2009; Va Vastrik et al. 2007), WikiPathways (Pico et al. 2008; Kelder et al. 2009), KEGG pathways (http://www.genome.jp/kegg/pathway.html), EntrezGene (http://www.ncbi.nlm.nih.gov/gene/), and UniProtKB/Swiss-Prot (http://www.uniprot.org/uniprot/) into four groups: (1) replication, repair, and recombination (RRR); (2) checkpoint; (3) regulation (translation and transcription regulation excluded); and (4) transition.

7.2.3 Repeat Search and Representation

Repeat search program SPUTNIK (http://espressosoftware.com/sputnik/index.html), which looks for di-, tri-, tetra-, and penta-nucleotide repeats, was used for analysis of cell cycle gene sequences of all nine mammals. Heat map was generated to represent repeat motif frequencies by using web interface of "Matrix2png" (Pavlidis and Noble 2003).

7.2.4 SSR CG Richness and Length

For calculation of SSR lengths, total numbers of nucleotides for each SSR were counted. Further, this length was adjusted to the repeat-divisible value – i.e., if the length of a dinucleotide repeat was given as 13nt by SPUTNIK, this was adjusted to 12nt repeat length and for trinucleotide repeat, if length was given as 16nt, it was adjusted to 15nt.

7.2.5 Repeat Position

3′ and 5′ FS positions in genes were identified based on the positions obtained from Ensembl. Repeats that were present in 3′ and 5′ FS but also extended to either exon or intron of the gene were named as 3′ FS_H and 5′ FS_H, respectively. Repeat positions obtained from SPUTNIK were then compared with positions of 5′ and 3′ FS.

7.2.6 Conservation of Repeats

Ensembl version 55 was used for downloading human cell cycle genes and their aligned (PECAN) orthologues in eight mammals (if present). Each nucleotide of repeats present in 5′ and 3′ FS of human genes was compared with aligned orthologue sequences. Web interface of "Matrix2png" (Pavlidis and Noble 2003) was used to generate heat map to represent repeat motif conservation.

7.2.7 Statistical Analysis

One way ANOVA (analysis of variance) followed by Tukey's HSD (honestly significant difference and Bonferroni correction) at 95 and 99 % confidence levels was done with the help of SPSS (version 16.0) to gauge significant differences between the nine mammals as well as differences between cell cycle genes within and between species.

Similarly, ANOVA followed by Tukey's HSD (honestly significant difference and Bonferroni correction) at 95 and 99 % confidence levels was done to seek significance of differences between repeat types as well as different cell cycle gene groups in each mammal.

7.3 Results

7.3.1 Cell Cycle Genes 5′ and 3′ Flanking Sequences and Repeats

Repeat search shows more repeats in 5′ FS compared to 3′ FS in genes of all mammals except human genes. However, there is no consistency in distribution of repeat numbers in FS_H regions of all nine mammals (Fig. 7.1). Moreover, there are no significant differences between total repeats of nine mammals except between human and cow repeats ($P < 0.05$).

Distributions of SSRs types are different in different mammals (Fig. 7.2a and b). Trinucleotides are the most abundant repeat class in human 3′ FS but are not present in chimp, orangutan, horse, and cow genes. In 5′ FS, though tri- and penta-nucleotide repeats are present in all mammals, dinucleotide repeats are not present in dog genes, and tetranucleotide repeats are not present in human and horse genes. There are no significant differences between repeat types in nine mammals.

7.3.2 Cell Cycle Gene Groups and Repeats

Only regulation genes have repeats in all regions, i.e., 3′ and 5′ FS and FS_H of all mammals (Fig. 7.3). Distributions of repeats in different gene groups also show higher repeat numbers in FS of regulation genes in 5′ and 3′ FS compared to other gene groups. There are no significant differences in repeat numbers in gene groups of nine mammals except between regulation genes of human and cow ($P < 0.05$). Further, within each mammal, different gene groups do not show significant differences in repeat numbers.

Dinucleotide repeats are not present in 3′ FS of checkpoint genes in human, chimp, orangutan, and macaque and regulation genes of rat. Only human and orangutan RRR genes and transition genes of horse and mouse have dinucleotide repeats. 5′ FS has repeats only in macaque checkpoint genes and RRR genes of only orangutan. Human, horse, and dog regulation genes do not have dinucleotide repeats in 5′ FS. 3′ FS_H has dinucleotide repeats only in regulation genes of macaque, horse, and rat. 5′ FS_H has repeats only in macaque checkpoint genes, human and chimp regulation genes, and macaque and mouse transition genes (Fig. 7.4). Similarly, distributions of tri-, tetra-, and penta-nucleotide repeats are different in different gene groups of the nine mammals (Fig. 7.4). Trinucleotide repeats compared to other repeat types are more in regulation genes of all mammals (in particular non-primate). It is interesting to note that 5′ FS of checkpoint genes do not have tetranucleotide repeats in all mammals. Repeat types show no significant differences in each mammal.

7.3.3 Motifs in Cell Cycle Genes

Distribution of repeat motifs varies in different gene groups of all nine mammals (Fig. 7.5a and b). It is interesting to note that GC repeat motif in 3′ FS is present only in human RRR genes. CG dinucleotide repeats are present only in 5′ FS of orangutan regulation genes. Among trinucleotide repeats GC-rich motifs like CCG,

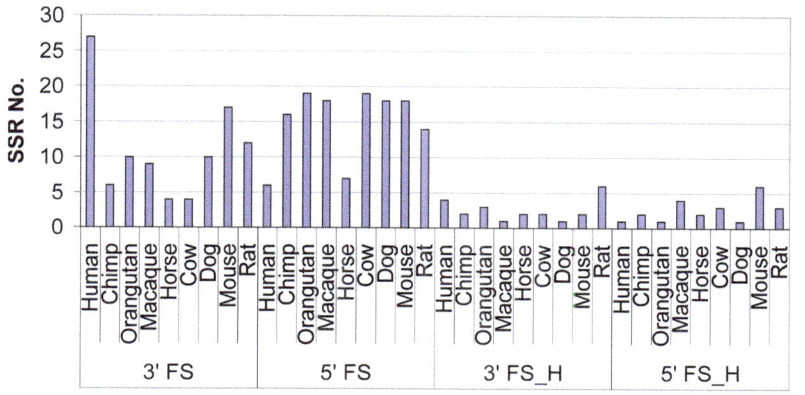

Fig. 7.1 Total repeats in flanking sequences (*FS*) of cell cycle genes in nine mammals. *FS_H* repeats that extend from either 3′ or 5′ flanking sequences to either exons or introns of gene sequences

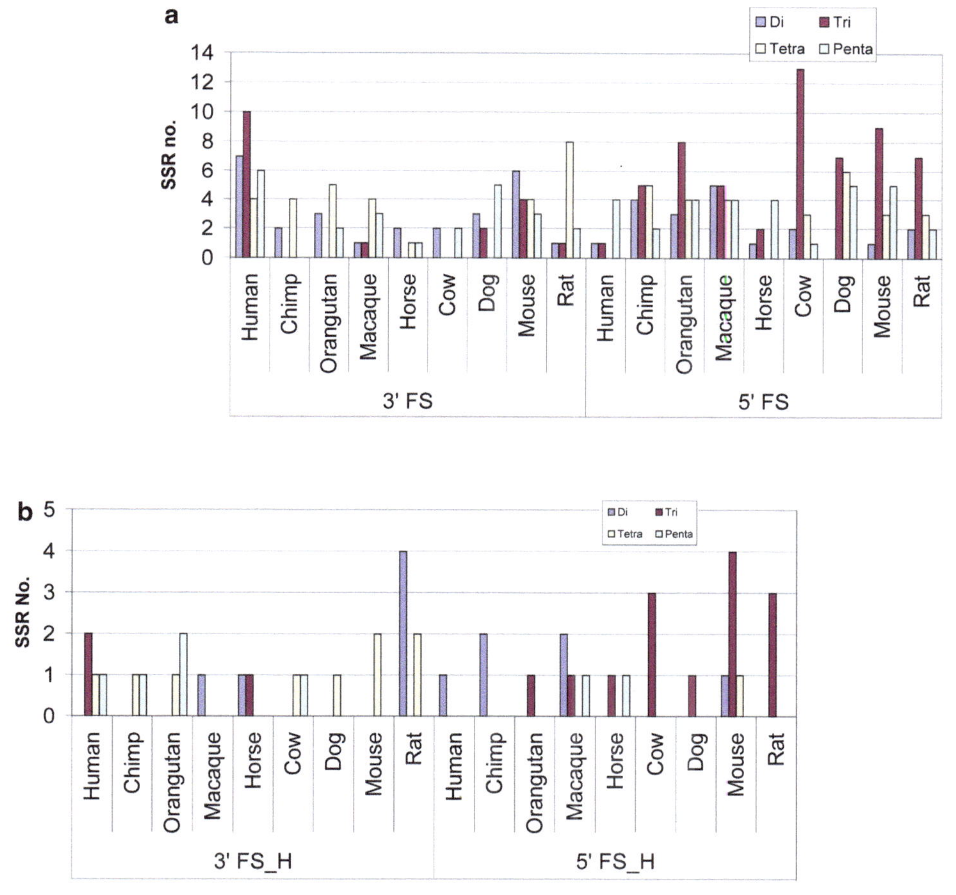

Fig. 7.2 (**a**) Repeat types in flanking sequences (*FS*) of cell cycle genes in nine mammals. *Di* – dinucleotide, *Penta* – penta-nucleotide, *Tri* – trinucleotide, *Tetra* – tetranucleotide. (**b**) Repeat types that extend from either 3′ or 5′ flanking sequences to either exons or introns of cell cycle gene sequences (*FS_H*) in nine mammals. *Di* – dinucleotide, *Penta* – penta-nucleotide, *Tri* – trinucleotide, *Tetra* – tetranucleotide

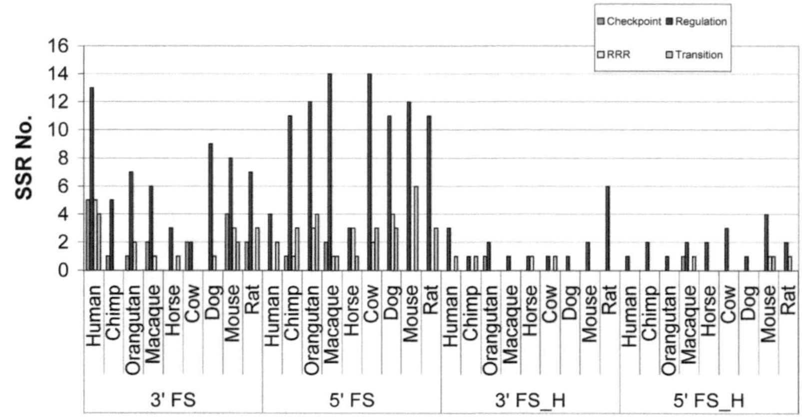

Fig. 7.3 Repeats in flanking sequences (*FS*) of different groups of cell cycle genes in nine mammals. *FS_H* repeats that extend from either 3′ or 5′ flanking sequences to either exons or introns of gene sequences, *RRR* replication, repair, and recombination

CCT, CGC, GCG, GGA, and GGC are more common in 5′ FS of regulation genes in nine mammals (with exceptions). Similarly, tetra- and penta-nucleotide repeat motifs have different distribution in 5′ and 3′ FS of different cell cycle genes in nine mammals (Fig. 7.5a and b).

7.3.4 Conservation of Repeats

In 5′ FS, only regulation and transitions genes show conservation of repeat motifs (CCTG and CCT, respectively). In 3′ FS GC motif is conserved in RRR genes of all mammals except horse. GA (except dog), TC (except macaque), and TG repeat motifs are conserved in regulation genes of all mammals. Dinucleotide repeats are not conserved in checkpoint and transition genes. Among trinucleotide repeat motifs, ATA, CCG, and TTC are conserved in checkpoint genes, CGC and TCC are conserved only in regulation genes, but GCG motifs are conserved in all gene groups except checkpoint genes. Tetra- and penta-nucleotide motifs show differences in conservation in different groups. Further, some motifs are not conserved in all mammals (Fig. 7.6). In 5′ FS_H only CG dinucleotide repeat is conserved (regulation genes) in all mammals except horse. In 3′ FS_H only trinucleotide motifs are conserved in regulation genes where CGC is conserved in all mammals except dog and CGG is conserved only in mouse and rat (data not shown).

7.4 Discussion

During DNA replication, strand slippage often leads to SSR flux which is corrected by replication repair and the checkpoint machinery (Chambers and MacAvoy 2000; Lahiri et al. 2004).

The present analysis shows repeats in human FS of cell cycle genes as well as in eight eutherian orthologues. Moreover, repeat frequency is higher in 5′ FS in genes of all mammals except human genes (3′ FS). Though many repeats may be neutral in nature, it is known that SSRs can form alternative non-B DNA structures and affect normal DNA replication or MMR system, leading to enhanced cancer susceptibility and neurodegenerative disorders (Lukusa and Fryns 2008; Bacolla and Wells 2009; Eckert and Hile 2009). Longer (AAAG)(*n*) repeats serve as binding site of many transcription factors in 5′-UTRs of the estrogen-related receptor gamma gene (ERR-γ) in breast cancer patients (Galindo et al. 2011).

It is known that repeat length alterations in CDKN2A and CCND1 result in dysplastic head and neck lesions (Tripathi Bhar et al. 2003). The present study finds penta-nucleotide repeat in 3′ FS of human and macaque CDKN2A gene besides repeats in other regions of the gene. Among human genes in the present study that contain repeats, some are listed in the Mendelian Inheritance in Man morbid (MIM) database (http://www.ncbi.nlm.nih.gov/omim/) (obtained

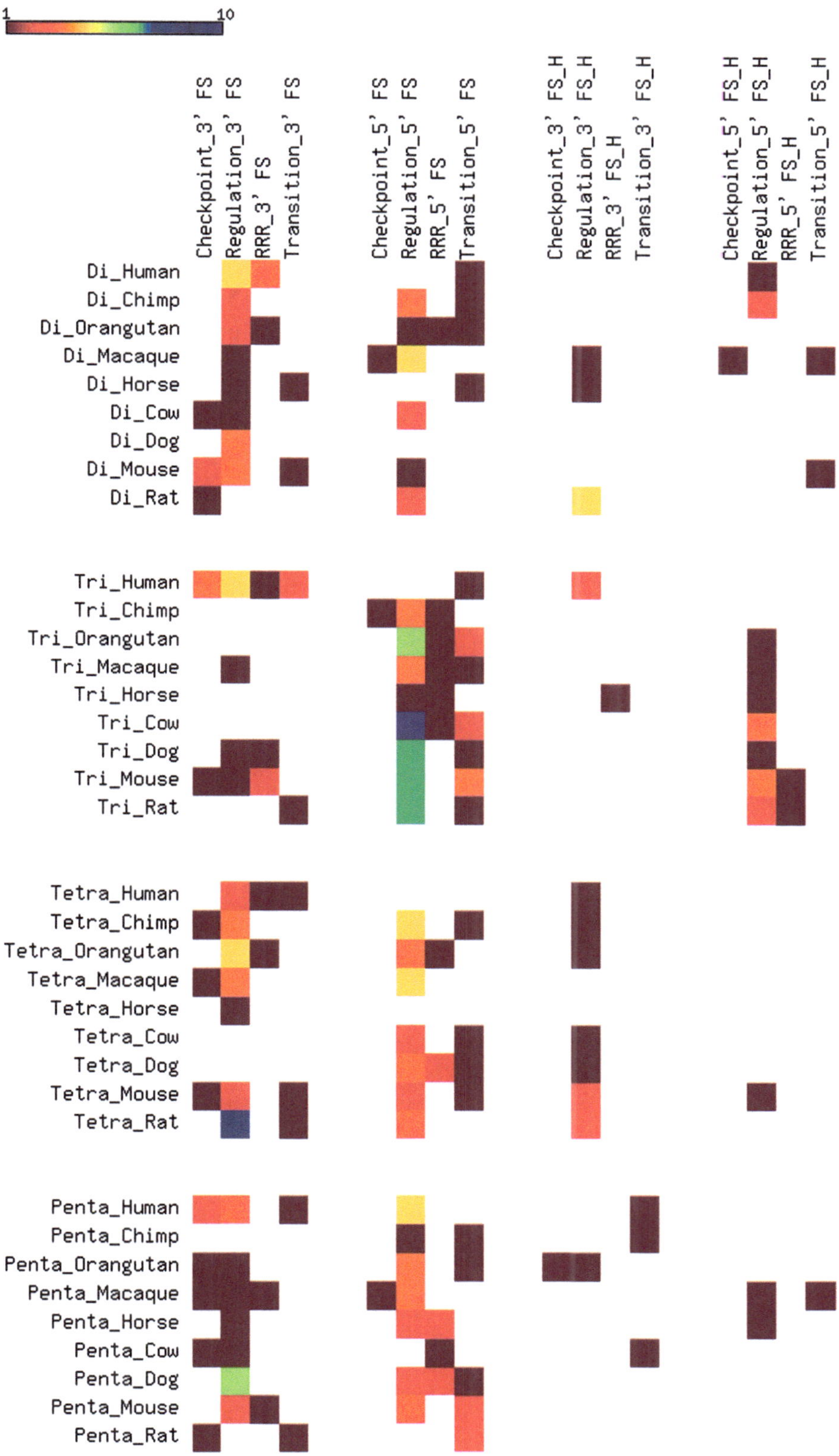

Fig. 7.4 Repeat types in flanking sequences of cell cycle gene groups

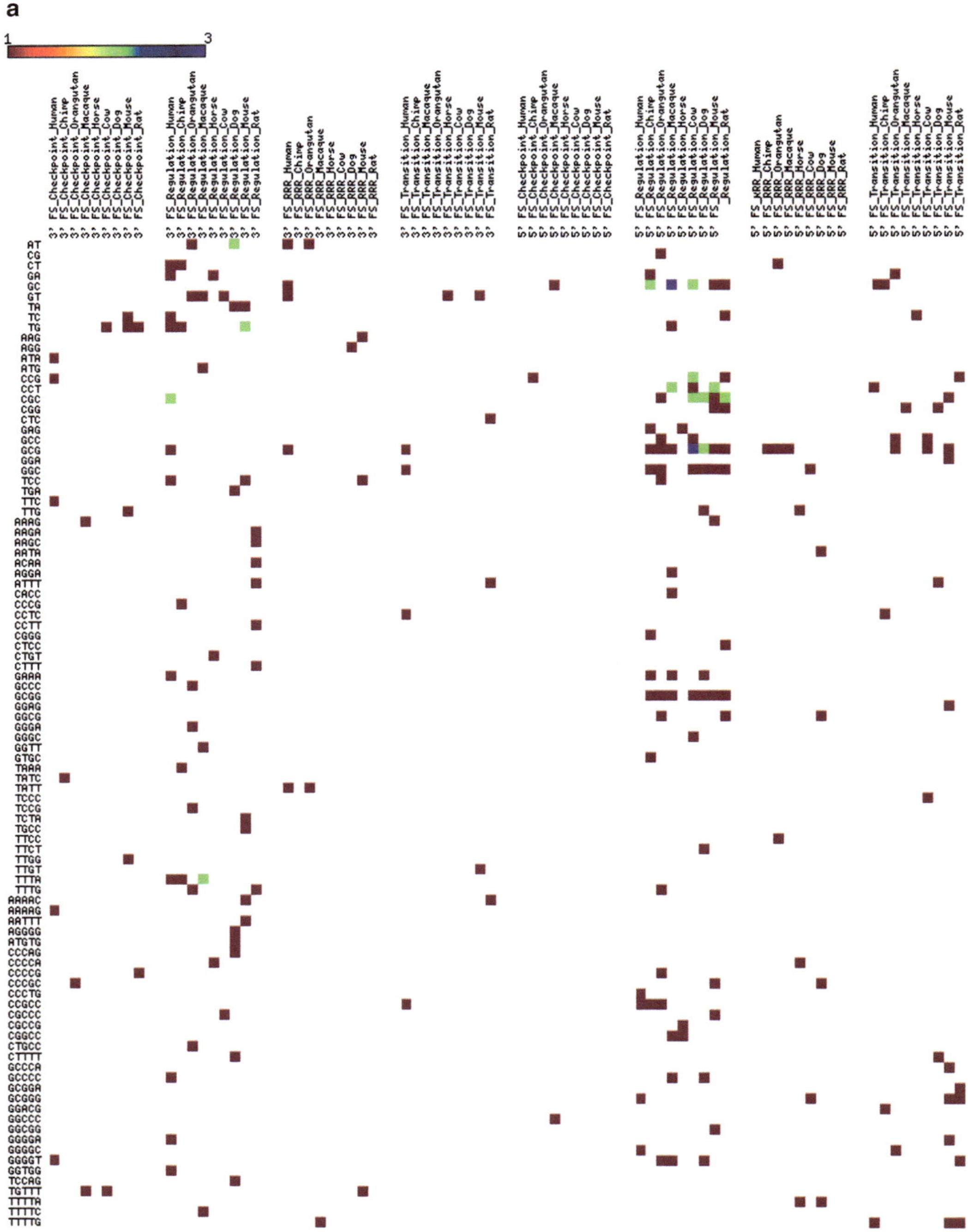

Fig. 7.5 (**a**) Repeat motifs in 3′ and 5′ flanking sequences of cell cycle genes in nine mammal. (**b**) Repeat motifs in flanking and overlapping sequences of cell cycle genes

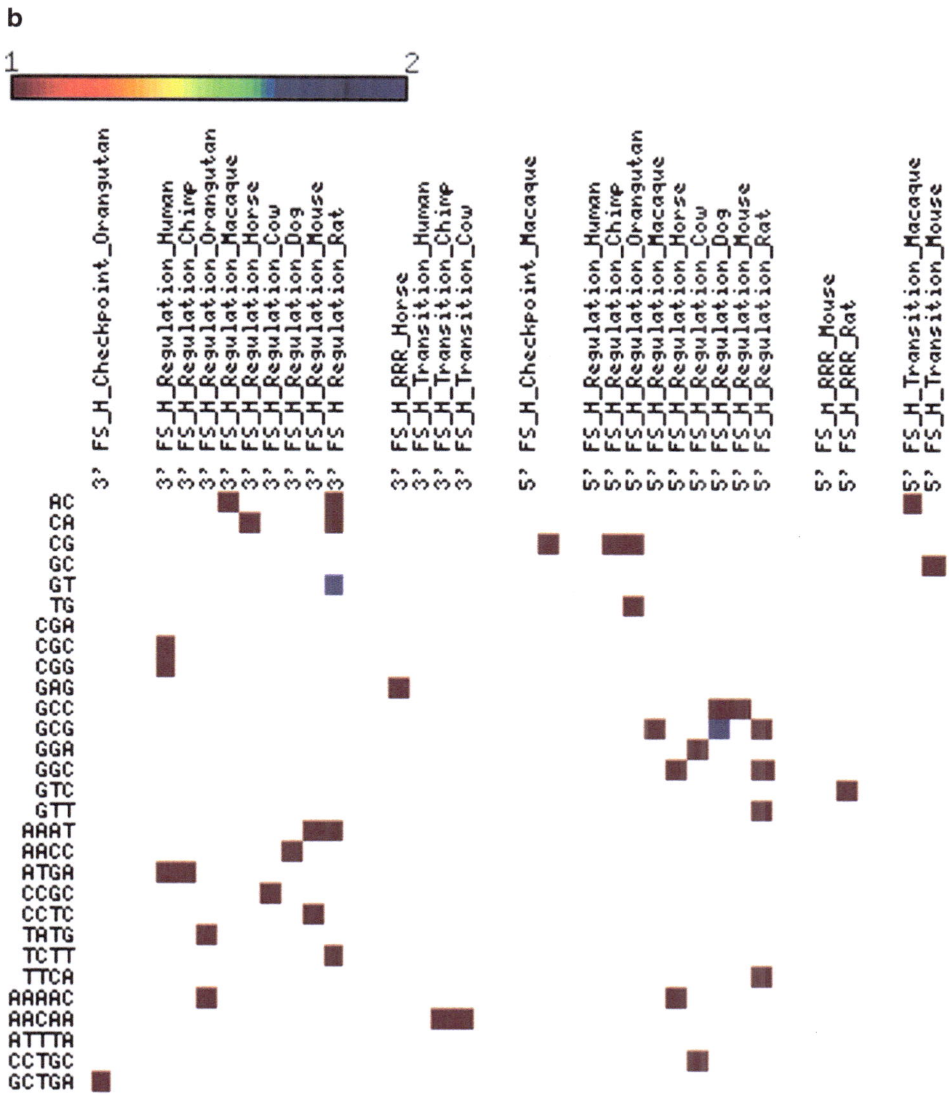

Fig. 7.5 (continued)

through Ensembl biomart version 55) (Table 7.1). Many disorders including different types of cancers are associated with these genes. These facts point to the possibility that SSRs in FS of cell cycle genes may contribute to disorders due to SSR mutations that may affect gene regulation.

Importance of SSRs in cell cycle 5′ and 3′ FS is further confirmed by establishment of association of mutations in SSRs present in 5′ and 3′-UTRs (that may be part of FS) with different types of cancers. Mutations in coding regions or methylation of promoters of MMR genes may lead to certain cancers like hematological malignancies though not always detected in all patients. In such cases, MMR deficiency may be due to mutation in the MLH1 3′-untranslated region (3′-UTR), though the exact mechanism is unknown (Mao et al. 2008). Poly (T)8 repeat deletion within the 3′-UTR of the CDK2-AP1 gene results in its decreased expression due to reduced mRNA stability and is associated with MSI human colorectal cancer (Shin et al.

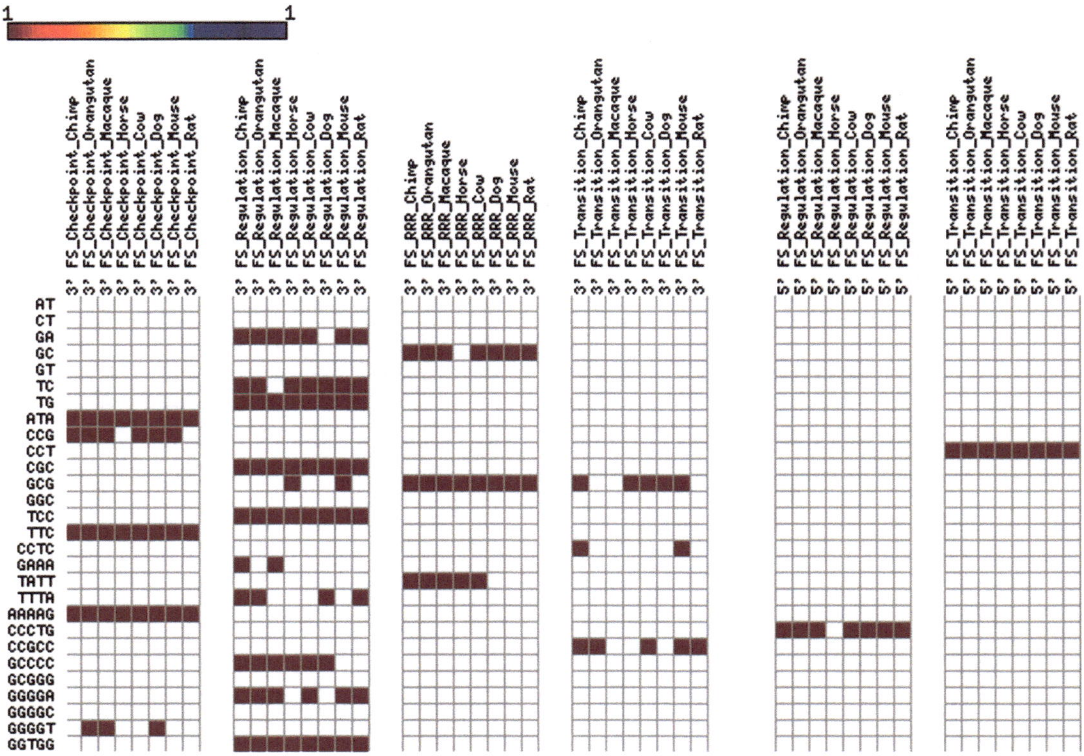

Fig. 7.6 Conserved motifs in human cell cycle genes flanking sequences. Blank cells indicate no conservation

Table 7.1 Repeat (in flanking sequences) containing human cell cycle gene names and MIM morbid description

Gene name	MIM morbid description
MCM6	Lactase persistence
TGFB1	Camurati-Engelmann disease
ACVR1	Fibrodysplasia ossificans progressiva
BMP4	Microphthalmia, syndromic 6
MTUS1	Hepatocellular carcinoma
MEN1	Hyperparathyroidism 1, multiple endocrine neoplasia, Type I
CDC73	Hyperparathyroidism 1 and 2, parathyroid carcinoma
AKT1	Breast cancer, breast-ovarian cancer, familial, colorectal cancer
CDKN2A	Li-Fraumeni syndrome 1, melanoma, cutaneous malignant, uveal, melanoma-astrocytoma syndrome, melanoma-pancreatic cancer syndrome
PTEN	Bannayan-Riley-Ruvalcaba syndrome, Cowden disease, endometrial cancer, glioma of brain familial, macrocephaly/autism syndrome, prostate cancer, Proteus syndrome, squamous cell carcinoma, head and neck, Vacterl association with hydrocephalus
EXT1	Chondrosarcoma, exostoses, multiple, Type I; trichorhinophalangeal syndrome, Type II
SEPT6	Amyotrophy, hereditary neuralgic

2007). Dinucleotide deletion in the 3′-UTR of CD24 also causes mRNA instability that may result in multiple sclerosis (MS) and systemic lupus erythematosus (SLE) (Wang et al. 2007). Microsatellite instability-high (MSI-H) tumors (in endometrial and colorectal carcinomas) show deletions of 3′-UTR polyA in epidermal growth factor receptor (EGFR) (Deqin et al. 2012), and its association is also seen in gastric cancer (Corso et al. 2011) and colon cancers (Yuan et al. 2009).

It is possible that despite risks of disorders, SSRs may exist in FS of cell cycle genes due to the possible involvement of repeats in processes like gene regulation and chromatin organization, or act as source of genetic variability that may be useful for rapid adaptation (Chang et al. 2001; Li et al. 2002; Fondon and Garner 2004; Kashi and King 2006). Repeats that can form loops and other secondary structures or cause unfolding of DNA can be advantageous for transcription (Li et al. 2002). Compared with CAG and CUG tracts, there is higher degree of stability of structure due to CGG repeats (Kiliszek et al. 2011). It is possible that some repeats found in the present study like CGG in CDKN2D and AKT1 are also associated with normal binding of transcription factors or other DNA binding proteins with or without formation of non-B DNA structures.

Single nucleotide polymorphism in dinucleotide repeat (TA)(*n*) in the promoter region of IL-28B affects transcriptional activity in length-dependent manner (Sugiyama et al. 2011). Therefore, it is possible that repeats in FS of cell cycle genes may also facilitate transcription during the division cycle especially during chromatin condensation. Z-DNA conformation is formed due to dinucleotide repeats present in the negative regulatory element (NRE, a transcriptional repressor) at the 5′-UTR of ADAM-12 gene (member of the multifunctional ADAM family of proteins linked to cancer, arthritis, and cardiac hypertrophy) and is essential for interaction with Z-DNA-binding protein that in turn repress transcription of ADAM-12 gene (Ray et al. 2011). In the present study, more dinucleotide repeats are present in 3′ FS compared to 5′ FS in human cell cycle gene but no motif type is particularly more in number. But the distribution is different in other mammals. Few genes in the present study contain CG/GC motifs or CG-rich repeats in FS. This could be because methylation and/or deamination of polymerase slippages is high in CG-rich motifs (Tian et al. 2011; Li and Chen 2011); thus, GC-rich SSRs are more unstable (Zahra et al. 2007; Tian et al. 2011), and, therefore, only essential CG-rich motifs may be retained in genes.

It is also possible that during G0 phase when activation of cell cycle genes (except recruitment for DNA damage) may not be necessary, SSRs in 5′ and 3′ FS may play a role in keeping these genes repressed until the cell cycle is reinitiated.

The present study indicates that the nine mammals are similar in terms of the repeat numbers in 5′ and 3′ FS of cell cycle genes, as there are no significant differences between them. Furthermore, many human repeats show conservation in FS of cell cycle genes all mammals studied here. The present study does not show presence of long repeats in primates except dinucleotide repeat GT (28nt) in 3′ FS of human RRR genes and pentanucleotide repeat GCCCC (35nt) in regulation genes. In 5′ FS also repeats are not long in primates except dinucleotide TG (44nt) in macaque regulation genes (data not shown). It is known that mutation rates are higher in long SSRs compared to shorter repeats. This is because the likelihood of substitutions that can interrupt repeat length is more in long repeats and can curtail their infinite growth (Kruglyak et al. 1998; Ellegren 2000; Xu et al. 2000; Dieringer and Schlotterer 2003). Further, short motifs are compared to motifs like tetra- and penta-nucleotide repeats are more unstable (Jacob and Eckert 2007; Eckert and Hile 2009). Some functional roles of tetranucleotide repeats are known (Li et al. 2004; Csink and Henikoff 1998); it is also known that repeat instability in tetranucleotide repeats may be a cause of cancer (Li et al. 2004). Possibly this could be the reason for conservation of very few tetranucleotide repeats in the present study.

7.5 Conclusion

The present study shows presence of repeats in 5′ and 3′ FS of cell cycle genes. SSRs in FS of regulation genes are present in all nine mammals studied but significance remains untested. There is no significant difference in total repeats between humans and the other eight mammals, except cow, and many repeats are conserved. The fact that some of these repeat-associated genes are in the MIM morbid database indicates that SSRs may act as “chink in the armor” for these critical genes. In future, it would be useful for investigators to recognize the potential role of instability of repeats and identify cycle-related disorders.

Acknowledgments I am grateful to Mr. Abhay Pendse for help with computational work. I am indebted to Ensembl workgroup especially Dr. Javier Herrero (Ensembl Compara Project Leader, European Bioinformatics Institute (EMBL-EBI), Wellcome Trust Genome Campus, Hinxton, Cambridge, UK) for their help in obtaining multiple aligned sequences. Further, I am obliged to all open-source journals, databases, and scientists who provided reprints and information related to this work.

References

Bacolla A, Wells RD (2009) Non-B DNA conformations as determinants of mutagenesis and human disease. Mol Carcinog 48(4):273–285

Chambers GK, MacAvoy ES (2000) Microsatellites: consensus and controversy. Comp Biochem Physiol B Biochem Mol Biol 126(4):455–476

Chang DK, Metzgar D, Wills C, Boland CR (2001) Microsatellites in the eukaryotic DNA mismatch repair genes as modulators of evolutionary mutation rate. Genome Res 11(7):1145–1146

Choudhary OP, Trivedi S (2010) Microsatellite or simple sequence repeat (SSR) instability depends on repeat characteristics during replication and repair. J Cell Molec Biol 8(2):21–34

Corso G, Velho S, Paredes J, Pedrazzani C, Martins D, Milanezi F, Pascale V, Vindigni C, Pinheiro H, Leite M, Marrelli D, Sousa S, Carneiro F, Oliveira C, Roviello F, Seruca R (2011) Oncogenic mutations in gastric cancer with microsatellite instability. Eur J Cancer 47(3):443–451

Csink AK, Henikoff S (1998) Something from nothing: the evolution and utility of satellite repeats. Trends Genet 14(5):200–204

Deqin M, Chen Z, Nero C, Patel KP, Daoud EM, Cheng H, Djordjevic B, Broaddus RR, Medeiros LJ, Rashid A, Luthra R (2012) Somatic Deletions of the PolyA Tract in the 3′ Untranslated Region of Epidermal Growth Factor Receptor Are Common in Microsatellite Instability-High Endometrial and Colorectal Carcinomas. Arch Pathol Lab Med 136(5):510–516

Dere R, Napierala M, Ranum LP, Wells RD (2004) Hairpin structure-forming propensity of the (CCTG.CAGG) tetranucleotide repeats contributes to the genetic instability associated with myotonic dystrophy type 2. J Biol Chem 279(40): 41715–41726

Dieringer D, Schlotterer C (2003) Two distinct modes of microsatellite mutation processes: evidence from the complete genomic sequences of nine species. Genome Res 13:2242–2251

Eckert KA, Hile SE (2009) Every microsatellite is different: Intrinsic DNA features dictate mutagenesis of common microsatellites present in the human genome. Mol Carcinog 48(4):379–388

Eisen JA, Hanawalt PC (1999) A phylogenomic study of DNA repair genes, proteins, and processes. Mut Res 435:171–213

Ellegren H (2000) Heterogeneous mutation processes in human microsatellite DNA sequences. Nat Genet 24:400–402

Fondon JW 3rd, Garner HR (2004) Molecular origins of rapid and continuous morphological evolution. Proc Natl Acad Sci USA 101(52):18058–18063

Galindo CL, McCormick JF, Bubb VJ, Abid Alkadem DH, Li LS, McIver LJ, George AC, Boothman DA, Quinn JP, Skinner MA, Garner HR (2011) A long AAAG repeat allele in the 5′-UTR of the ERR-γ gene is correlated with breast cancer predisposition and drives promoter activity in MCF-7 breast cancer cells. Breast Cancer Res Treat 130(1):41–48

Gauthier NP, Larsen ME, Wernersson R, de Lichtenberg U, Jensen LJ, Brunak S, Jensen TS (2008) Cyclebase.org-a comprehensive multi-organism online database of cell-cycle experiments. Nucleic Acids Res 36(Database issue):D854–9

Jacob KD, Eckert KA (2007) Escherichia coli DNA polymerase IV contributes to spontaneous mutagenesis at coding sequences but not microsatellite alleles. Mut Res 619(1–2):93–103

Joshi-Tope G, Vastrik I, Gopinath GR, Matthews L, Schmidt E, Gillespie M, D'Eustachio P, Jassal B, Lewis S, Wu G, Birney E, Stein L (2003) The genome knowledgebase: a resource for biologists and bioinformaticists. Cold Spring Harb Symp Quant Biol 68: 237–243

Kashi Y, King DG (2006) Simple sequence repeats as advantageous mutators in evolution. Trends Genet 22(5):253–259

Kelder T, Pico AR, Hanspers K, van Iersel MP, Evelo C, Conklin BR (2009) Mining biological pathways using WikiPathways web services. PLoS One 4(7)

Kiliszek A, Kierzek R, Krzyzosiak WJ, Rypniewski W (2011) Crystal structures of CGG RNA repeats with implications for fragile X-associated tremor ataxia syndrome. Nucleic Acids Res 39(16):7308–7315

Kruglyak S, Durrett RT, Schug MD, Aquadro CF (1998) Equilibrium distributions of microsatellite repeat length resulting from a balance between slippage events and point mutations. Proc Natl Acad Sci USA 95:10774–10778

Lahiri M, Gustafson TL, Majors ER, Freudenreich CH (2004) Expanded CAG repeats activate the DNA damage checkpoint pathway. Mol Cell 15(2):287–293

Levinson G, Gutman GA (1987) Slipped-strand mispairing: a major mechanism for DNA sequence evolution. Mol Biol Evol 4:203–221

Li M, Chen SS (2011) The tendency to recreate ancestral CG dinucleotides in the human genome. BMC Evol Biol 11:3

Li YC, Korol AB, Fahima T, Beiles A, Nevo E (2002) Microsatellites: genomic distribution, putative functions and mutational mechanisms: a review. Mol Ecol 11(12):2453–2465

Li YC, Korol AB, Fahima T, Nevo E (2004) Microsatellites within genes: structure, function, and evolution. Mol Biol Evol 21(6):991–1007

Lukusa T, Fryns JP (2008) Human chromosome fragility. Biochim Biophys Acta 1779(1):3–16

Mao G, Pan X, Gu L (2008) Evidence that a mutation in the MLH1 3′-untranslated region confers a mutator phenotype and mismatch repair deficiency in patients with relapsed leukemia. J Biol Chem 283(6): 3211–3216

Matthews L, D'Eustachio P, Gillespie M, Croft D, de Bono B, Gopinath G, Jassal B, Lewis S, Schmidt E, Vastrik I, Wu G, Birney E, Stein L (2007) An introduction to the reactome knowledgebase of human biological pathways and processes. Bioinform Primer NCI/Nat Pathway Interact Datab. doi:10.1038/pid.2007.3

Matthews L, Gopinath G, Gillespie M, Caudy M, Croft D, de Bono B, Garapati P, Hemish J, Hermjakob H, Jassal B, Kanapin A, Lewis S, Mahajan S, May B, Schmidt E, Vastrik I, Wu G, Birney E, Stein L, D'Eustachio P (2009) Reactome knowledgebase of biological pathways and processes. Nucleic Acids Res 37(Database issue):D619–D622

Metzgar D, Bytof J, Wills C (2000) Selection against frameshift mutations limits microsatellite expansion in coding DNA. Genome Res 10(1):72–80

Pavlidis P, Noble WS (2003) Matrix2png: a utility for visualizing matrix data. Bioinformatics 19:295–296. doi:10.1093/bioinformatics/19.2.295

Pico AR, Kelder T, van Iersel MP, Hanspers K, Conklin BR, Evelo C (2008) WikiPathways: pathway editing for the people. PLoS Biol 6(7)

Ray BK, Dhar S, Shakya A, Ray A (2011) Z-DNA-forming silencer in the first exon regulates human ADAM-12 gene expression. Proc Natl Acad Sci USA 108(1):103–108

Regelson M, Eller CD, Horvath S, Marahrens Y (2006) A link between repetitive sequences and gene replication time. Cytogenet Genome Res 112(3–4):184–193

Russell L, Forsdyke DR (1991) A human putative lymphocyte G0/G1 switch gene containing a CpG-rich island encodes a small basic protein with the potential to be phosphorylated. DNA Cell Biol 10(8):581–591

Shin J, Yuan Z, Fordyce K, Sreeramoju P, Kent TS, Kim J, Wang V, Schneyer D, Weber TK (2007) A del T poly T (8) mutation in the 3′ untranslated region (UTR) of the CDK2-AP1 gene is functionally significant causing decreased mRNA stability resulting in decreased CDK2-AP1 expression in human microsatellite unstable (MSI) colorectal cancer (CRC). Surgery 142(2):222–227

Strand M, Prolla TA, Liskay RM, Petes TD (1993) Destabilization of tracts of simple repetitive DNA in yeast by mutations affecting DNA mismatch repair. Nature 365:274–276

Sugiyama M, Tanaka Y, Wakita T, Nakanishi M, Mizokami M (2011) Genetic variation of the IL-28B promoter affecting gene expression. PLoS One 6(10):e26620

The Gene Ontology Consortium (2000) Gene Ontology: tool for the unification of biology. Nature Genet 25:25–29. http://amigo.geneontology.org/cgi-bin/amigo/browse.cgi

Tian X, Strassmann JE, Queller DC (2011) Genome nucleotide composition shapes variation in simple sequence repeats. Mol Biol Evol 28(2):899–909

Toth G, Gaspari Z, Jurka J (2000) Microsatellites in different eukaryotic genomes: survey and analysis. Genome Res 10:967–981

Tripathi Bhar A, Banerjee S, Chunder N, Roy A, Sengupta A, Roy B, Roychowdhury S, Panda CK (2003) Differential alterations of the genes in the CDKN2A-CCND1-CDK4-RB1 pathway are associated with the development of head and neck squamous cell carcinoma in Indian patients. J Cancer Res Clin Oncol 129(11):642–650

Trivedi S (2003) Do microsatellites have biased associations? Nucleus 46:61–76

Trivedi S (2006) Comparison of simple sequence repeats in 19 Archaea. Genet Mol Res 5(4):741–772

Trivedi S (2010) Do simple sequence repeats in replication, repair and recombination genes of mycoplasmas provide genetic variability? J Cell Mole Biol 7(2) & 7(2 & 8(1)):53–70

Va Vastrik I, D'Eustachio P, Schmidt E, Joshi-Tope G, Gopinath G, Croft D, de Bono B, Gillespie M, Jassal B, Lewis S, Matthews L, Wu G, Birney E, Stein L (2007) Reactome: a knowledge base of biologic pathways and processes. Genome Biol 8:R39

Wang L, Lin S, Rammohan KW, Liu Z, Liu JQ, Liu RH, Guinther N, Lima J, Zhou Q, Wang T, Zheng X, Birmingham DJ, Rovin BH, Hebert LA, Wu Y, Lynn DJ, Cooke G, Yu CY, Zheng P, Liu Y (2007) A dinucleotide deletion in CD24 confers protection against autoimmune diseases. PLoS Genet 3(4):e49

Xu X, Peng M, Fang Z (2000) The direction of microsatellite mutations is dependent upon allele length. Nat Genet 24:396–399

Yuan Z, Shin J, Wilson A, Goel S, Ling YH, Ahmed N, Dopeso H, Jhawer M, Nasser S, Montagna C, Fordyce K, Augenlicht LH, Aaltonen LA, Arango D, Weber TK, Mariadason JM (2009) An A13 repeat within the 3′-untranslated region of epidermal growth factor receptor (EGFR) is frequently mutated in microsatellite instability colon cancers and is associated with increased EGFR expression. Cancer Res 69(19): 7811–7818

Zahra R, Blackwood JK, Sales J, Leach DR (2007) Proofreading and secondary structure processing determine the orientation dependence of CAG × CTG trinucleotide repeat instability in Escherichia coli. Genetics 176(1): 27–41

Mechanisms of Chemopreventive Activity of Sulforaphane

8

Yogesh C. Awasthi, Shailesh Jaiswal, Mukesh Sahu, Abha Sharma, and Rajendra Sharma

Abstract

D, L-Sulforaphane (SFN) found in cruciferous vegetables is a highly promising anticancer and chemopreventive agent. SFN has been shown to exhibit cytostatic and cytotoxic activities against a number of cancer cell types in vitro and inhibit chemically induced carcinogenesis in rodent models in vivo. SFN also prevents metastasis in mouse models of different cancer types. Cytostatic and cytotoxic activities of SFN have been attributed to several mechanisms including the reactive oxygen species (ROS)-dependent cell cycle arrest and apoptosis. Recent studies discussed in this chapter strongly suggest that 4-hydroxynonenal (HNE), the most abundant end product of ROS-induced lipid peroxidation of ω-6 fatty acids, is a major contributor to the chemopreventive activity of SFN. The chemopreventive activity of SFN, and perhaps its analogs found in cruciferous plants, may be attributed to HNE-induced selective apoptosis in cancer cells and simultaneous protection of neighboring normal cells from carcinogenic insult through the induction of defense mechanisms such as the activation of Nrf2 and Hsf1.

Keywords

Carcinogenesis • Sulforaphane • Chemoprevention • 4-Hydroxynonenal • Lipid peroxidation

8.1 Introduction

Cancer leads to immense human suffering as it is one of the major causes of mortality in the world. Cancer is caused due to the genetic and epigenetic alterations leading to disruption in pathways responsible for controlling normal cellular homeostasis. While a significant progress has been achieved in therapy and the management

Y.C. Awasthi (✉) • S. Jaiswal • M. Sahu • A. Sharma • R. Sharma
Department of Molecular Biology and Immunology, University of North Texas Health Science Center, 3500 Camp Bowie Blvd., Fort Worth, TX 76107, USA
e-mail: yogesh.awasthi@unthsc.edu

P.R. Sudhakaran (ed.), *Perspectives in Cancer Prevention – Translational Cancer Research*, DOI 10.1007/978-81-322-1533-2_8, © Springer India 2014

of cancer, this disease still remains a leading cause of death and suffering. The approaches to prevent initiation and progression of cancer are therefore very important in our war against cancer. Effective chemoprevention would require the use of GRAS (generally regarded as safe) micronutrients that could prevent initiation, progression, and proliferation of cancer. It has been generally believed for long time that vegetarian diet may be an important source of phytochemicals that may prevent carcinogenesis and in recent years, a multitude of phytochemicals present in vegetables, fruits, green tea, etc. have been shown to possess significant anticancer activity (Fahey et al. 1997; Wang et al. 2004; Brennan et al. 2005; Fowke et al. 2003). Many of the cruciferous vegetables such as broccoli, cauliflower, and cabbage have been identified as a rich source of cancer-preventing isothiocyanates that inhibit chemically induced carcinogenesis in animal models (Fahey et al. 1997; Wang et al. 2004; Brennan et al. 2005; Fowke et al. 2003; Conaway et al. 2002; Chung et al. 2000). Isothiocyanates occur in these plants as glucosinolates that yield respective isothiocyanates upon hydrolysis catalyzed by myrosinase. The major constituent glucosinolate of broccoli is hydrolyzed by myrosinase to yield sulforaphane (SFN) that is perhaps the most widely studied anticancer compound among these isothiocyanates. SFN has been shown to decrease the incidence, initiation, progression, and severity of chemical carcinogenesis induced by dimethylbenz(*a*)anthracene (DMBA) and azoxymethane (AOM) in a number of animal models (Fahey et al. 1997; Wang et al. 2004; Brennan et al. 2005; Fowke et al. 2003; Conaway et al. 2002; Chung et al. 2000). SFN has also been shown to selectively inhibit proliferation of cancer cells by specifically targeting the factors that provide growth advantage to cancer cells (Huang et al. 1999; Chandel et al. 1998; Yao et al. 2008; Shan et al. 2009). For example, the hypoxia-inducible factor-1α (HIF-1α), that is known to provide advantage to the growth and motility of cancer cells, is downregulated by SFN in Tca8113 cell line. In another study it has been shown that in human bladder cancer cells, SFN induces apoptosis by inhibiting the activation of NF-κB and cyclooxygenase-2 (Shan et al. 2009). These and many other studies attest to the validity of SFN as a promising GRAS (generally regarded as safe) anticancer natural product that can inhibit not only the initiation of chemical carcinogenesis but also the progression of cancer.

8.2 An Overview of the Mechanisms of Anticancer Activities of SFN

In general, the chemopreventive activities of many of the anticancer agents including SFN can be attributed to their two pronged effect on biotransformation enzymes. First, the anticancer agents inhibit Phase I enzymes to prevent the formation of activated "ultimate carcinogens" from xenobiotics, e.g., formation of benzo[*a*]pyrene diol-epoxide (BAPD) from benzo[*a*]pyrene (Caldwell 1986), and second, these agents induce Phase II enzymes such as glutathione S-transferases (GSTs) to accelerate the detoxification of "ultimate electrophilic carcinogens." Recent studies suggest that the overall cancer preventive activities of SFN may be due to its capability to induce defense mechanisms that protects normal cells from carcinogenic insult along with its simultaneous proapoptotic effects specifically on cancer cells that prevent their proliferation (Brooks et al. 2001; Zhang et al. 2004, 2006; Juge et al. 2007; Basten et al. 2002; Büchler et al. 2002). SFN exhibits both these activities as it has been shown to inhibit the expression as well as the activity of various Phase I CYP 450 enzymes (Barcelo et al. 1996, 1998; Maheo et al. 1997; Yoxall et al. 2005; Skupinska et al. 2009) and is also a strong inducer of Phase II enzymes such as GSTs and NAD[P]H quinone oxidoreductase (NQO) (Brooks et al. 2001; Zhang et al. 2004, 2006; Juge et al. 2007; Basten et al. 2002). The induction of Phase II enzymes by SFN has been shown to be both in vivo and in vitro (Basten et al. 2002; Scharf et al. 2003; Zhang 2000; Dinkova-Kostova et al. 2002). Among these enzymes, GSTs and NQO1 may perhaps be particularly important because collectively these enzymes can reduce the concentration of the "ultimate carcinogens" and also provide protection against oxidative stress generated during the biotransformation. The suppression of Phase I enzymes and induction of Phase II enzymes by SFN is not selective to normal cells and cancer cells. It appears SFN exerts its selective toxicity to cancer cells by targeting the growth advantage of cancer cells. In these mechanisms, the reactive oxygen species (ROS) generated by SFN exposure and subsequently formed lipid peroxidation products, particularly HNE, play a major role.

8.3 Role of ROS-Induced LPO in the Chemopreventive Activity of SFN

ROS are generated in cells upon exposure to SFN, and it has been suggested that the ROS-mediated signaling may contribute to its chemopreventive activities (Simon et al. 2000; Pham et al. 2004; Singh et al. 2005). For example, it has been shown that ROS generated due to SFN treatment leads to apoptosis in U937 cells through different mechanisms (Choi et al. 2008) and that it could be prevented by antioxidants. Our recent studies show that SFN-induced apoptosis in cancer cells can be inhibited by the overexpression of GSTA4-4 that specifically detoxifies HNE and attenuates its intracellular accumulation (Sharma et al. 2010). These findings strongly suggest an obligatory role of HNE in ROS-mediated signaling and the selective toxicity of SFN to cancer cells (Choi et al. 2008; Singh et al. 2004a, b; Choi and Singh 2005). A multitude of studies in the last decade (reviewed in references Sharma et al. 2012 and Awasthi et al. 2008a, b) have shown that ROS-induced signaling is at least in part mediated via lipid peroxidation products particularly lipid hydroperoxides and HNE (Awasthi et al. 2004; Yang et al. 2003; Cheng et al. 2001; Dwivedi et al. 2007). It has been shown that apoptosis induced by hydrogen peroxide, superoxide anion, UV, and xenobiotics such as naphthalene can be inhibited by attenuating lipid peroxidation and formation of HNE caused by these agents (Sharma et al. 2010; Yang et al. 2003; Cheng et al. 2001).

It has also been shown that HNE plays a major role in ROS-induced signaling for apoptosis, cell cycle arrest, proliferation, angiogenesis, and tyrosine kinase receptor-mediated signaling (Sharma et al. 2004; Vatsyayan et al. 2011; Awasthi et al. 2003a, b, 2005; Cheng et al. 1999; Yang et al. 2001, 2002). This role of lipid peroxidation products in stress signaling is corroborated by many of our studies showing that ROS-induced signaling is amplified by lipid peroxidation products and that it can be inhibited by interrupting LPO and minimizing the formation of the end product HNE (reviewed in Awasthi et al. 2008a, b and Dwivedi et al. 2007).

In recent years, the role of HNE in the mechanisms of the chemopreventive activity of SFN has been thoroughly examined (reviewed in Sharma et al. 2012). SFN activates Nrf2 and induces its target genes such as GSTs, gamma-glutamyl cysteine synthetase, and NQO1 that contribute to its chemopreventive properties (Jeong et al. 2006; Thimmulappa et al. 2002). HNE can also stimulate these defense mechanisms against oxidative stress via Nrf2, HSF1, the EGFR-related proliferative pathways, and angiogenesis (Vatsyayan et al. 2011) and activate p53-mediated mechanisms for preserving genome integrity (Sharma et al. 2008a, b, 2010; Chaudhary et al. 2010). HNE induces apoptosis in all cancer cell lines studied so far in our laboratory (Awasthi et al. 2008a, b; Singhal et al. 2006, 2007, 2009). Likewise, many of the biological activities of SFN listed in Table 8.1 are also exhibited by HNE. The studies summarized in following sections indicate that many of the effects of SFN can be blocked by transfecting cells with GSTA1-1 or GSTA4-4 that attenuate the formation and accumulation HNE and strongly suggest a role of HNE in the biological activities of SFN (Fig. 8.1).

Table 8.1 Biological effects of sulforaphane

	Biological effects	References
1	Apoptosis	Zhang et al. (2006), Pham et al. (2004), Singh et al. (2004a, b, 2005); Choi et al. (2008), Sharma et al. (2010), Xu and Thornalley (2000), Pledgie-Tracy et al. (2007), Fawzy and Nehad (2011), Myzak et al. (2006), Kaminski et al. (2011)
2	Induction of Bax, p21, caspase3	Sharma et al. (2010), Kaminski et al. (2011), Kallifatidis et al. (2009)
3	Loss of membrane potential	Choi et al. (2008), Sharma et al. (2010), Kallifatidis et al. (2009)
4	Cell cycle arrest	Zhang et al. (2006), Choi et al. (2008), Singh et al. (2004a, b), Shan et al. (2006), Jackson et al. (2006), Kallifatidis et al. (2009), Fawzy and Nehad (2011)
5	Interaction with NfkB	Zhang et al. (2006), Wagner et al. (2010), Ho et al. (2009)
6	Inhibition of HDAC[a]	Clarke et al. (2011), Kallifatidis et al. (2009), Gan et al. (2010)
7	Activation of Nrf2	Zhang et al. (2006), Sharma et al. (2008a, b), Myzak et al. (2006), Ho et al. (2009)
8	Activation of HSF1[b]	Singh et al. (2004a, b), Gamet-Payrastre (2006)
9	Activation of p53	Meeran et al. (2010)
10	Induction of HSP70	Gamet-Payrastre (2006)
11	Repression of hTERT[c]	Moon et al. (2010), Kong et al. (2001)
12	Induction of oxidative stress	Pham et al. (2004), Singh et al. (2004a, b, 2005), Choi et al. (2008), Sharma et al. (2010)
13	Activation of MAPK[d]	Thejass and Kuttan (2006)
14	Inhibition of angiogenesis	Asakage et al. (2006), Rose et al. (2005), Bertl et al. (2006), Talalay (2000)

[a]Histone deacetylases
[b]Heat shock factor 1
[c]Human telomerase reverse transcriptase
[d]Mitogen-activated protein (MAP) kinases

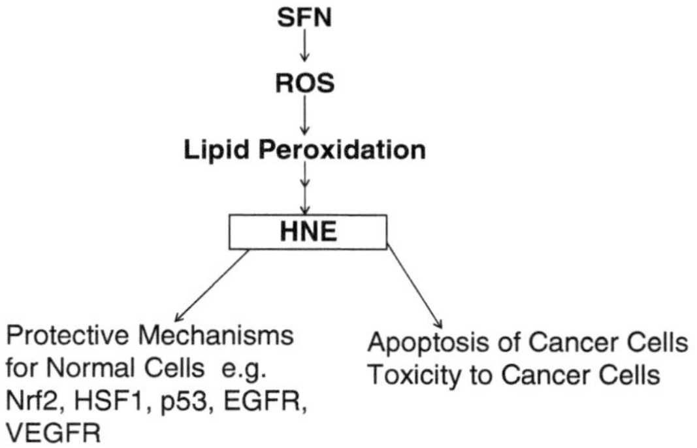

Fig. 8.1 Proposed mechanism for the chemopreventive activity of sulforaphane

8.4 Overlap in SFN and 4-HNE-Induced Signaling

It has been shown that HNE signals for cell proliferation, cell cycle arrest, differentiation, and apoptosis, and, in a concentration-dependent manner, regulates the expression of many genes in various types of cells (Dianzani 2003; Esterbauer et al. 1991; Awasthi et al. 2004, 2005, 2008a, b; Yang et al. 2003; Cheng et al. 2001; Dwivedi et al. 2007; Sharma et al. 2004; Vatsyayan et al. 2011; Cheng et al. 1999; Yang et al. 2001, 2002). At low concentration, HNE can limit its own toxicity by activating mechanisms for cell survival (Sharma et al. 2008a, b; Chaudhary et al. 2010) and is known to induce stress-responsive pro-survival factors, such as Nrf2, heat shock factor 1 (HSF1), and its client heat shock proteins, EGFR, VEGFR, and the transcription repressor Daxx that can inhibit Fas-mediated apoptosis (Sharma et al. 2004, 2008a, b; Vatsyayan et al. 2011; Awasthi et al. 2005; Cheng et al. 1999; Yang et al. 2001; Chaudhary et al. 2010). Many of the biological activities of SFN listed in Table 8.1 are shared by HNE. ROS-induced generation of HNE upon SFN exposure seems to contribute to its protective effects against cancer through two mechanisms. First, it activates the survival mechanisms to protect normal cells against electrophilic insult, and, second, it promotes apoptosis in cancer cells and inhibits their proliferation. In this model initially generated low levels of HNE may induce survival mechanisms beneficial for the normal cells, but sustained oxidative stress caused by SFN and increase in HNE levels may selectively kill cancer cells and prevent their proliferation by targeting the factors that provide advantage to cancer cells in their proliferation (Sharma et al. 2012). Our studies (Sharma et al. 2011) with human erythroleukemic cells are in line with this idea. These studies show that some of the biological activities associated with the chemoprotective properties of SFN are mediated through HNE generated during SFN-induced ROS formation, and that these activities of SFN could be inhibited by the overexpression of alpha class GST isozymes that attenuate HNE levels in cells (Sharma et al. 2011). It has been demonstrated that SFN-induced cytotoxicity, cell cycle arrest, and apoptosis in HL60 and K562 cells is inhibited by forced overexpression of GSTA1-1 that attenuates LPO and suppresses the accumulation of HNE. This would strongly suggest that at least some of the biological activities of SFN are being mediated via HNE. This contention finds further support from many previous studies showing that HNE is a common denominator in the mechanisms of ROS-mediated signaling (Sharma et al. 2010; Jeong et al. 2006). HNE per se is known to induce cell cycle arrest and cause cytotoxicity to cells via necrosis and apoptosis (Awasthi et al. 2003a, b, 2008a, b; Zhang and Forman 2009) and these effects are common with SFN. While the observed inhibition of the biological activities of SFN accompanied with the suppression of HNE levels in GSTA1-1 overexpressing cells (Sharma et al. 2010) implicate HNE in the mechanisms of the chemopreventive effects of SFN, it is possible that the increased SFN-conjugating activity in GSTA1-1-overexpressing cells may lower the actual concentration of SFN by its accelerated conjugation with GSH. However, no significant alterations in the GSH levels of SFN-treated cells transfected with either empty vector or h*GSTA* were observed in these studies (Sharma et al. 2010) suggesting that the protective effect of GSTA1-1 against SFN toxicity was preferentially imparted through the inhibition of SFN-induced LPO and consequent lowering of HNE levels, rather than GST-mediated detoxification of SFN.

The effects of SFN similar to those in HL60 and K562 cells have also been reported for colon and prostate cancer cells (Singh et al. 2005; Choi et al. 2008; Gamet-Payrastre et al. 1998). These effects include the induction of cell cycle arrest and apoptosis. It has been shown that SFN can arrest cell cycle at different stages of its progression, a mechanism by which it can inhibit growth of cancer cells. Arrest of cells in G0/G1, G2/M, and S phases upon treatment with SFN have been reported in leukemia, breast, bladder, colon, and prostate cancer cells (Singh et al. 2004a, b; Gamet-Payrastre et al. 2000; Fowke et al. 2003; Xu and Thornalley 2000; Fimognari et al. 2002; Tang and Zhang 2004; Herman-Antosiewicz et al. 2006). A number of mechanisms have been proposed for the SFN-induced cell cycle arrest in different cell types. Cyclins and cyclin-dependent kinase complexes play an important role in the mechanisms of cell cycle progression (Sherr 1996; Sherr and Roberts 1999). By binding to Cdk1/2, cyclin B1 can activate Cdk1/2 (cdc2) to facilitate its nuclear accumulation for mitotic initiation in the late G2 phase of mammalian cells. It has been suggested that while SFN-induced cell cycle arrest in the G2/M phase appears to be regulated by cell cycle-related proteins cyclin B1 and Cdk1, the arrest in G1 phase is mediated by the inhibition of cyclin D1 and DNA synthesis (Shen et al. 2006; Singh et al. 2004a, b; Shan et al. 2006). Another suggested mechanism through which SFN induces cell cycle arrest is via the upregulation of CDKI, p21, and p27 (Singh et al. 2005; Choi et al. 2008; Sharma et al. 2010). SFN-induced cell cycle arrest has also been attributed to the disruption of normal mitotic microtubule polymerization and histone acetylation (Jackson et al. 2006; Myzak et al. 2004). Many of these effects of SFN on cell cycle progression can be attenuated by the overexpression of GSTA1-1 or GSTA4-4 in cells (Sharma et al. 2010; Singh et al. 2004a, b). HNE may be a causative factor for

SFN-induced apoptosis via mitochondrial apoptotic pathways as well because in GSTA1-1-overexpressing cells, SFN fails to induce apoptosis and, unlike the wild-type cells HNE levels, do not increase in these cells upon SFN treatment. In GSTA1-1-overexpressing cells, SFN-induced translocation of Bax to mitochondria, a proapoptotic signal, is inhibited, and antiapoptotic signaling is activated as indicated by activation of Bcl-xL (Sharma et al. 2010). Furthermore, in GSTA1-1-overexpressing cells, SFN-induced release of cytochrome c to the cytosol and nuclear accumulation of AIF is also inhibited [29]. These studies suggest that caspase3-independent apoptosis by SFN is also HNE dependent further indicating a role of HNE in the biological activities of SFN (Sharma et al. 2010).

8.5 Contributions of SFN and HNE Toward the Defense of Normal Cells

Both SFN and HNE promote nuclear translocation of HSF1 and induction of the expression of Hsp70, the mechanisms involved in defense against stress. SFN-induced upregulation of heat shock proteins (Sharma et al. 2010) most likely results from the reverse nuclear-cytoplasmic trafficking of the transcription factor HSF1 and its repressor protein Daxx (Sharma et al. 2010). HNE also induces translocation of Daxx from nucleus to cytoplasm and that of HSF1 from cytoplasm to nucleus (Sharma et al. 2008a, b). Both HNE and SFN induce the nuclear translocation and activation of Nrf2 (Sharma et al. 2010). However, it has been shown that SFN-induced nuclear translocation of Nrf2 is more pronounced in GSTA1-1 overexpressing HL60 and K562 cells as compared to the empty vector-transfected cells (Sharma et al. 2010). The question then arises that if HNE is the causative factor for such translocation, why a lesser nuclear translocation of Nrf2 and HSF1 is not seen in SFN-treated GSTA1-1 over expressing cells? This apparent anomaly could perhaps be due to the concentration-dependent opposite effects of HNE on signaling for survival at low concentration and apoptosis at higher concentration (Sharma et al. 2012) discussed above. It is possible that initial low levels of HNE generated during SFN exposure act as a sensor to induce translocation of Nrf2 and HSF1 in both the vector and GSTA1-1 overexpressing cells as a survival mechanism. Whereas in GSTA1-1 overexpressing cells, low levels of HNE that are required for the translocation are maintained, in vector-transfected cells, sustained higher accumulation of HNE leads to apoptosis and apparently a lesser nuclear accumulation of Nrf2 and HSF1. This postulate however remains to be confirmed through further studies and the constitutive levels of HNE in cells that would promote either proliferation or cell death need to be clearly established. Nevertheless, so far available evidence strongly suggests that HNE plays a crucial role in the mechanisms of the biological activities of SFN including its chemoprotective properties, namely, (1) the protection of normal cells against oxidative/electrophilic stress by upregulating defense mechanisms and (2) specific killing of cancer cells by targeting signaling of pathways that provide selective growth advantage to cancer cells. Further studies to validate these conjectures may help in further refining of the approaches for the search of more effective chemoprotective agents.

Acknowledgment Supported in part by NEIHS grants ES 012171 and Patricia Rogers Joslin Foundation for Pancreatic Cancer Research, Arlington, Texas.

References

Asakage M, Tsuno NH, Kitayama J, Tsuchiya T, Yoneyama S, Yamada J, Okaji Y, Kaisaki S, Osada T, Takahashi K, Nagawa H (2006) Sulforaphane induces inhibition of human umbilical vein endothelial cells proliferation by apoptosis. Angiogenesis 9:83–91

Awasthi S, Singhal SS, Sharma R, Zimniak P, Awasthi YC (2003a) Transport of glutathione – conjugates and chemotherapeutic drugs by RLIP76 (RalBP1): a novel link between G-protein and tyrosine kinase signaling and drug resistance. Int J Cancer 106:635–646

Awasthi YC, Sharma R, Cheng JZ, Yang Y, Sharma A, Singhal SS, Awasthi S (2003b) Role of 4-hydroxynonenal in stress-mediated apoptosis signaling. Mol Aspects Med 24:219–230

Awasthi YC, Yang Y, Tiwari NK, Patrick B, Sharma A, Li J, Awasthi S (2004) Regulation of 4-hydroxynonenal-mediated signaling by glutathione S-transferases. Free Radic Biol Med 37(5):607–619

Awasthi YC, Ansari GA, Awasthi S (2005) Regulation of 4-hydroxynonenal mediated signaling by glutathione S-transferases. Methods Enzymol 401:379–407

Awasthi S, Singhal SS, Awasthi YC, Martin B, Woo JH, Cunningham CC, Frankel AE (2008a) RLIP76 and Cancer. Clin Cancer Res 14(14):4372–4377

Awasthi YC, Sharma R, Sharma A, Yadav S, Singhal SS, Chaudhary P, Awasthi S (2008b) Self-regulatory role of 4-hydroxynonenal in signaling for stress-induced programmed cell death. Free Radic Biol Med 45(2):111–118

Barcelo S, Gardiner JM, Gescher A, Chipman JK (1996) CYP2E1-mediated mechanism of anti-genotoxicity of the broccoli constituent sulforaphane. Carcinogenesis 17:277–282

Barcelo S, Mace K, Pfeifer AM, Chipman JK (1998) Production of DNA strand breaks by N-nitrosodimethylamine and 2-amino-3-methylimidazo[4,5-f]quinoline in THLE cells expressing human CYP isoenzymes and inhibition by sulforaphane. Mutat Res 402:111–120

Basten GP, Bao Y, Williamson G (2002) Sulforaphane and its glutathione conjugate but not sulforaphane nitrile induce UDP-glucuronosyl transferase (UGT1A1) and glutathione transferase (GSTA1) in cultured cells. Carcinogenesis 23:1399–1404

Bertl E, Bartsch H, Gerhauser C (2006) Inhibition of angiogenesis and endothelial cell functions are novel sulforaphane-mediated mechanisms in chemoprevention. Mol Cancer Ther 5:575–585

Brennan P, Hsu CC, Moullan N, Szeszenia-Dabrowska N, Lissowska J, Zaridze D, Rudnai P, Fabianova E, Mates D, Bencko V, Foretova L, Janout V, Gemignani F, Chabrier A, Hall J, Hung RJ, Boffetta P, Canzian F (2005) Effect of cruciferous vegetables on lung cancer in patients stratified by genetic status: a Mendelian randomization approach. Lancet 366:1558–1560

Brooks JD, Paton VG, Vidanes G (2001) Potent induction of phase 2 enzymes in human prostate cells by sulforaphane. Cancer Epidemiol Biomarkers Prev 10:949–954

Büchler M, Salnikov A, Herr I (2011) Sulforaphane increases drug-mediated cytotoxicity toward cancer stem-like cells of pancreas and prostate. Mol Ther 19:188–195

Caldwell JA (1986) Xenobiotic metabolism: mammalian aspects. ACS Symp Ser Am Chem Soc 299:2–28

Chandel NS, Maltepe E, Goldwasser E, Mathieu CE, Simon MC, Schumacker PT (1998) Mitochondrial reactive oxygen species trigger hypoxia-induced transcription. Proc Natl Acad Sci USA 95: 11715–11720

Chaudhary P, Sharma R, Sharma A, Vatasyayan A, Yadav R, Singhal S, Awasthi SS, Awasthi YC (2010) Mechanisms of 4-hydroxy-2-nonenal induced pro and anti apoptotic signaling. Biochemistry 49:6263–6275

Cheng JZ, Singhal SS, Saini MK, Singhal J, Piper JT, van Kujik FJGM, Zimniak P, Awasthi YC, Awasthi S (1999) Effects of mGST A4 transfection on 4-hydroxynonenal-mediated apoptosis and differentiation of K562 human erythroleukemia cells. Arch Biochem Biophys 372:29–36

Cheng JZ, Sharma R, Yang Y, Singhal SS, Sharma A, Saini MK, Singh SV, Zimniak P, Awasthi S, Awasthi YC (2001) Accelerated metabolism and exclusion of 4-hydroxynonenal through induction of RLIP76 and hGST5.8 is an early adaptive response of cells to heat and oxidative stress. J Biol Chem 276(44):41213–41223

Choi S, Singh SV (2005) Bax and Bak are required for apoptosis induction by sulforaphane, a cruciferous vegetable-derived cancer chemopreventive agent. Cancer Res 65:2035–2043

Choi WY, Choi BT, Lee WH, Choi YH (2008) Sulforaphane generates reactive oxygen species leading to mitochondrial perturbation for apoptosis in human leukemia U937 cells. Biomed Pharmacother 62(9):637–644

Chung FL, Conaway CC, Rao CV, Reddy BS (2000) Chemoprevention of colonic aberrant crypt foci in Fischer rats by sulforaphane and phenethyl isothiocyanate. Carcinogenesis 21:2287–2291

Clarke J, Hsu A, Yu Z, Dashwood R, Ho E (2011) Differential effects of sulforaphane on histone deacetylases, cell cycle arrest and apoptosis in normal prostate cells versus hyperplastic and cancerous prostate cells. Mol Nutr Foods Res 55:999–1009

Conaway CC, Yang YM, Chung FL (2002) Isothiocyanates as cancer chemopreventive agents: their biological activities and metabolism in rodents and humans. Curr Drug Metab 3:233–255

Dianzani UM (2003) 4-Hydroxynonenal from pathology to physiology. Mol Aspects Med 24:263–272

Dinkova-Kostova AT, Holtzclaw WD, Cole RN, Itoh K, Wakabayashi N, Katoh Y, Yamamoto M, Talalay P (2002) Direct evidence that sulfhydryl groups of Keap1 are the sensors regulating induction of phase 2 enzymes that protect against carcinogens and oxidants. Proc Natl Acad Sci USA 99:11908–11913

Dwivedi S, Sharma A, Patrick B, Sharma R, Awasthi YC (2007) Role of HNE and its Metabolites in Signaling. Redox Report 12(1):4–10

Esterbauer H, Zollner H, Schaur RJ (1991) Chemistry and biochemistry of 4-hydroxynonenal, malonaldehyde and related aldehydes. Free Redic Biol Med 11:81–128

Fahey JW, Zhang Y, Talalay P (1997) Broccoli sprouts: an exceptionally rich source of inducers of enzymes that protect against chemical carcinogens. Proc Natl Acad Sci USA 94(19):10367–10372

Fawzy E, Nehad E (2011) Potential health benefits of sulforaphane: a review of the experimental, clinical and epidemiological evidences and underlying mechanisms. J Med Plants Res 5:473–484

Fimognari C, Nusse M, Cesari R, Iori R, Cantelli-Forti G, Hrelia P (2002) Growth inhibition, cell-cycle arrest and apoptosis in human T-cell leukemia by the isothiocyanate sulforaphane. Carcinogenesis 23:581–586

Fowke JH, Chung FL, Jin F, Qi D, Cai Q, Conaway C, Cheng JR, Shu XO, Gao YT, Zheng W (2003) Urinary isothiocyanate levels, brassica, and human breast cancer. Cancer Res 63:3980–3986

Gamet-Payrastre L (2006) Signaling pathways and intracellular targets of sulforaphane mediating cell cycle arrest and apoptosis. Curr Cancer Drug Targets 6:135–145

Gamet-Payrastre L, Lumeau S, Gasc N, Cassar G, Rollin P, Tulliez J (1998) Selective cytostatic and cytotoxic effects of glucosinolates hydrolysis products on human colon cancer cells in vitro. Anticancer Drugs 9: 141–148

Gamet-Payrastre L, Li P, Lumeau S, Cassar G, Dupont MA, Chevolleau S, Gasc N, Tulliez J, Terce F (2000) Sulforaphane, a naturally occurring isothiocyanate, induces cell cycle arrest and apoptosis in HT29 human colon cancer cells. Cancer Res 60:1426–1433

Gan N, Wu Y, Brunet C, Chung F, Dai C, Mi L (2010) Sulforaphane activates heat shock response and enhances proteasome activity through up-regulation of Hsp27. J Biol Chem 285:35528–35536

Herman-Antosiewicz A, Johnson DE, Singh SV (2006) Sulforaphane causes autophagy to inhibit release of cytochrome C and apoptosis in human prostate cancer cells. Cancer Res 66:5828–5835

Ho E, Clarke J, Dashwood R (2009) Dietary sulforaphane, a histone deacetylase inhibitor for cancer prevention. J Nutr 139:2393–2396

Huang LE, Willmore WG, Gu J, Goldberg MA, Bunn HF (1999) Inhibition of hypoxia-inducible factor 1 activation by carbon monoxide and nitric oxide. Implications for oxygen sensing and signaling. J Biol Chem 274:9038–9044

Jackson SJ, Singletary KW, Venema RC (2006) Sulforaphane suppresses angiogenesis and disrupts endothelial mitotic progression and microtubule polymerization. Vascul Pharmacol 46:77–84

Jeong WS, Jun M, Kong AN (2006) Nrf2: a potential molecular target for cancer chemoprevention by natural compounds. Antioxid Redox Signal 8:99–106

Juge N, Mithen RF, Traka M (2007) Molecular basis for chemoprevention by sulforaphane: a comprehensive review. Cell Mol Life Sci 64:1105–1127

Kallifatidis G, Rausch V, Baumann B, Apel A, Beckermann B, Groth A, Mattern J, Li Z, Kolb A, Moldenhauer G, Altevogt P, Wirth T, Werner J, Schemmer P, Büchler M, Salnikov A, Herr I (2009) Sulforaphane targets pancreatic tumour-initiating cells by NF-kappaB-induced antiapoptotic signalling. Gut 58:949–963

Kaminski B, Weigert A, Brüne B, Schumacher M, Wenzel U, Steinhilber D, Stein J, Ulrich S (2011) Sulforaphane potentiates oxaliplatin-induced cell growth inhibition in colorectal cancer cells via induction of different modes of cell death. Cancer Chemother Pharmacol 67:1167–1178

Kong A, Yu R, Hebbar V, Chen C, Owuor E, Hu R, Ee R, Mandlekar S (2001) Signal transduction events elicited by cancer prevention compounds. Mutat Res 480–481:231–241

Maheo K, Morel F, Langouet S, Kramer H, Le Ferrec E, Ketterer B, Guillouzo A (1997) Inhibition of cytochromes P-450 and induction of glutathione S-transferases by sulforaphane in primary human and rat hepatocytes. Cancer Res 57:3649–3652

Meeran S, Patel S, Tollefsbol T (2010) Sulforaphane causes epigenetic repression of hTERT expression in human breast cancer cell lines. PLoS One 5:e11457

Moon D, Kang S, Kim K, Kim M, Choi Y, Kim G (2010) Sulforaphane decreases viability and telomerase activity in hepatocellular carcinoma Hep3B cells through the reactive oxygen species-dependent pathway. Cancer Lett 295:260–266

Myzak MC, Karplus PA, Chung FL, Dashwood RH (2004) A novel mechanism of chemoprotection by sulforaphane: inhibition of histone deacetylase. Cancer Res 64:5767–5774

Myzak MC, Dashwood WM, Orner GA, Ho E, Dashwood RH (2006) Sulforaphane inhibits histone deacetylase in vivo and suppresses tumorigenesis in Apcmin mice. FASEB J 20:506–508

Pham NA, Jacobberger JW, Schimmer AD, Cao P, Gronda M, Hedley DW (2004) The dietary isothiocyanate sulforaphane targets pathways of apoptosis, cell cycle arrest, and oxidative stress in human pancreatic cancer cells and inhibits tumor growth in severe combined immunodeficient mice. Mol Cancer Ther 3: 1239–1248

Pledgie-Tracy A, Sobolewski M, Davidson N (2007) Sulforaphane induces cell type-specific apoptosis in human breast cancer cell lines. Mol Cancer Ther 6:1013–1021

Rose P, Huang Q, Ong CN, Whiteman M (2005) Broccoli and watercress suppress matrix metalloproteinase-9 activity and invasiveness of human MDA-MB-231 breast cancer cells. Toxicol Appl Pharmacol 209: 105–113

Scharf G, Prustomersky S, Knasmuller S, Schulte-Hermann R, Huber WW (2003) Enhancement of glutathione and gamma-glutamylcysteine synthetase, the rate limiting enzyme of glutathione synthesis, by chemoprotective plant derived food and beverage components in the human hepatoma cell line HepG2. Nutr Cancer 45:74–83

Shan Y, Sun C, Zhao X, Wu K, Cassidy A, Bao Y (2006) Effect of sulforaphane on cell growth, G0/G1 phase cell progression and apoptosis in human bladder cancer T24 cells. Int J Oncol 29:883–888

Shan Y, Wu K, Wang W, Wang S, Lin N, Zhao R, Cassidy A, Bao Y (2009) Sulforaphane down-regulates COX-2 expression by activating p38 and inhibiting NF-kappaB-DNA-binding activity in human bladder T24 cells. Int J Oncol 34(4):1129–1134

Sharma R, Brown D, Awasthi S, Yang Y, Sharma A, Patrick B, Saini MK, Singh SP, Zimniak P, Singh SV, Awasthi YC (2004) Transfection with 4-hydroxynonenal-metabolizing glutathione S-transferase isozymes leads to phenotypic transformation and immortalization of adherent cells. Eur J Biochem 271:1690–1701

Sharma A, Sharma R, Chaudhary P, Vatsyayan R, Pearce V, Jeyabal PV, Zimniak P, Awasthi S, Awasthi YC (2008a) 4-Hydroxynonenal induces p53-mediated apoptosis in retinal pigment epithelial cells. Arch Biochem Biophys 480:85–94

Sharma R, Sharma A, Dwivedi S, Zimniak P, Awasthi S, Awasthi YC (2008b) 4-Hydroxynonenal self limits Fas-mediated DISC independent apoptosis by promoting export of Daxx from nucleus to cytosol and its binding to Fas. Biochemistry 47:143–156

Sharma R, Sharma A, Chaudhary P, Vatsyayan R, Pearce V, Singh SV, Awasthi S, Awasthi YC (2010) Role of lipid peroxidation in cellular responses to D, L-sulforaphane, a promising cancer chemopreventive agent. Biochemistry 49:3191–3202

Sharma R, Ellis B, Sharma A (2011) Role of alpha class glutathione transferases in chemoprevention: Human leukemia (HL60) cells overexpression GSTA1and GSTA4 resist sulphorphane and curcumin induced cytotoxicity. Phytother Res 25(4):563–568

Sharma R, Sharma A, Chaudhary P, Sahu M, Jaiswal S, Awasthi S, Awasthi YC (2012) Role of 4-hydroxynonenal in chemopreventive activities of sulforaphane. Free Radic Biol Med 52(11–12):2177–2185

Shen G, Xu C, Chen C, Hebbar V, Kong AN (2006) p53-independent G1 cell cycle arrest of human colon carcinoma cells HT-29 by sulforaphane is associated with induction of p21CIP1 and inhibition of expression of cyclin D1. Cancer Chemother Pharmacol 57: 317–327

Sherr CJ (1996) Cancer cell cycles. Science 274: 1672–1677

Sherr CJ, Roberts JM (1999) CDK inhibitors: positive and negative regulators of G1-phase progression. Genes Dev 13:1501–1512

Simon HU, Haj-Yehia A, Levi-Schaffer F (2000) Role of reactive oxygen species (ROS) in apoptosis induction. Apoptosis 5:415–418

Singh AV, Xiao D, Lew KL, Dhir R, Singh SV (2004a) Sulforaphane induces caspase-mediated apoptosis in cultured PC-3 human prostate cancer cells and retards growth of PC-3 xenografts in vivo. Carcinogenesis 25:83–90

Singh SV, Herman-Antosiewicz A, Singh AV, Lew KL, Srivastava SK, Kamath R, Brown KD, Zhang L, Baskaran R (2004b) Sulforaphane-induced G2/M phase cell cycle arrest involves checkpoint kinase 2-mediated phosphorylation of cell division cycle 25C. J Biol Chem 279:25813–25822

Singh SV, Srivastava SK, Choi S, Lew KL, Antosiewicz J, Xiao D, Zeng Y, Watkins SC, Johnson CS, Trump DL, Lee YJ, Xiao H, Herman- Antosiewicz A (2005) Sulforaphane-induced cell death in human prostate cancer cells is initiated by reactive oxygen species. J Biol Chem 280:19911–19924

Singhal SS, Awasthi YC, Awasthi S (2006) Regression of melanoma in a murine model by RLIP76 depletion. Cancer Res 66(4):2354–2360

Singhal SS, Singhal J, Yadav S, Dwivedi S, Boor PJ, Awasthi YC, Awasthi S (2007) Regression of lung and colon cancer xenografts by depleting or inhibiting RLIP76 (Ral-binding protein 1). Cancer Res 67(9):4382–4389

Singhal SS, Singhal J, Yadav S, Sahu M, Awasthi YC, Awasthi S (2009) RLIP76: a target for kidney cancer therapy. Cancer Res 69(10):4244–4251

Skupinska K, Misiewicz-Krzeminska I, Stypulkowski R, Lubelska K, Kasprzycka-Guttman T (2009) Sulforaphane and its analogues inhibit CYP1A1 and CYP1A2 activity induced by benzo[a]pyrene. J Biochem Mol Toxicol 23:18–28

Talalay P (2000) Chemoprotection against cancer by induction of phase 2 enzymes. Biofactors 12:5–11

Tang L, Zhang Y (2004) Dietary isothiocyanates inhibit the growth of human bladder carcinoma cells. J Nutr 134:2004–2010

Thejass P, Kuttan G (2006) Antimetastatic activity of sulforaphane. Life Sci 78:3043–3050

Thimmulappa RK, Mai KH, Srisuma S, Kensler TW, Yamamoto M, Biswal S (2002) Identification of Nrf2-regulated genes induced by the chemopreventive agent sulforaphane by oligonucleotide microarray. Cancer Res 62:5196–5203

Vatsyayan R, Chaudhary P, Sharma A, Sharma R, Rao Lelsani PC, Awasthi S, Awasthi YC (2011) Role of 4-hydroxynonenal in epidermal growth factor receptor-mediated signaling in retinal pigment epithelial cells. Exp Eye Res 92(2):147–154

Wagner A, Ernst I, Iori R, Desel C, Rimbach G (2010) Sulforaphane but not ascorbigen, indole-3-carbinole and ascorbic acid activates the transcription factor Nrf2 and induces phase-2 and antioxidant enzymes in human keratinocytes in culture. Exp Dermatol 19: 137–144

Wang LI, Giovannucci EL, Hunter D, Neuberg D, Su L, Christiani DC (2004) Dietary intake of cruciferous vegetables, glutathione S-transferase (GST) polymorphisms and lung cancer risk in a Caucasian population. Cancer Causes Control 15:977–985

Xu K, Thornalley PJ (2000) Studies on the mechanism of the inhibition of human leukaemia cell growth by dietary isothiocyanates and their cysteine adducts in vitro. Biochem Pharmacol 60: 221–231

Yang Y, Cheng JZ, Singhal SS, Saini M, Pandya U, Awasthi S, Awasthi YC (2001) Role of glutathione S-transferases in protection against lipid peroxidation. Overexpression of hGSTA2-2 in K562 cells protects against hydrogen peroxide-induced apoptosis and inhibits JNK and caspase 3 activation. J Biol Chem 276(22):19220–19230

Yang Y, Sharma R, Zimniak P, Awasthi YC (2002) Role of alpha class glutathione S-transferases as antioxidant enzymes in rodent tissues. Toxicol Appl Pharmacol 182:105–115

Yang Y, Sharma A, Sharma R, Patrick B, Singhal SS, Zimniak P, Awasthi S, Awasthi YC (2003) Cells preconditioned with mild, transient UVA irradiation acquire resistance to oxidative stress and UVA-induced apoptosis: role of 4-hydroxynonenal in UVA-mediated signaling for apoptosis. J Biol Chem 278(42):41380–41388

Yao H, Wang H, Zhang Z, Jiang BH, Luo J, Shi X (2008) Sulforaphane inhibited expression of hypoxia-inducible factor-1alpha in human tongue squamous cancer cells and prostate cancer cells. Int J Cancer 15:123(6):1255–1261

Yoxall V, Kentish P, Coldham N, Kuhnert N, Sauer MJ, Ioannides C (2005) Modulation of hepatic cytochromes P450 and phase II enzymes by dietary doses of sulforaphane in rats: implications for its chemopreventive activity. Int J Cancer 117:356–362

Zhang Y (2000) Role of glutathione in the accumulation of anticarcinogenic isothiocyanates and their glutathione conjugates by murine hepatoma cells. Carcinogenesis 21:1175–1182

Zhang H, Forman HJ (2009) Signaling pathways involved in Phase II gene induction by alpha beta unsaturated aldehydes. Toxicol Ind Health 4–5:269–278

Zhang Y, Marshall JR, Ambrosone CB (2004) Cruciferous vegetables, genetic polymorphisms in glutathione S-transferases M1 and T1, and prostate cancer risk. Nutr Cancer 50:206–213

Zhang Y, Munday R, Jobson HE, Munday CM, Lister C, Wilson P, Fahey JW, Mhawech-Fauceglia P (2006) Induction of GST and NQO1 in cultured bladder cells and in the urinary bladders of rats by an extract of broccoli (Brassica oleracea italica) sprouts. J Agric Food Chem 54:9370–9376

Reciprocal Relationship Between VE-Cadherin and Matrix Metalloproteinases Expression in Endothelial Cells and Its Implications to Angiogenesis

9

A.P. Athira, M.S. Kiran, and P.R. Sudhakaran

Abstract

Angiogenesis, the process of new blood vessel formation from preexisting ones, is critical in the development and progression of tumor. Since metastasis is favored by increased neovascularization, understanding the molecular mechanism governing angiogenesis gains utmost importance. Endothelial cells respond to numerous angiogenic factors like VEGF and switch over to angiogenic phenotype. Apart from VEGF, another key molecule involved is matrix metalloproteinases which are the enzymes involved in pericellular proteolysis, a process critically important in initiating angiogenesis. But during the later stages, when cell–cell contact formation occurs, MMP expression is downregulated. Regulation of MMPs by cell–cell contact formation was found. This article focuses on a reciprocal relationship between the expression of cell adhesion molecules that modulates cell–cell contact formation and MMP expression.

Keywords

Matrix metalloproteinases • VE-cadherin • β-Catenin • Angiogenesis • Pericellular proteolysis • Cell adhesion molecules

9.1 Introduction

Angiogenesis, the formation of new blood vessels from preexisting ones, is one of the most pervasive and fundamentally essential biological processes required for the maintenance of

A.P. Athira
Department of Biochemistry, University of Kerala, Kariavattom, Thiruvananthapuram 695 581, Kerala, India

M.S. Kiran
Department of Biochemistry, University of Kerala, Kariavattom, Thiruvananthapuram 695 581, Kerala, India

Biomaterials Division, Central Leather Research Institute, Adyar, Chennai 600 020, Tamil Nadu, India

P.R. Sudhakaran (✉)
Computational Biology & Bioinformatics, University of Kerala, Kariavattom, Thiruvananthapuram 695 581, Kerala, India
e-mail: prslab@gmail.com

P.R. Sudhakaran (ed.), *Perspectives in Cancer Prevention – Translational Cancer Research*, DOI 10.1007/978-81-322-1533-2_9, © Springer India 2014

functional and structural integrity of organism. Endothelial cells are the key players in angiogenesis. All tissues develop a vascular network that provides cells with nutrients and oxygen. The vascular network, once formed, is a stable system that regenerates slowly. Normal angiogenesis is an essential process during wound healing, fetal development, ovulation, as well as growth and development. When angiogenesis is deranged, pathological problems often follow. Angiogenesis-dependent diseases result when new blood vessels either grow excessively or insufficiently. Insufficient angiogenesis occurs in diseases such as coronary artery disease, stroke, and chronic wounds. In these conditions, blood vessel growth is less due to inadequate production of angiogenic growth factors; hence circulation is not properly restored, leading to the risk of tissue death. Excessive angiogenesis occurs when abnormal amounts of angiogenic growth factors are produced by the diseased cells which overwhelm the effects of natural angiogenesis inhibitors. Excessive angiogenesis occurs in diseases such as cancer (Charlesworth and Harres 2006), inflammation (Chade et al. 2004), atherosclerosis (Hermann et al. 2006; Lip and Blann 2004), diabetic blindness, age-related macular degeneration, rheumatoid arthritis, and psoriasis (Folkman 1997).

Angiogenesis plays a critical role in the development of cancer. Vascularization is not observed in solid tumors which are smaller than 1–2 mm^3. To metastasize, they need to be supplied by blood vessels that bring oxygen and nutrients and remove metabolic wastes. Beyond the critical volume of 2 mm^3, oxygen and nutrients have difficulty in diffusing to the cells in the center of the tumor, causing a state of cellular hypoxia, which is an important factor stimulating the production of proangiogenic molecules (Shweiki et al. 1992). It is the shifting of balance from the anti- to the proangiogenic factors, which causes the transition from the dormant to the angiogenic phase (Hanahan and Folkman 1996). New blood vessel development is an important process in tumor progression, which favors its transition from hyperplasia to neoplasia, i.e., the passage from a state of cellular multiplication to a state of uncontrolled proliferation. Neovascularization also influences the spreading of cancer cells throughout the entire body eventually leading to metastasis formation. The vascularization level of a solid tumor is an indicator of its metastatic potential.

For angiogenesis to proceed, first the diseased or injured tissues must produce and release angiogenic growth factors that diffuse into the nearby tissues. The angiogenic growth factors bind to specific receptors located on the endothelial cells of nearby preexisting blood vessels. Once they bind to their receptors, the endothelial cells become activated. Signals sent from the cell's surface to the nucleus trigger the production of new molecules including enzymes like MMPs, which degrade the basement membrane surrounding existing blood vessels that helps the endothelial cells to proliferate and migrate toward the diseased tissue (Folkman 1997; Risau 1997).

9.2 Role of Proteases in Angiogenesis

Three major groups of endoproteases participate in the processes that regulate angiogenesis, including the remodeling of the extracellular matrix, cell migration and invasion, and the liberation and modification of growth factors. They comprise the metalloproteinases, in particular the matrix metalloproteinases, the cathepsin cysteine proteases, and the serine proteases. The activities of these proteases are controlled by specific activation mechanisms and specific inhibitors, particularly tissue inhibitor of matrix metalloproteinases, cystatins, and inhibitors of serine proteases called serpins (Victor et al. 2006).

Of these endopeptidases, matrix metalloproteinases play a major role in angiogenesis. MMPs are a diverse family of enzymes capable of degrading various components of the extra cellular matrix. They require zinc for catalytic activity and are synthesized as inactive zymogens which have to be proteolytically cleaved to be active. Normally, MMPs are expressed only when and where needed for tissue remodeling. However, aberrant expression of various MMPs has been correlated with pathological conditions, such as tumor cell invasion and metastasis, periodontitis, and rheumatoid arthritis (Woessner 1991). Matrix metalloproteinase can be classified into two groups: as soluble MMPs and membrane-type MMPs. The soluble MMPs consist of collagenases (MMP 1, MMP 8, and MMP 13), gelatinases (MMP 2 and MMP 9), stromelysins (MMP 3, MMP 10 and MMP 11), matrilysins (MMP 7 and MMP 25), and MMP 12 and MMP 26 (Visse and Nagase 2003). The membrane-type MMPs encompass 6 members, MT1-MMP to MT6-MMP, that are activated intracellularly by furin-like enzymes. The MT-MMP family members were first identified as activators of soluble MMPs and subsequently also shown to be able to degrade extracellular matrix components such as fibrillar collagen, laminin-1 and laminin-5, aggrecan and fibronectin, and the plasma-derived matrix proteins vitronectin and fibrin (Visse and Nagase 2003; Seiki et al. 2003). The MMPs are inhibited by their endogenous inhibitors, the TIMPs (TIMP 1, 2, 3, 4), each capable of inhibiting virtually all members of the MMP family (Herriet et al. 1999). The equilibrium between TIMPs and MMPs is important in localized proteolysis.

MMPs not only degrade basement membrane and other ECM components allowing endothelial cells to detach and migrate into the tissues but also release ECM-bound proangiogenic factors like bFGF, VEGF, and TGF β. They also trigger integrin intracellular signaling by degrading ECM components, thereby generating fragments with integrin binding site. However, MMP 2 also generates endogenous angiogenic inhibitors from larger precursors. Cleavage of plasminogen by MMPs releases angiostatin; endostatin is the COOH terminal fragment of the basement membrane collagen XVIII, which can be generated by cleavage by cathepsins and MMPs; and generation of the hemopexin domain of MMP-2 from MMP-2 may be through autocatalysis. Thus, the MMPs have both pro- and antiangiogenic functions. On the whole, however, MMPs are required for angiogenesis, and inhibitors of MMPs have been shown to inhibit angiogenesis in animal models (Naglich et al. 2001).

Reports suggest that cultures of endothelial cells, which are used as model cell systems to study angiogenesis, expressed MMP 1, 2, 3, 9, and 14 and TIMP 1, 2 (Moses 1997). The requirement of MMPs produced by endothelial cells for angiogenesis is evidenced by the studies where naturally occurring (Moses et al. 1990; Fisher et al. 1994; Schnaper et al. 1993; Anand-Apte et al. 1997) or synthetic inhibitors (Montesano and Orci 1985; Hass et al. 1998; Maekawa et al. 1999) of MMPs caused inhibition of angiogenesis or various events thereof. Additional evidence for the requirement of MMPs during angiogenesis comes from genetic studies in mice. With regard to the MMP knockout mice deficient in MMP-2, tumor-induced angiogenesis was markedly reduced in dorsal sac assay with B16-BL6 melanoma cells, and in MMP-9-deficient mice, there was reduced bone growth plate angiogenesis (Itoh et al. 1998; Vu et al. 1998).

Recent reports suggest a temporal relationship between MMP production and angiogenic process in HUVEC in culture. When endothelial cells establish cell–cell contact formation resembling angiogenic process, downregulation in the production of MMP-2 and MMP-9 occurs, which suggests that MMPs are produced during initial stages of angiogenesis before cell–cell contacts are established (Kiran et al. 2006). Agents that promote angiogenesis such as curcumin (in serum free conditions) induces capillary network-like structure formation and cell–cell contact formation at a faster rate (within 48 h for curcumin) compared to control cells. We observed an inverse relation between cell–cell contact formation and MMP expression. There are increasing number of reports demonstrating that, apart from requirement of MMPs in proteolysis of extracellular matrix, endothelial cell requires MMPs for cell movement, proliferation, migration, and attachment to one another as well as to the ECM (Gingras et al. 2001; Qian et al. 1997; Yu and Stamenkovic 1999). Further, MMPs have been reported to alter with change in endothelial cell shape where maximum activity was reported when the cells were spherical in shape (Yan et al. 2000).

9.3 Cell Adhesion Molecules and Angiogenesis

Apart from MMPs, cell adhesion molecules are also important regulators of angiogenesis. They give endothelium the ability to control the passage of solute and circulating cells by forming intercellular junction between endothelial cells (Simionescu and Simionescu 1991). They also provide endothelial surface polarity and regulate initiation and maturation of newly formed vessels during angiogenesis (Muller and Gimbrone 1986). During the initiation phase of angiogenesis, the continuity of endothelial layers is interrupted due to loosening of cell–cell contacts enabling the endothelial cells to proliferate and migrate to free area (Schwartz et al. 1978; Sholley et al. 1977). But during the maturation phase, the endothelial cells establish the intercellular contacts in order to maintain the morphological integrity and quiescence of newly formed vessel (Yang et al. 1999; Lampugnani et al. 1992). Hence, the molecular mechanism that governs the formation and stabilization of cell–cell contacts and pericellular proteolysis must be suitably coordinated and regulated.

Cell adhesion molecules can be classified into four families depending on their biochemical and structural characteristics. These include the cadherins, selectins, immunoglobulin supergene family, and the integrins. Members of each family are implicated in neovascularization. Endothelial cells express several distinct types of integrins, allowing attachment to a wide variety of ECM proteins (Eliceiri and Cheresh 1999). It is reported that $\alpha v\beta 3$ binds to MMP 2, thereby localizing MMP-2-mediated matrix degradation to the endothelial cell surface (Brooks et al. 1996). It is nearly undetectable on quiescent endothelium but is highly upregulated during cytokine or tumor-induced angiogenesis. Besides integrins, members of immunoglobulin superfamily also mediate heterophilic cell–cell adhesion. ICAM-1 and VCAM-1 are expressed on quiescent endothelium but are upregulated after stimulation with TNF-α, IL-1, or interferon-α (Brooks et al. 1996). VCAM-1 can induce chemotaxis in endothelial cells in vitro and angiogenesis in vivo. Members of the selectin family, in particular P-selectin and E-selectin, promote adhesion of leukocytes to cytokine-activated vascular endothelium, which plays a major role in angiogenesis (Koch et al. 1995). E-selectin induces endothelial migration and tube formation in vitro and angiogenesis in vivo (Nguyen et al. 1993).

Recent reports indicate that the components of the intercellular adherence junctions also function in intracellular signaling during angiogenesis (Bazzoni and Dejana 2004). Cadherin is the major endothelial specific cell adhesion molecule that plays important role in vascular morphogenesis and growth control (Lampugnani and Dejana 1997). They establish direct molecular connections with cytoplasmic partners that bind to different and specific domains of their cytoplasmic region. Classical cytoplasmic partners of cadherins are the catenins, namely, α, β, and p120 catenin (Anastasiadis and Reynolds 2000), which, besides promoting anchorage to actin cytoskeleton, when released into the cytoplasm, may translocate to the nucleus and influence gene transcription (Ben-Ze'ev and Geiger 1998). Moreover, cadherins associate to growth factor receptors (Carmeliet et al. 1999; Pece and Gutkind 2000) and some components of their signaling cascade such as Shc (Xu et al. 1997) phosphatidylinositol 3-kinase (Carmeliet et al. 1999; Pece et al. 1999) and various protein phosphatases (Zondag et al. 2000). These types of interactions may play a role in controlling growth factor signaling. VE-cadherin is exclusively expressed in the endothelium and regulates fundamental activities of this tissue (Dejana et al. 1999). Inactivation of VE-cadherin expression by gene targeting results in early embryonic lethality due to impairment of vascular organization and remodeling (Carmeliet et al. 1999). Antibodies blocking VE-cadherin adhesion and clustering strongly affect formation of new vascular structures in adult animals (Liao et al. 2000) and increase permeability of constitutive vessels (Corada et al. 1999).

We examined the molecular mechanisms involved in cell–cell contact-dependent regulation of MMPs in endothelial cells undergoing angiogenic process using HUVECs in culture and the results showed a reciprocal change in the expression of MMPs (MMP 2 and MMP 9) and VE-cadherin as the cells undergo angiogenic transition. A significant decrease in the production and secretion of MMP 2 and MMP 9 was seen with the progression of culture, when grouping of cells and tubular network-like structure developed. Development of extensive tubular network-like structure involves cell–cell contact formation, which correlated with the expression of endothelial cell markers like CD 31, ICAM 1, and E-selectin, which mediates cell adhesion, and VEGF and FGF, which are the biochemical markers of angiogenesis. Thus, a reciprocal relationship between the expression of markers of angiogenesis, cell adhesion molecules, and MMPs was evident. Further proof for the relationship between MMP 2, MMP 9, and angiogenesis came from the results of the experiments where endothelial cells were treated with curcumin and ursolic acid. Angiogenic effect of ursolic acid was shown by upregulation of the expression of angiogenic markers ICAM-1 and angiogenic factors like VEGF and fibroblast growth factor-2 by endothelial cells (Kiran et al. 2008a). Opposing effects of curcumin on angiogenesis was shown using different model systems and the proangiogenic effect was mediated through VEGF and PI3K-Akt pathway (Kiran et al. 2008b). Treatment of endothelial cells with substances which promote angiogenesis caused downregulation of MMP 2 and MMP 9. But such downregulation was not produced by aspirin which inhibited angiogenesis and reduced the production of cell adhesion molecules that promote cell–cell contact formation (Kiran et al. 2006).

During the initial stages when cells remained mostly as individual ones, there was more MMP-2 and MMP-9 and less VE-cadherin, and at later stages, when grouping of cells and network-like structures developed, increase in VE-cadherin and decrease in MMP-2 and MMP-9 production were observed. In serum-free conditions, curcumin accelerated angiogenic phenotype, which caused a significant upregulation of VE-cadherin and downregulation of MMPs. Further investigations on the signaling pathway downstream to VE-cadherin suggested the involvement of β catenin. During the initial stages of the culture, β-catenin was less in the cytosol, but there was a rapid translocation of β-catenin to the cytosol during the later stages, when cell–cell contacts were established. The activity of β-catenin is regulated by its phosphorylation status. We observed an increased tyrosine phosphorylation, when catenin remained in the nucleus during the initial stages, and relative increase in serine phosphorylation during the later stages of the culture, when cell–cell contact formation occurred and β-catenin was translocated to the cytosol. A correlation between nuclear localization of β-catenin and MMPs was observed, i.e., when β-catenin remained in the nucleus, there was an upregulation in the production of MMPs, and when β-catenin was translocated to cytosol, MMP expression was downregulated. Agents which cause inhibition of angiogenesis (curcumin in presence of FCS) affect the downregulation of MMPs as well as the phosphorylation of beta catenin. Such downregulation of MMP was not seen in cells treated with lithium chloride and SB 216763, which caused increased nuclear localization of β-catenin. The downregulation of MMP 2 and MMP 9 caused by curcumin was also reversed by lithium (Kiran et al. 2011). Lithium and SB 216763 inhibits GSK 3β, which is involved in the serine phosphorylation of β-catenin. Since serine phosphorylation was inhibited, catenin remained in the nucleus which correlated with the upregulation of MMPs and decreased cell–cell contact formation. MMP genes are under the influence of the transcriptional activity of β-catenin as β-catenin responsive elements are reported to be present in the MMP genes (Munshi and Stack 2006; Overall and Lopez-Otin 2002). We observed the downregulation of MMPs when the level of VE-cadherin increased and β-catenin remained in the nucleus. This suggests the possibility that VE-cadherin modulates MMP expression through β-catenin-dependent mechanism.

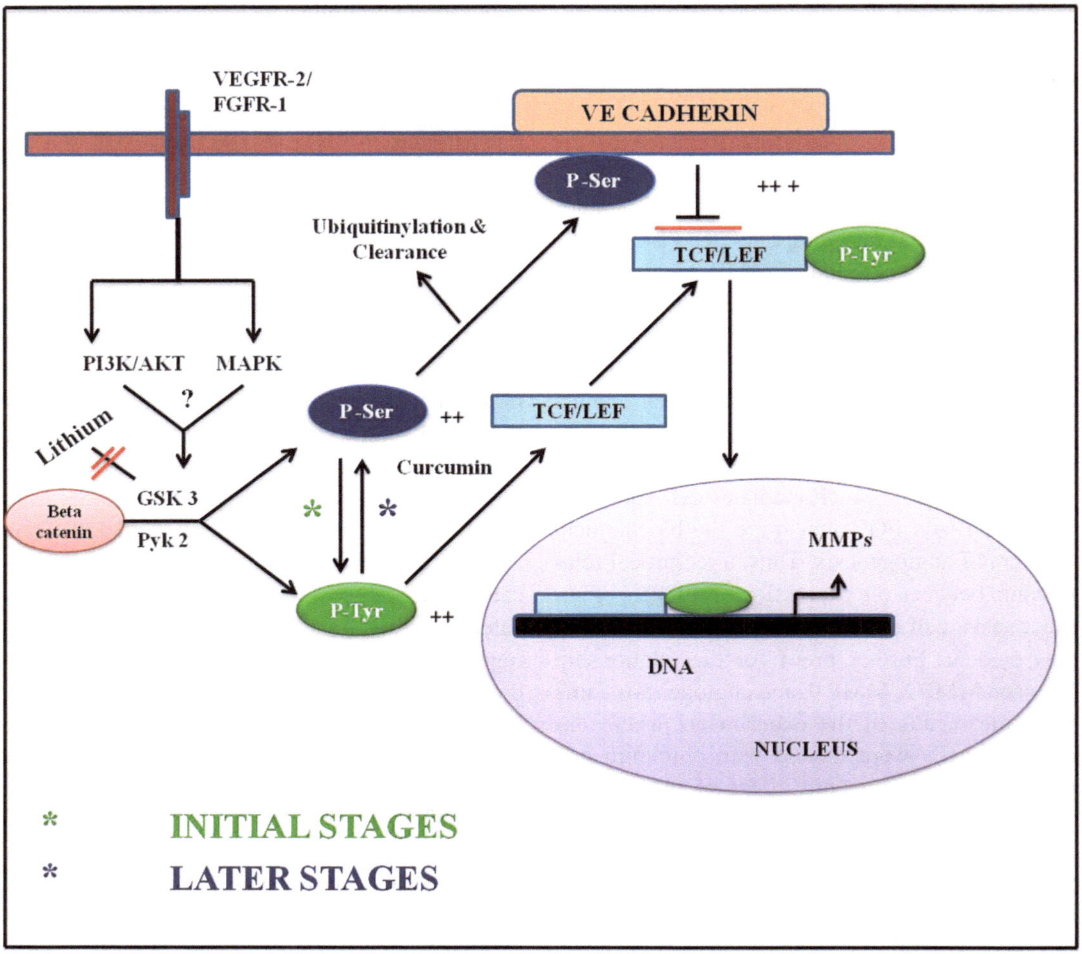

Fig. 9.1 *Scheme showing VE-cadherin–β-catenin signaling in the regulation of MMPs*. The transcriptional activity of β-catenin is regulated by its phosphorylation status. Serine phosphorylation increases its affinity to VE-cadherin and prevents its nuclear translocation. In the absence of VE-cadherin Ser-phosphorylated β-catenin is cleared from the cytosol by ubiquitinylation. Tyrosine phosphorylation reduces its affinity to VE-cadherin, and it binds with Tcf/Lef protein and translocates into the nucleus and regulates gene expression. Higher levels of VE-cadherin inhibit the translocation of Tyr-phosphorylated β-catenin. The role of PI3K-AKT and MAPK pathways (as was observed to be involved in mediating the angiogenesis) in regulating the activities of GSK-3 and Pyk2 is unknown. We observed higher levels Tyr-phosphorylated β-catenin during the initial 48 h when the level of VE-cadherin was significantly low and concomitantly MMP levels were high. During the later stages, high levels of Ser-phosphorylated β-catenin was observed when the levels of VE-cadherin increased and a significantly low level of MMPs

9.4 Conclusion

Our results suggested a reciprocal relationship between VE-cadherin and MMP production. The production and secretion of MMP-2 and MMP-9 was high in the initial stages of HUVECs in culture, when they remained as individual cells, which was associated with the decreased expression of VE-cadherin and increased nuclear localization of β-catenin. But during the later stages, when cell–cell contact formation was established, there was a downregulation in the production of MMPs, which was associated with increased expression of VE-cadherin and decreased nuclear localization of β-catenin. These results suggest that VE-cadherin may mediate the expression of MMP production through a β-catenin-dependent mechanism (Fig. 9.1).

Acknowledgments Financial assistance received from CSIR, New Delhi (MSK), and (KSCSTE), Trivandrum (AAP) is gratefully acknowledged.

References

Anand-Apte B, Pepper M, Voest E, Iwata K, Montesano R, Olsen BR (1997) Inhibition of angiogenesis by tissue inhibitors of matrix metalloproteinases-3. Invest Ophthalmol Vis Sci 38:817–823

Anastasiadis PZ, Reynolds AB (2000) The p120 catenin family: complex roles in adhesion, signaling and cancer. J Cell Sci 113:1319–1334

Bazzoni G, Dejana E (2004) Endothelial cell to cell junctions: molecular organization and role in vascular homeostasis. Physiol Rev 84:869–901

Ben-Ze'ev A, Geiger B (1998) Differential molecular interactions of beta-catenin and plakoglobin in adhesion, signaling and cancer. Curr Opin Cell Biol 10:629–639

Brooks PC, Stromblad S, Sanders LC, von Schalscha TL, Aimes RT, Stetler-Stevenson WG, Quigley JP, Cheresh DA (1996) Localization of matrix metalloproteinase MMP-2 to the surface of invasive cells by interaction with integrin αvβ3. Cell 85:683–693

Carmeliet P, Lampugnani MG, Moons L, Breviario F, Lupu F, Herbert JM, Collen D (1999) Dejana E Targeted deficiency or cytosolic truncation of the VE-cadherin gene in mice impairs VEGF-mediated endothelial survival and angiogenesis. Cell 98: 147–157

Chade AR, Bentley HD, Zhu X, Rodriguez-Porcel M, Niemeyer S, Amores-Arriaga B, Napolic C, Ritman EL, Lerman A, Lerman LO (2004) Antioxidant intervention prevents renal neovascularization in hypercholesterolemic pigs. J Am Soc Nephrol 15:1816–1825

Charlesworth PJ, Harres AL (2006) Mechanisms of disease: angiogenesis in urologic malignancies. Nat Clin Pract Urol 3:157–169

Corada M, Mariotti M, Thurston G, Smith K, Kunkel R, Brockhaus M, Lampugnani MG, Martin-Padura I, Stoppacciaro A, Ruco L, McDonald DM, Ward PA, Dejana E (1999) Vascular endothelial-cadherin is an important determinant of microvascular integrity *in vivo*. Proc Natl Acad Sci USA 96:9815–9820

Dejana E, Bazzoni G, Lampugnani MG (1999) Vascular endothelial (VE)-cadherin: only an intercellular glue? Exp Cell Res 252:13–19

Eliceiri BP, Cheresh DA (1999) The role of alphaV integrins during angiogenesis: insights into potential mechanisms of action and clinical development. J Clin Invest 103:1227–1230

Fisher C, Gilbertsonbeadling S, Powers EA, Petzold G, Poorman R, Mitchell MA (1994) Interstitial collagenase is required for angiogenesis *in vitro*. Dev Biol 162:499–510

Folkman J (1997) Angiogenesis in cancer, vascular, rheumatoid and other disease. Nat Med 1:27–31

Gingras D, Bousquet-Gagnon N, Langois S, Lachambre MP, Annabi B, Beliveau R (2001) Activation of the extracellular signal regulated protein kinase (ERK) cascade by membrane type-1matrix metalloproteinase (MT1-MMP). FEBS Lett 507:231–236

Hanahan D, Folkman J (1996) Patterns and emerging mechanisms of the angiogenic switch during tumorigenesis. Cell 86:353–364

Hass TL, Davis SJ, Madri JA (1998) Three-dimensional type I collagen lattices induce co ordinate expression of matrix metalloproteinases MT1 MMP and MMP-2 in microvascular endothelial cells. J Biol Chem 273:3604–3610

Henriet P, Blavier L, Declerck YA (1999) Tissue inhibitors of matrix metalloproteinases in invasion and proliferation. APMIS 107:111–119

Hermann J, Lerman LO, Mukhopadhyay D, Napoli C, Lerman A (2006) Angiogenesis in atherogenesis. Thromb Vasc Biol 26:1948–1957

Itoh T, Tanioka M, Yoshida H, Yoshioka T, Nishimoto H, Itohara S (1998) Reduced angiogenesis and tumor progression in gelatinase A deficient mice. Cancer Res 58:1048–1051

Kiran MS, Sameer Kumar VB, Viji RI, Sudhakaran PR (2006) Temporal relationship between MMP production and angiogenic process in HUVECs. Cell Biol Inter 30:704–713

Kiran MS, Viji RI, Kumar VB, Sudhakaran PR (2008a) Modulation of angiogenic factors by ursolic acid. Biochem Biophys Res Commun 371:556–560

Kiran MS, Kumar VB, Viji RI, Sherin GT, Rajasekharan KN, Sudhakaran PR (2008b) Opposing effects of curcuminoids on serum stimulated and unstimulated angiogenic response. J Cell Physiol 215:251–264

Kiran MS, Viji RI, Kumar VB, Athira AP, Sudhakaran PR (2011) Changes in expression of VE-cadherin and MMPs in endothelial cells: Implications for angiogenesis. Vascular Cell 3:6

Koch AE, Halloran MM, Haskell CJ (1995) Angiogenesis mediated by soluble form of E selectin and vascular cell adhesion molecule 1. Nature 376:517–519

Lampugnani MG, Dejana E (1997) Interendothelial junctions: structure, signaling and functional roles. Curr Opin Cell Biol 9:674–682

Lampugnani MG, Resnati M, Raiteri M, Pigott R, Pisacane A, Houen G, Ruco LP, Dejana E (1992) A novel endothelial-specific membrane protein is a marker of cell-cell contacts. J Cell Biol 118:1511–1522

Liao F, Li Y, O'Connor W, Zanetta L, Bassi R, Santiago A, Overholser J, Hooper A, Mignatti P, Dejana E, Hicklin DJ, Bohlen P (2000) Monoclonal antibody to vascular endothelial (VE)-cadherin is a potent inhibitor of angiogenesis, tumor growth, and metastasis. Cancer Res 60:6805–6810

Lip GY, Blann AD (2004) Thrombogenesis, atherosclerosis, angiogenesis in vascular disease: a new "Vascular triad". Ann Med 36:119–125

Maekawa R, Maki H, Yoshida H, Hojo K, Tanaka H, Wada T (1999) Correlation of anti angiogenic and anti tumor efficacy of N-biphenylsulfonyl phenylalanine hydroxamic acid (BPHA), an orally active, selective matrix metalloproteinase inhibitor. Cancer Res 59:1231–1235

Montesano R, Orci L (1985) Tumor promoting phorbol esters induced angiogenesis *in vitro*. Cell 42: 469–477

Moses MA (1997) The regulation of neovascularization by matrix metalloproteinases and their inhibitors. Stem Cells 15:180–189

Moses MA, Sudhalter J, Langer R (1990) Identification of inhibitor of neovascularization from cartilage. Science 248:1408–1410

Muller WA, Gimbrone MA (1986) Plasmalemmal proteins of cultured vascular endothelial cells exhibit apical-basal polarity: analysis by surface-selective iodination. J Cell Biol 103:2389–2402

Munshi HG, Stack MS (2006) Reciprocal interactions between adhesion receptor signaling and MMP regulation. Cancer Metastasis Rev 25: 45–56

Naglich JG, Jure-Kunkel M, Gupta E, Fargnoli J, Henderson AJ, Lewin AC, Talbott R, Baxter A, Bird J, Savopoulos R, Wills R, Kramer RA, Trail PA (2001) Inhibition of angiogenesis and metastasis in two murine models by the matrix metalloproteinase inhibitor. Cancer Res 61:8480–8485

Nguyen M, Strubel NA, Bischoff J (1993) A role of sialyl Lewis X/A glycoconjugates in capillary morphogenesis. Nature 365:267–269

Overall CM, Lopez-Otin C (2002) Strategies for MMP inhibition in cancer: innovations for the post-trial era. Nat Rev Cancer 2:657–672

Pece S, Chiariello M, Murga C, Gutkind J (1999) Activation of the protein kinase Akt/PKB by the formation of E-cadherin-mediated cell-cell junctions. Evidence for the association of phosphatidylinositol 3-kinase with the E-cadherin adhesion complex. J Biol Chem 274:19347–19351

Pece S, Gutkind JS (2000) Signaling from E-cadherin to MAPK pathway by the recruitment and activation of epidermal growth factor receptors upon cell-cell contact formation. J Biol Chem 275:41227–41233

Qian X, Wang TN, Rothman VL, Nicosia RF, Tuszynski GP (1997) Thrombospondin-1 modulates angiogenesis in vitro by up regulation of matrix metalloproteinase-9 in endothelial cells. Exp Cell Res 235:403–412

Risau W (1997) Mechanisms of angiogenesis. Nature 386:671–674

Schnaper HW, Grant DS, Stetler Stevenson WG, Fridman R, D'Orazi G, Murphy AN (1993) Type IV collagenase(s) and TIMPs modulate endothelial cell morphogenesis in vitro. J Cell Physiol 156:235–246

Schwartz SM, Haudenschild CC, Eddy EM (1978) Endothelial regeneration. Quantitative analysis of initial stages of endothelial regeneration in rat aortic intima. Lab Invest 38:568–580

Seiki M, Naohiko Koshikawa, Ikuo Yana (2003) Role of pericellular proteolysis by membrane-type 1 matrix metalloproteinase in cancer invasion and angiogenesis. Cancer Metastasis Rev 22:129–143

Sholley MM, Gimbrone MA, Cotran RS (1977) Cellular migration and replication in endothelial regeneration: a study using irradiated endothelial cultures. Lab Invest 36:18–25

Shweiki D, Itin A, Soffer D, Keshet E (1992) Vascular endothelial growth factor induced by hypoxia may mediate hypoxia-initiated angiogenesis. Nature 359:843–845

Simionescu M, Simionescu N (1991) Endothelial transport of macromolecules: transcytosis and endocytosis. A look from cell biology. Cell Biol Rev 25:1–78

Victor WM, van Hinsbergh MA, Engelse PHA (2006) Pericellular proteases in angiogenesis and vasculogenesis. Arter Thromb Vasc Biol 26:716–720

Visse R, Nagase H (2003) Matrix metalloproteinases and tissue inhibitors of metalloproteinases: structure, function, and biochemistry. Circ Res 92(8):827–839

Vu TH, Shipley JM, Bergers G, Berger JE, Helms JA, Hanahan D et al (1998) MMP-9/gelatinase B is a key regulator of growth plate angiogenesis and apoptosis of hypertrophic chondrocytes. Cell 93: 411–422

Woessner JF (1991) Matrix metalloproteinases and their inhibitors in connective tissue remodeling. FASEB J 5:2145–2154

Xu Y, Guo DF, Davidson M, Inagami T, Carpenter G (1997) Interaction of the adaptor protein Shc and the adhesion molecule cadherin. J Biol Chem 272:13463–13466

Yan L, Moses MA, Huang S, Ingber DE (2000) Adhesion dependent control of matrix metalloproteinases-2 activation in human capillary endothelial cells. J Cell Sci 113:3979–3987

Yang S, Graham J, Kahn JW, Schwartz EA, Gerritsen ME (1999) Functional roles for PECAM-1 (CD31) and VE-cadherin (CD144) in tube assembly and lumen formation in three-dimensional collagen gels. Am J Pathol 155:887–895

Yu Q, Stamenkovic I (1999) Localization of matrix metalloproteinase 9 to the cell surface provides a mechanism for CD44-mediated tumor invasion. Genes Dev 13:35–48

Zondag GC, Reynolds AB, Moolenaar WH (2000) Receptor protein-tyrosine phosphatase RPTPmu binds to, and dephosphorylates the catenin p120(ctn). J Biol Chem 275:11264–11269

10 Androgen Receptor Expression in Human Thyroid Cancer Tissues: A Potential Mechanism Underlying the Gender Bias in the Incidence of Thyroid Cancers

Jone A. Stanley, Ramalingam Neelamohan, Esakky Suthagar, Kannan Annapoorna, Sridharan Sharmila, Jayaraman Jayakumar, Narasimhan Srinivasan, Sakhila K. Banu, Maharajan Chandrasekaran, and Michael M. Aruldhas

Abstract

Sex difference in the incidence of thyroid cancer with predominance of the disease in women is well known, whereas the underlying mechanism remains obscure. Research performed during the last four decades points out that sex steroids may underlie this bias in thyroid cancer incidence. This review attempts to compile the available information in the area. The authors have taken care to include all relevant publications. If any of the important reports is not included, it is inadvertent and not intentional. A series of reports from our laboratory have established that testosterone stimulates the proliferation and growth of normal thyroid gland in rats of either sex, whereas estradiol has a specific stimulatory effect in females and an inhibitory effect in males. Early experimental studies in rats revealed that sex steroids may promote thyroid tumorigenesis;

J.A. Stanley
Doctoral student, Department of Endocrinology, Dr. ALM. Post Graduate Institute of Basic Medical Sciences, University of Madras, Taramani Campus, Chennai 600113, TN, India

Post Doctoral Fellow, Department Integrative Biosciences, College of Veterinary Medicine & Biomedical Sciences, Texas A&M University, College Station, TX 77843, USA

R. Neelamohan • E. Suthagar • K. Annapoorna • S. Sharmila
Doctoral Students, Department of Endocrinology, Dr. ALM. Post Graduate Institute of Basic Medical Sciences, University of Madras, Taramani Campus, Chennai 600113, TN, India

J. Jayakumar
Post Graduate Student in Medicine, Department of Endocrine Surgery, Madras Medical College, Chennai 600003, TN, India

N. Srinivasan • M.M. Aruldhas (✉)
Professor, Department of Endocrinology, Dr. ALM. Post Graduate Institute of Basic Medical Sciences, University of Madras, Taramani Campus, Chennai 600113, TN, India
e-mail: aruldhasmm@gmail.com

S.K. Banu
Clinical Assistant Professor, Department Integrative Biosciences, College of Veterinary Medicine & Biomedical Sciences, Texas A&M University, College Station, TX 77843, USA

M. Chandrasekaran
Professor, Department of Endocrine Surgery, Madras Medical College, Chennai 600003, TN, India

P.R. Sudhakaran (ed.), *Perspectives in Cancer Prevention – Translational Cancer Research*, DOI 10.1007/978-81-322-1533-2_10, © Springer India 2014

we have shown that testosterone may specifically promote malignancy. We have also shown the stimulatory effect of testosterone and estradiol in human thyroid cancer cell lines NPA-87-1 and WRO-82-1. In a recent paper we reported a positive correlation between AR ligand-binding activity and its protein expression level; AR mRNA expression had a positive correlation with its transcription factors Spl and a negative correlation with p53, its repressor in papillary thyroid carcinoma (PTC) or follicular adenoma (FTA) tissues of women. There was inconsistency between expression levels of AR mRNA and its protein, which was influenced by the expression level of the microRNA (miR)-124a. From our in vitro experiments using a human PTC cell line (NPA-87-1) transfected with either *miR-124a* or anti-*miR-124a* in the light of our findings from human thyroid tumor tissues, we have shown for the first time that *miR-124a* is a potent inhibitor of AR expression, and its expression pattern may determine the mitogenic effect of testosterone on thyroid cancer.

Keywords
Thyroid cancer • Estradiol • Tumorigenesis • Papillary thyroid carcinoma • Mitogenic effect • Testosterone

10.1 Introduction

Thyroid cancer has emerged as the most common endocrine malignancy. Broadly, thyroid tumors are classified into tumors of follicular and C cells origin. Benign follicular adenoma, well-differentiated papillary thyroid carcinoma (PTC), follicular thyroid carcinoma (FTC), and poorly differentiated anaplastic thyroid carcinoma (ATC) are tumors of follicular cells; medullary thyroid carcinoma (MTC) is the tumor of C cells (Hedinger et al. 1989). PTC is the major thyroid neoplasia, constituting more than 80 % of all thyroid cancers, followed by FTC, which constitutes 2–5 % thyroid cancers. Though carcinoma of the thyroid constitutes less than 2 % of total cancer cases (Landis et al. 1998; Colonna et al. 2010; Ward et al. 2010), it accounts for 90 % of all endocrine tumors and 63 % of all deaths due to endocrine malignancy (Franker 1995). The incidence of thyroid cancer has increased significantly in the past several decades (Chen et al. 2009). It is estimated that thyroid cancer accounts for approximately 140,000 of the 11 million annual global cancer cases (Nandakumar et al. 2005) and about 37,400 of the 1.5 million cases of cancers that are diagnosed annually in the USA (ACS 2012). It is the 6th most commonly diagnosed cancer among American women and the most common cancer of the endocrine system (ACS 2012).

The disease is relatively more prevalent in younger age group than adults, with almost two-thirds of the diagnosed cases being persons aged 20–55 years and the mortality rate increasing gradually by 40–45years of age (Dean and Hay 2000). Thyroid cancer had the fastest reported increase in the age-adjusted annual incidence rate, compared to other cancers recorded in the USA between 1980 and 2005 (Chen et al. 2009). In the last decade, the incidence of thyroid cancer in the USA had increased by 82 %, whereas the USA population grew at a rate of 12 % (ACS 2012). The pattern of thyroid cancer in India is different from that seen in Western countries. The Indian National Cancer Registry (INCR) reported 3,617 female and 2,007 male thyroid cancer cases between 1984 and 1993 (Rao 1999). The nationwide relative frequency of thyroid cancer among all the cancer cases was 0.1–0.2 % (Unnikrishnan and Menon 2011). In Mumbai, western India, the thyroid cancer incidence was found to be at the lowest level in both sexes but was about three times more frequent among women than in men (Rao 1999). The age-adjusted incidence rate of thyroid cancer per 100,000 is about 1 for males and 1.8 for females as per the Mumbai Cancer Registry, which covered a population of 9.81 million subjects (Unnikrishnan and Menon 2011). One report from Chennai, South India, showed that thyroid carcinoma constitutes about 1–2 % of all cancers (Dorairajan et al. 2002). Our study conducted during the period 2005–2007 recorded 125 cases of thyroid cancer, among 381 patients who were admitted for surgical treatment of different thyroid disorders at the Department of Endocrine Surgery, Rajiv Gandhi Government General Hospital, Madras Medical College, Chennai (one of the major referral center for endocrine surgeries in South India), with the female:male ratio of 5.2:1 (unpublished data). In Goa, the incidence of PTC was reported to be higher than other thyroid cancers with a low ratio of PTC to FTC in iodine-deficient areas, where iodized salts are not in use (Arora and Dias 2006).

10.2 Etiology of Thyroid Cancer

The thyroid gland is one of the most radiosensitive organs in the human body (Ron et al. 1998; Schonfeld et al. 2011). Exposure to radiation is by far the most well-established risk factor for thyroid cancer (Reiners 2009; Lukas et al. 2012; Mazonakis et al. 2012; Tronko et al. 2012; Veiga et al. 2012). The increased incidence of thyroid cancer from 1935 to 1975 observed in the USA was attributed to therapeutic radiation administered to the head and neck area of children for the treatment of benign abnormalities (Pottern et al. 1980). The Chernobyl nuclear reactor accident resulted in a marked increase (nearly 2,400 %) in the incidence of thyroid cancer in Belarus, affecting predominantly females (Demidchik et al. 2007; Tronko et al. 2012). Even in the adjoining Ukraine, there was marked increase in the incidence of thyroid cancer among men and women (Tronko et al. 2012; Demidchik et al. 2007). This dramatically increased the number of thyroid cancer in children living in Belarus, Ukraine, and Russia was related to the radioactive iodine contamination (Pacini et al. 1997; Stiller 2005; Demidchik et al. 2007; Kesminiene et al. 2012; Tronko et al. 2012). Memon et al. (2004) suggested that family history of benign thyroid diseases may be associated with an increased risk of thyroid cancer, particularly among first-degree female relatives. Epidemiological data have revealed a four- to ten fold increase in the incidence of PTC among the first-generation relatives of PTC patients (Pal et al. 2001), suggesting the possibility of familial predisposition to PTC. Several oncogenes and a series of genetic alterations are associated with thyroid cancer. Multiple lines of evidence suggest that *RET/PTC* rearrangements may be an early event in thyroid cancer development (Mishra et al. 2009). Involvement of the rat sarcoma (*RAS*) gene has been reported as an early and important event in thyroid tumorigenesis (Volante et al. 2009). Activation of *MYC* oncogene has been detected in human thyroid cancers. Living in volcanic areas (Duntas and Doumas 2009), iodine intake (Franceschi 1998), obesity (Schonfeld et al. 2011), and importantly the female sex (Rahbari et al. 2010) have also been associated with higher incidence of thyroid cancer.

10.3 Thyroid Cancer and Gender

Thyroid cancer is one of the cancers in which the incidence rate in women far exceeds that of men (Reynolds et al. 2005). Data from cancer registries of different countries show that more women than men are diagnosed with thyroid cancer (3–5.5:1) (Mack et al. 1999; Negri et al. 1999; Cook et al. 2009; Howlader et al. 2011), a patented phenomenon observed across geographic locations and ethnicity. Our earlier report also confirmed the gender disparity in thyroid cancer incidence as indicated by a sex ratio of 3:1 for PTC, 5:1 for FTC, and 5.4:1 for FTA between women and men (Stanley et al. 2012). The incidence of thyroid cancer in women increases with age (Reynolds et al. 2005), reaches the peak during pubertal age, and decreases after menopause (Preston-Martin et al. 1987; Farahati et al. 1998). Though females have the high incidence of thyroid tumors, men have a high rate of malignancy, usually with poor prognosis (LiVolsi 1996; Holzer et al. 2000; Wartofsky 2010). In 2012, among 56,000 adults diagnosed with thyroid cancer in the United States, 43,000 were women (ACS 2012). The difference in the incidence of thyroid cancer between men and women suggests a possible role of sex steroids in the incidence of thyroid cancer (Howlader et al. 2011). However, the exact relationship between thyroid cancer incidence and women's reproductive life remains unclear due to the great variability observed among different ethnic groups (Mack et al. 1999; Negri et al. 1999).

10.4 Specific Effects of Sex Steroids on Normal and Cancer Thyroid

A sex-specific difference in the ligand-binding activity (LBA) of AR in human thyroid with higher activity in males than in females was reported (Marugo et al. 1991). A series of reports from our laboratory on postnatal development/growth of thyroid gland in rats ascertained the sex-specific effects of testosterone and estradiol on thyrocytes proliferation. Banu et al. (2002) demonstrated that the peak in thyrocytes proliferation in normal male and female rats during the second postnatal week is associated with elevated levels of testosterone and estradiol and their receptors in the thyroid. Another in vitro study on thyrocytes of immature and adult rats revealed a direct mitogenic effect of sex steroids; while testosterone promoted the proliferation of thyrocytes isolated from either sex, estradiol specifically promoted the same in females, whereas it inhibited in males. The above study entrenched the role of sex steroids on thyrocytes proliferation by demonstrating the inhibitory effect of the antiestrogen tamoxifen and the antiandrogen flutamide on estradiol and testosterone-induced thyrocytes proliferation, respectively (Banu et al. 2002). Recently, we reported that the mitogenic effects of testosterone and estradiol on rat thyrocytes are associated with increased expression of IGF-1 (Stanley et al. 2010). Earlier, we reported the differential effect of testosterone and estradiol on the proliferation of human thyroid cancer cell lines; while testosterone promoted the proliferation of PTC (NPA-87-1) and FTC (WRO-82-1) cell lines, estradiol promoted the proliferation of NPA-87-1 alone, whereas it inhibited that of WRO-82-1 cell line (Banu et al. 2001b). The differential effects of estradiol and testosterone on the proliferation of thyroid cancer cell lines underscored the importance of these sex steroids in the sex-specific difference in thyroid cancer incidence. Thiruvengadam et al. (2003) from our laboratory provided evidence for the specific effects of estradiol and testosterone in the promotion of nonmalignant and malignant thyroid tumorigenesis in rat. The above study demonstrated that estradiol promotes the DHPN-induced development of thyroid adenoma in either sex, whereas excess testosterone favored the development of malignant thyroid tumors alone. The effects of testosterone in promoting the malignant thyroid tumors were obvious in gonad intact males and ovariectomized rats, suggesting a modulatory effect of endogenous estradiol on the effects of testosterone (Aruldhas et al. 1995; Thiruvengadam et al. 2003). In vitro studies from our laboratory also revealed the stimulatory effects of testosterone and estradiol on (^{3}H)-thymidine uptake by normal (Banu et al. 2001a, b; Stanley et al. 2010) and cancerous rat thyrocytes (Aruldhas et al. 1995) and human PTC and FTC cell lines (Banu et al. 2001a, b; Stanley et al. 2012), suggesting the direct action of sex steroids on the thyroid. Rossi et al. (1996) reported that 5α-dihydrotestosterone inhibited the proliferation of primary culture of goitrous thyrocytes and the PTC cell line TPC, which was associated with a reduction in the expression of *c-myc* gene, whereas thyroperoxidase and thyroglobulin genes remained unaltered. The exact reason for the inconsistency between our study and that of Rossi et al. is not clear. Probably, the difference in the cell lines used and the type of the androgen and doses employed in the two studies are the reasons for the inconsistency. Bahrami et al. (2009) reported that testosterone decreased thyroid enlargement and prevented the fall in serum free T_4 levels in castrated iodine-deficient rats. Testosterone decreased thyroxine binding globulin (TBG) and total iodothyronines (T_4 and T_3), indicating the direct effect of testosterone on the thyroid gland (Tahboub and Arafah 2009).

10.5 Sex Steroid Receptors and Thyroid Cancer

Androgen receptor (AR), estrogen receptor (ER), progesterone receptor (PR), glucocorticoid receptor, mineralocorticoid receptor, and thyroid hormone receptor (TR) are members of the nuclear receptor super family, a diverse group of transcription factors activated by the binding of a hormone ligand (Flamant et al. 2006). In general, these intracellular receptors undergo a conformational change upon ligand binding, which allows for separation of the receptor from its cytoplasmic chaperone proteins (exception, ERs and TRs). There is subsequent dimerization and binding of the receptor to a specific steroid response element located on the promoter region of target genes, recruiting and interacting with coactivators, co-repressors, or other *cis*-acting transcription factors to regulate gene expression and activate various intracellular pathways (Thakur and Paramanik 2009).

There are two distinct ER subtypes, ERα and ERß, which are coded by separate genes. ERα is expressed most abundantly in the female reproductive tract, in particular the uterus, vagina, and ovaries, while ERß has its highest expression in the prostate, ovaries, and lungs (Saunders and Critchley 2002). Endogenous ligands for AR are testosterone and its potent metabolite 5-α-dihydrotestosterone (DHT), as well as the adrenal pre-hormones dehydroepiandrosterone (DHEA) and DHEA sulfate (DHEAS); the male reproductive organs exhibit the highest level of AR expression (Cooke et al. 1991).

Thyroid tissue is responsive to sex steroids as AR and ERs are expressed in normal and cancer thyroid tissues (Marugo et al. 1991; Banu et al. 2001a, b, 2002; Banu and Aruldhas 2002; Thiruvengadam et al. 2003; Stanley et al. 2010, 2012). Though radiation exposure, low iodine diet, family history and previous history of thyroid goiter and sex chromosomes have been attributed for thyroid cancer incidence, AR and ER genes have emerged as the most significant candidates responsible for the sex-specific differences in thyroid cancer incidence (Rossi et al. 1996; Banu et al. 2001a, b; Thiruvengadam et al. 2003). Both testosterone and estradiol regulate the proliferation of thyrocytes by upregulating their respective receptors (Banu et al. 2001a, b; Stanley et al. 2010). The presence of AR, ERα, and ERß, and their regulation by respective ligands, suggests that these nuclear receptors might play an important role in the pathogenesis of thyroid tumors. We have shown that the stimulatory effect of testosterone on proliferation of human PTC (NPA-87-1) and FTC (WRO-82-1) cell lines is associated with homologous upregulation of AR, independent of thyroid-stimulating hormone (Banu et al. 2001a, b). The above study also reported homologous regulation of ER by estradiol in those cell lines. Recently, our laboratory investigated (Annapoorna et al. 2011; Annapoorna 2012) the expression pattern of ERα and ERß in 68 human PTC tissue samples (17 males, 51 females); the results from these studies revealed a varied expression pattern of ER subtypes with overexpression of ERα in 51 % of the female and the remaining subjects showing either normal (33 %) or decreased (16 %) expression; among the males 59 % showed overexpression, 24 % had decreased expression, and the remaining recorded normal expression level of ERα. The same study revealed an interesting picture of a general trend of decreased expression of ERß in most of the females (73 %) and increased expression in most of the PTC samples from males (88 %), suggesting a clear sex difference in the expression pattern. Using NPA-87-1 cell lines, Annapoorna (2012) has demonstrated that estradiol prefers ERα over ERß for its mitogenic activity, and the estradiol-induced cell proliferation is associated with activation of the MAP kinase pathway. Recently, we reported sex difference in AR status in human thyroid cancer tissues, i.e. increased expression level of AR mRNA in majority of PTC men and decreased expression in many of the women (Stanley et al. 2012). Magri et al. (2012) reported that increased expression of AR, ERα and ERß negativity may be associated with aggressive thyroid cancer phenotypes and may represent an additional criterion in deciding whether to perform radioiodine ablation in these tumors. In a recent review Yao et al. (2011) had given an elaborative account of these aspects, and interested readers may refer to the article for additional information.

10.6 Androgen Receptor in Thyroid Cancer

AR is expressed in many tissues, including normal and malignant thyroid tumors with the highest level observed in male reproductive organs (Magri et al. 2012; Stanley et al. 2012). *AR* gene is located on the X chromosome (q11-12) and the receptor protein is well known as a ligand-inducible transcription factor that regulates target gene expression (Heinlein and Chang 2002; Lee et al. 2003; Brinkmann 2011). As a member of the nuclear receptor superfamily, the *AR* gene consists of eight exons that encode four structurally and functionally distinct domains: the NH_2-terminal transactivation domain, the DNA-binding domain, a hinge region, and the COOH-terminal ligand-binding domain (Matsumoto et al. 2013). Upon ligand binding, the receptor undergoes transformation, homodimerization, and nuclear translocation and binds to specific AR-responsive elements located in the promoter region of its target genes; this is followed by recruitment of specific coregulators and basal transcriptional machinery including RNA polymerase II, leading to the transcription of target genes (Heinlein and Chang 2002; Brinkmann 2011).

The presence of AR in normal and cancer thyroid tissues of rodent, primate, and humans favors its role in the pathogenesis of thyroid cancer. A series of reports ascertained the presence of AR in human thyroid tissues (Table 10.1). The rate of thyroid malignancy is high in men with poor prognosis, compared to women. Marugo et al. (1991) showed the presence of higher nuclear AR concentration in the male rather than in the female thyroid cancer tissues. We have reported a varied pattern of AR expression in human thyroid tumor tissue, which could be categorized into subjects with increased, decreased, and unaltered expression (Stanley et al. 2012). These findings suggest that one cannot generalize about the expression pattern of AR in thyroid cancer, and it needs an individualized or categorized approach based on the tumor type, grade, and sex. Recently, based on their immunohistochemical observations of AR in 122 of thyroid cancer tissues, Magri et al. (2012) reported that AR(+) tumors are more aggressive than the AR(−) tumors due to a significantly higher prevalence of capsular invasion. The capsular invasion is a major factor increasing the risk of nodal metastasis in PTC (Pisanu et al. 2009).

All these studies pointed out that androgens have a regulatory role on thyroid tumorigenesis and sex disparity in the incidence and aggressiveness of thyroid cancer. However, the exact mechanism underlying the effect of AR on thyroid cancer and the factors responsible for its varied expression among subjects afflicted with the disease remain obscure. With this background in mind, we investigated 125 thyroid tumor tissue samples excised during surgery for PTC ($n=68$; 17 males and 51 females), FTC ($n=6$; 1 male and 5 females), and FTA ($n=51$; 8 males and 43 females) at the Department of Endocrine Surgery, Madras Medical College, Chennai, India; the parameters studied include testosterone concentration, AR ligand-binding activity, *AR* expression using real-time PCR and western blot techniques, and expression pattern of a few specific regulators of AR mRNA expression (Stanley et al. 2012). The following were the salient features of our report: (1) Peripheral and thyroid tissue concentration increased in women with thyroid tumors, whereas the same decreased in male subjects with the disease. (2) AR ligand-binding activity increased in a majority of male subjects (41 % PTC, 100 % FTC, 88 % FTA) and in carcinoma tissues of females (51 % PTC and 80 % FTC), whereas in 75 % of FTA tissues from females, it decreased. Interestingly, it remained unaltered in 35 % and decreased in 24 % of PTC tissues from males and decreased in 35 %

Table 10.1 List of reports on androgen receptor expression in human thyroid tissues

	Author	Tissue type	Notes
1	Prinz et al. (1984)	PTC, FTA, NTG	AR was detected in 4/5 malignant and 9/20 nonmalignant human thyroid tissues. No significant difference between sex.
2	Miki et al. (1990)	PTC, ATC, FTA, NTG	AR was detected in 8/29 nonneoplastic and 4/26 neoplastic tissues. No data on sex or sex disparity.
3	Ruizeveld de Winter et al. (1991)	No detail provided	Immunostaining of AR in thyroid tissues ($n = 2$). No data on sex or sex disparity.
4	Marugo et al. (1991)	NTG	*AR* expression detected in 12 female and 6 male thyroid tissues. *AR* expression was higher in men than women.
5	Kimura et al. (1993)	No detail provided	AR immunostaining detected in human thyroid follicular cells. No data on sex or sex disparity.
6	Rossi et al. (1996)		AR was detected in all the noncancerous ($n = 7$) and few of the cancerous samples ($n = 3$) studied. No data on sex or sex disparity.
7	Zhai et al. (2003)	MTC	AR was detected in 12/16 male and 7/9 female thyroid tissues.
8	Bléchet et al. (2007)	MTC, CCH	*AR* expression was detected mainly in men and lower expression in women. No sex disparity observed.
9	Magri et al. (2012)	PTC	*AR* expression detected in 16/78 female, 3/13 male tissues. No data on sex or sex disparity.
10	Stanley et al. (2012)	PTC, FTC, FTA	*AR* expression was detected in all the 125 samples analyzed; *AR* expression increased in men and decreased in women. Varied *AR* expression and the testosterone levels might contribute for the sex disparity.

and remained unaltered in 14 % of PTC females. (3) Western blot analysis revealed normal pattern of AR protein expression level in a majority of cancer tissues from males. However, a majority of cancer tissues from female subjects recorded decreased expression level of AR protein; a few samples from either sex recorded increased expression of AR protein. When we subjected the data on AR ligand-binding activity and western blot to Pearson's correlation coefficient analysis, there was a positive correlation between the two parameters in PTC and FTA females and males. (4) In an attempt to comprehend the mechanism underlying the expression AR gene, we determined AR mRNA expression by real-time PCR analysis which showed either increased or normal expression (41 % in each) in males, but decreased expression was evident in a majority of thyroid tumor tissues from women. Pearson's correlation coefficient analysis revealed a positive correlation between AR mRNA and protein in malignant and nonmalignant tissues of women and only in PTC tissues of men. In general, our findings revealed the existence of a sex-specific difference in the expression and ligand-binding activity of AR in thyroid cancer. As discussed earlier, AR is a ligand-mediated transcription factor (Lee and Chang 2003; Flamant et al. 2006) and undergoes homologous upregulation in response to testosterone stimulation (Banu et al. 2001a, b). Therefore, based on the findings of correlation analysis of thyroidal concentration of testosterone and AR ligand-binding activity, and expression levels of AR mRNA and protein, we suggested that the tissue level of testosterone in the thyroid may be an important marker for the prognosis of thyroid cancer in men and women (Stanley et al. 2012).

The *AR* 5′ upstream promoter region lacks a typical TATA box and CAAT box but contains binding sites for key regulatory elements like specificity protein 1 (Sp1) (Mizokami et al. 1994), cAMP response element-binding protein (CBP) (Takane and McPhaul 1996), and p53 (Alimirah et al. 2007). Both Sp1 and CBP were reported to enhance *AR* expression (Faber et al. 1993; Aarnisalo et al. 1998), while p53 was reported to repress it (Alimirah et al. 2007) Increased p53 decreased the expression of AR mRNA and protein in 22Rv1 and LNCaP prostate cancer cell lines (Cronauer et al. 2004; Alimirah et al. 2007). Cyclin D1 was reported to function as a strong corepressor of *AR* in LNCaP cell line (Petre-Draviam et al. 2003).

We also detected the expression level of *AR* transcription factors CBP and SP1 by western blot, in an attempt to understand the regulation of AR transcription. There was no significant correlation between AR mRNA and CBP expression in thyroid tumor tissues from females and males. However, there was a positive correlation between AR mRNA and SP1expressions in PTC tissues of women alone. Increased level of testosterone is known to suppress AR expression via inhibition of Sp1 in rat prostate (Beklemisheva et al. 2007), suggesting that Sp1 and increased testosterone bioavailability could contribute to the downregulation of *AR* in a majority of thyroid tumors in females. Based on the above findings, we suggested that (1) SP1 may be the major positive regulator of *AR* expression in thyroid cancer, and (2) it may be one of the putative factors contributing for the specific decrease in AR expression in PTC women (Stanley et al. 2012).

As there was no consistency between AR mRNA and the positive regulators of its transcription in males, we looked for the expression of repressors of *AR* transcription, P53 and cyclin D1; there was a negative correlation between (decreased) expression of AR mRNA and P53/cyclin D1 proteins in females and an opposite trend between AR mRNA and P53 in males. We also reported a positive association between tissue testosterone level and cyclin D1 expression in PTC tissues from women and an opposite trend in males. An important finding in our study was an inconsistency between AR mRNA and protein expressions in a number of thyroid cancer tissues, particularly in males. Therefore, we looked for the existence of a specific microRNA (miRNA) that may decrease the translation of AR mRNA into its protein. miRNAs regulate translation and stability of particular target mRNAs by imperfect base pairing (Olsen and Ambros 1999). miRNAs are noncoding single-stranded RNAs of about 22 nucleotides. A large number of miRNAs are involved in almost every major cellular function like proliferation, differentiation, and apoptosis, and as a consequence, deregulation of miRNAs has also been linked to a broad variety of cancers (Ha 2011). The role of miRNAs in thyroid cancer is incompletely understood. Several studies have analyzed miRNA expression in numerous and different types of thyroid tumors, suggesting a deregulation of miRNAs in cancer tissues, compared with their normal counterparts (Ricarte-Filho et al. 2009; Abraham et al. 2011; Marini et al. 2011; Leonardi et al. 2012; Vriens et al. 2012). Using bioinformatics analysis we predicted the presence of a binding site (GUGCCUU) for miR-124a at the nucleotide position 88–94 of *AR* 3′ UTR. We found an increase in miR-124a expression in all women who had decreased expression of AR protein, suggesting a negative correlation between the two parameters in those cases that had an inconsistency between AR mRNA and protein. The finding of negative correlation between AR protein and miR-124a in PTC and FTA tissues from women alone also pointed out the sex-specific variation in the regulation of AR in thyroid cancers. We also confirmed the negative effect of miR-124a on AR protein and, thus, on testosterone-mediated proliferation of thyroid cancer cells in NPA-87-1 PTC cell line transfected with miR-124a and anti-miR-124a. *miR-124a* also decreased the AR reporter luciferase activity and the thyroid cancer cell proliferation, suggesting that *miR-124a* can be a potential candidate that determines *AR* gene expression pattern in human thyroid tumors, which could be a putative mechanism underlying the sex bias in the incidence of thyroid cancers. Thus, for the first time, to the best of our knowledge, we provided evidence that *AR* gene is the direct target for miR-124a, and its expression level determines the expression pattern of *AR* in thyroid tumor tissues. Our study also reported for the first time the existence of a sex-specific relation between testosterone bioavailability and *AR* expression pattern in thyroid tumors (Stanley et al. 2012).

10.7 Conclusion

Based on our findings and existing literature, it is concluded that the varying pattern of testosterone level and AR status in thyroid tissues of men and women might contribute to the sex-specific incidence of thyroid tumors. *miR-124a* plays a significant role in determining *AR* gene expression pattern and may direct AR influence on sex-specific thyroid cancer incidence.

Acknowledgments This study was supported by the Government of India, Department of Biotechnology (DBT) in the form of a major research project (BT/PR4841/Med/12/187/2004) to Prof. M. Michael Aruldhas, and financial support from University Grants Commission under the Special Assistance Programme and the Department of Science and Technology under FIST Programme is gratefully acknowledged.

References

Aarnisalo P, Palvimo JJ, Janne OA (1998) CREB-binding protein in androgen receptor-mediated signaling. Proc Natl Acad Sci USA 95:2122

Abraham D, Jackson N, Gundara JS, Zhao J, Gill AJ et al (2011) MicroRNA profiling of sporadic and hereditary medullary thyroid cancer identifies predictors of nodal metastasis, prognosis, and potential therapeutic targets. Clint Cancer Res 17:4772–4781

ACS (2012) Cancer facts and figures. American Cancer Society, Atlanta, pp 1–66

Alimirah F, Panchanathany R, Cheny J, Zhang X, Ho S, Choubey D (2007) Expression of androgen receptor is negatively regulated by p53. Neoplasia 9:1152–1159

Annapoorna K (2012) Mitogenic effect of estradiol on human papillary thyroid carcinoma is mediated through MAPK signaling downstream of estrogen receptor alpha. PhD thesis, University of Madras, India

Annapoorna K, Stanley J, Neelamohan R, Aruldhas MM (2011) Estradiol-induced proliferation of human papillary thyroid cancer by activating Mitogen-activated protein kinase (MAPK) signaling is mediated through its specific receptor subtype. In: AACR International conference on New Horizons in Cancer Research: Biology to Prevention to Therapy, December 13–16, 2011. The Leela Kempinski Gurgaon, Gurgaon, Delhi (NCR), India. Poster No. B29

Arora R, Dias A (2006) Iodine and Thyroid Cancer in Goa. J Health Allied Sci 5:1–3

Aruldhas MM, Thiruvengadam A, Banu SK, Govindarajulu P (1995) Thyroidal concentration of testosterone and estradiol determines the promotion of thyroid tumours in N-nitrosodiisopropanolamine (DHPN) treated Wistar rats. In: 12th Asia Pacific Cancer Conference: towards total cancer control, Singapore, p 43

Bahrami Z, Hedayati M, Taghikhani M, Azizi F (2009) Effect of testosterone on thyroid weight and function in iodine deficient castrated rats. Horm Metab Res 41:762–766

Banu KS, Aruldhas MM (2002) Sex steroids regulate TSH-induced thyroid growth during sexual maturation in Wistar rats. Exp Clint Endocrinol Diabetes 110:37–42

Banu SK, Arosh JA, Govindarajulu P, Aruldhas MM (2001a) Testosterone and estradiol differentially regulate thyroid growth in Wistar rats from immature to adult age. Endocr Res 27:447–463

Banu SK, Govindarajulu P, Aruldhas MM (2001b) Testosterone and estradiol have specific differential modulatory effect on the proliferation of human thyroid papillary and follicular carcinoma cell lines independent of TSH action. Endocr Pathol 12:315–327

Banu SK, Govindarajulu P, Aruldhas MM (2002) Testosterone and estradiol up-regulate androgen and estrogen receptors in immature and adult rat thyroid glands in vivo. Steroids 67:1007–1014

Beklemisheva AA, Feng J, Yeh YA, Wang LG, Chiao JW (2007) Modulating testosterone stimulated prostate growth by phenethyl isothiocyanate via Sp1 and androgen receptor down-regulation. Prostate 67: 863–870

Bléchet C, Lecomte P, De Calan L, Beutter P, Guyétant S (2007) Expression of sex steroid hormone receptors in C cell hyperplasia and medullary thyroid carcinoma. Virchows Arch 450:433–439

Brinkmann AO (2011) Molecular mechanisms of androgen action – a historical perspective. Methods Mol Biol 776:3–24

Chen AY, Jemal A, Ward EM (2009) Increasing incidence of differentiated thyroid cancer in the United States, 1988–2005. Cancer 115:3801–3807

Colonna M, Bossard N, Guizard AV, Remontet L, Grosclaude P (2010) Descriptive epidemiology of thyroid cancer in France: incidence, mortality and survival. Ann Endocrinol (Paris) 71:95–101

Cook MB, Dawsey SM, Freedman ND, Inskip PD, Wichner SM et al (2009) Sex disparities in cancer incidence by period and age. Cancer Epidemiol Biomarkers Prev 18:1174–1182

Cooke PS, Young P, Cunha GR (1991) Androgen receptor expression in developing male reproductive organs. Endocrinology 128:2867–2873

Cronauer MV, Schulz WA, Burchardt T, Ackermann R, Burchardt M (2004) Inhibition of p53 function diminishes androgen receptor-mediated signaling in prostate cancer cell lines. Oncogene 23:3541–3549

Dean DS, Hay ID (2000) Prognostic indicators in differentiated thyroid carcinoma. Cancer Control 7:229–239

Demidchik YE, Saenko VA, Yamashita S (2007) Childhood thyroid cancer in Belarus, Russia, and Ukraine after Chernobyl and at present. Arq Bras Endocrinol Metabol 51:748–762

Dorairajan N, Pandiarajan R, Yuvaraja S (2002) A descriptive study of papillary thyroid carcinoma in a teaching hospital in Chennai, India. Asian J Surge 25:300–303

Duntas LH, Doumas C (2009) The "rings of fire" and thyroid cancer. Hormones 8:249–253

Farahati J, Parlowsky T, Mader U, Reiners C, Bucsky P (1998) Differentiated thyroid cancer in children and adolescents. Langenbecks Arch Surge 383:235–239

Flamant F, Baxter JD, Forrest D, Refetoff S, Samuels H et al (2006) International Union of Pharmacology. LIX. The pharmacology and classification of the nuclear receptor superfamily: thyroid hormone receptors. Pharmacol Rev 58:705–711

Franceschi S (1998) Iodine intake and thyroid carcinoma – a potential risk factor. Exp Clint Endocrinol Diabetes 106(Suppl 3):S38–S44

Franker DL (1995) Radiation exposure and other factors that predispose to human thyroid neoclassic. Surge Clint North Am 75:365–375

Ha T (2011) Micro RNAs in human diseases: from cancer to cardiovascular disease. Immune Netw 11:135–154

Hedinger C, Williams ED, Sobin LH (1989) The WHO histological classification of thyroid tumors: a commentary on the second edition. Cancer 63:908–911

Heinlein CA, Chang C (2002) Androgen receptor (AR) coregulators: an overview. Endocri Rev 23:175–200

Holzer S, Reiners C, Mann K, Bamberg M, Rothmund M et al (2000) Patterns of care for patients with primary differentiated carcinoma of the thyroid gland treated in Germany during 1996. U.S. and German Thyroid Cancer Group. Cancer 89:192–201

Howlader N, Noone AM, Krapcho M, Neyman N, Aminou R, Waldron W, Altekruse SF, Kosary CL, Ruhl J, Tatalovich Z, Cho H, Mariotto A, Eisner MP, Lewis DR, Chen HS, Feuer EJ, Cronin KA, Edwards BK (2011) SEER Cancer Statistics Review, 1975–2008, National Cancer Institute. Bethesda. http://seer.cancer.gov/csr/1975_2008

Kesminiene A, Evrard AS, Ivanov VK, Malakhova IV, Kurtinaitise J et al (2012) Risk of thyroid cancer among Chernobyl liquidators. Radiat Res 178:425–436

Kimura N, Mizokami A, Oonuma T, Sasano H, Nagura H (1993) Immunocytochemical localization of androgen receptor with polyclonal antibody in paraffin-embedded human tissues. J Histochem Cytochem 41:671–678

Landis SH, Murray T, Bolden S, Wingo PA (1998) Cancer statistics. CA Cancer J Clin 48:6–29

Lee Y, Ahn C, Han J, Choi H, Kim J, Yim J et al (2003) The nuclear RNase III Drosha initiates microRNA processing. Nature 425:415–419

Lee HJ, Chang C (2003) Recent advances in androgen receptor action. Cell Mol Life Sci 60:1613–1622

Leonardi GC, Candido S, Carbone M, Colaianni V, Garozzo SF et al (2012) MicroRNAs and thyroid cancer: biological and clinical significance (Review). Int J Mol Med 30:991–999

LiVolsi VA (1996) Well differentiated thyroid carcinoma. Clin Oncol (R Coll Radiol) 8:281–288

Lukas J, Drabek J, Lukas D, Dusek L, Gatek J (2012) The epidemiology of thyroid cancer in the Czech Republic in comparison with other countries. Biomed Pap Med Fac Univ Palacky Olomouc Czech Repub 2012 Nov 2. doi: 10.5507/bp.2012.086. [Epub ahead of print]

Mack WJ, Preston-Martin S, Bernstein L, Qian D, Xiang M (1999) Reproductive and hormonal risk factors for thyroid cancer in Los Angeles County females. Cancer Epidemiol Biomarkers Prev 8:991–997

Magri F, Capelli V, Rotondi M, Leporati P, La Manna L et al (2012) Expression of estrogen and androgen receptors in differentiated thyroid cancer: an additional criterion to assess the patient's risk. Endocr Relat Cancer 19:463–471

Marini F, Luzi E, Brandi ML (2011) MicroRNA role in thyroid cancer development. J Thyroid Res 2011:12 p. Article ID 407123. doi:10.4061/2011/407123

Marugo M, Torre G, Bernasconi D, Fazzuoli L, Cassulo S et al (1991) Androgen receptors in normal and pathological thyroids. J Endocrinol Invest 14:31–35

Matsumoto T, Sakari M, Okada M, Yokoyama A, Takahashi S et al (2013) The androgen receptor in health and disease. Annu Rev Physiol 75:201–224

Mazonakis M, Kourinou K, Lyraraki E, Varveris H, Damilakis J (2012) Thyroid exposure to scattered radiation and associated second cancer risk from paediatric radiotherapy for extracranial tumours. Radiat Prot Dosimetry 152:317–322

Memon A, Berrington De Gonzalez A, Luqmani Y, Suresh A (2004) Family history of benign thyroid disease and cancer and risk of thyroid cancer. Eur J Cancer 40:754–760

Miki H, Oshimo K, Inoue H, Morimoto T, Monden Y (1990) Sex hormone receptors in human thyroid tissues. Cancer 66:1759–1762

Mishra A, Agrawal V, Krishnani N, Mishra SK (2009) Prevalence of RET/PTC expression in papillary thyroid carcinoma and its correlation with prognostic factors in a north Indian population. J Postgrad Med 55:171–175

Mizokami A, Yeh SY, Chang C (1994) Identification of 3′,5′-cyclic adenosine monophosphate response element and other cis-acting elements in the human androgen receptor gene promoter. Mol Endocrinol 8:77–88

Nandakumar A, Gupta PC, Gangadharan P, Visweswara RN, Parkin DM (2005) Geographic pathology revisited: development of an atlas of cancer in India. Int J Cancer 116:740–754

Negri E, Ron E, Franceschi S, Dal Maso L, Mark SD et al (1999) A pooled analysis of case–control studies of thyroid cancer. I. Methods. Cancer Causes Control 10:131–142

Olsen PH, Ambros V (1999) The lin-4 regulatory RNA controls developmental timing in Caenorhabditis elegans by blocking LIN-14 protein synthesis after the initiation of translation. Dev Biol 216:671–680

Pacini F, Vorontsova T, Demidchik EP, Molinaro E, Agate L et al (1997) Post-Chernobyl thyroid carcinoma in Belarus children and adolescents: comparison with naturally occurring thyroid carcinoma in Italy and France. J Clint Endocrinol Metab 82:3563–3569

Pal T, Hamel N, Vesprini D, Sanders K, Mitchell M et al (2001) Double primary cancers of the breast and thyroid in women: molecular analysis and genetic implications. Fam Cancer 1:17–24

Petre-Draviam CE, Cook CL, Burd CJ, Marshall TW, Wetherill YB, Knudsen KE (2003) Specificity of cyclin D1 for androgen receptor regulation. Cancer Res 63:4903–4913

Pisanu A, Reccia I, Nardello O, Uccheddu A (2009) Risk factors for nodal metastasis and recurrence among patients with papillary thyroid microcarcinoma: differences in clinical relevance between nonincidental and incidental tumors. World J Surg 33:460–468

Pottern LM, Stone BJ, Day NE, Pickle LW, Fraumeni JF Jr (1980) Thyroid cancer in Connecticut, 1935–1975: an analysis by cell type. Am J Epidemiol 112: 764–774

Preston-Martin S, Bernstein L, Pike MC, Maldonado AA, Henderson BE (1987) Thyroid cancer among young women related to prior thyroid disease and pregnancy history. Br J Cancer 55:191–195

Prinz RA, Sandberg L, Chaudhari PK (1984) Androgen receptors in human thyroid tissue. Surgery 96:996–1000

Rahbari R, Zhang L, Kebebew E (2010) Thyroid cancer gender disparity. Future Once 11:1771–1779

Rao DN (1999) Epidemiological observations of thyroid cancer. In: Shah AH, Samuel AM, Rao RS (eds) Thyroid cancer – an Indian perspective. Quest Publications, Mumbai, pp 3–16

Reiners C (2009) Radioactivity and thyroid cancer. Hormones (Athens) 8:185–191

Reynolds RM, Weir J, Stockton DL, Brewster DH, Sandeep TC et al (2005) Changing trends in incidence and mortality of thyroid cancer in Scotland. Clint Endocrinol (Oxf) 62:156–162

Ricarte-Filho JC, Fuziwara CS, Yamashita AS, Rezende E, da-Silva MJ et al (2009) Effects of let-7 microRNA on cell growth and differentiation of papillary thyroid cancer. Transl Once 2:236–241

Ron E, Doody MM, Becker DV, Brill AB, Curtis RE et al (1998) Cancer mortality following treatment for adult hyperthyroidism. Cooperative Thyrotoxicosis Therapy Follow-up Study Group. JAMA 280:347–355

Rossi R, Zatelli MC, Franceschetti P, Maestri I, Magri E et al (1996) Inhibitory effect of dihydrotestosterone on human thyroid cell growth. J Endocrinol 151:185–194

Ruizeveld de Winter JA, Trapman J, Vermey M, Mulder E, Zegers ND, van der Kwast TH (1991) Androgen receptor expression in human tissues: an immunohistochemical study. J Histochem Cytochem 39:927–936

Saunders PTK, Critchley HOD (2002) Estrogen receptor subtypes in the female reproductive tract. Reprod Med 10:149–164

Schonfeld SJ, Ron E, Kitahara CM, Brenner A, Park Y, et al (2011) Hormonal and reproductive factors and risk of postmenopausal thyroid cancer in the NIH-AARP Diet and Health Study. Cancer Epidemiol 35:e85–e90

Stanley JA, Aruldhas MM, Yuvaraju PB, Banu SK, Anbalagan J et al (2010) Is gender difference in postnatal thyroid growth associated with specific expression patterns of androgen and estrogen receptors? Steroids 75:1058–1066

Stanley JA, Aruldhas MM, Chandrasekaran M, Neelamohan R, Suthagar E et al (2012) Androgen receptor expression in human thyroid cancer tissues: a potential mechanism underlying the gender bias in the incidence of thyroid cancers. J Steroid Biochem Mol Biol 130:105–124

Stiller CA (2005) Thyroid cancer in Belarus. Int J Epidemiol 34:714

Tahboub R, Arafah BM (2009) Sex steroids and the thyroid. Best Pract Res Clin Endocrinol Metab 23:769–780

Takane KK, McPhaul MJ (1996) Functional analysis of the human androgen receptor promoter. Mol Cell Endocrinol 119:83–93

Thakur MK, Paramanik V (2009) Role of steroid hormone coregulators in health and disease. Hor Res 71:194–200

Thiruvengadam A, Govindarajulu P, Aruldhas MM (2003) Modulatory effect of estradiol and testosterone on the development of N-nitrosodiisopropanolamine induced thyroid tumors in female rats. Endocr Res 29:43–51

Tronko M, Mabuchi K, Bogdanova T, Hatch M, Likhtarev I et al (2012) Thyroid cancer in Ukraine after the Chernobyl accident (in the framework of the Ukraine-US Thyroid Project). J Radiol Prot 32:N65–N69

Unnikrishnan A, Menon U (2011) Thyroid disorders in India: an epidemiological perspective. Indian J Endocr Metab 15:S78–S81

Veiga LH, Lubin JH, Anderson H, de Vathaire F, Tucker M et al (2012) A pooled analysis of thyroid cancer incidence following radiotherapy for childhood cancer. Radiat Res 178:365–376

Volante M, Rapa I, Gandhi M, Bussolati G, Giachino D, Papotti M, Nikiforov YE (2009) RAS mutations are the predominant molecular alteration in poorly differentiated thyroid carcinomas and bear prognostic impact. J Clint Endocrinol Metab 94:4735–4741

Vriens MR, Weng J, Suh I, Huynh N, Guerrero MA et al (2012) MicroRNA expression profiling is a potential diagnostic tool for thyroid cancer. Cancer 118:3426–3432

Ward EM, Jemal A, Chen A (2010) Increasing incidence of thyroid cancer: is diagnostic scrutiny the sole explanation? Future Once 6:185–188

Wartofsky L (2010) Increasing world incidence of thyroid cancer: Increased detection or higher radiation exposure? Hormones 9:103–108

Yao R, Chiu G, Strugnell SS, Gill S, Wiseman SM (2011) Gender differences in thyroid cancer. Expert Rev Endocrinol Metab 6:215–243

Zhai QH, Ruebel K, Thompson GB, Lloyd RV (2003) Androgen receptor expression in C-cells and in medullary thyroid carcinoma. Endocr Pathol 14(Summer):159–165, PubMed PMID: 12858007

Novel Coordination Complexes of a Few Essential Trace Metals: Cytotoxic Properties and Lead Identification for Drug Development for Cancer

11

Anvarbatcha Riyasdeen, Rangasamy Loganathan, Mallayan Palaniandavar, and Mohammad A. Akbarsha

Abstract

Metals and metal compounds have been used in medicine since ancient times. Transition metals, which exhibit different oxidation states and can interact with biomolecules, have an important place in the field of medicinal chemistry. This property of transition metals facilitated the development of metal-based drugs with promising pharmacological applications and unique therapeutic opportunities. Discovery of antitumor activity of a transition metal complex, *cis*-diamminedichloroplatinum(II) (cisplatin), during the 1960s has been a milestone in metal-based cancer chemotherapeutics and provided leads for the synthesis of many more transition metal complexes for treatment of cancer. In our laboratories, we synthesize, isolate, and characterize transition metal coordination complexes such as iron(II), cobalt(II), nickel(II), and copper(II), which are all among the essential metals and so could be potentially producing little or less side effects, and study the DNA-binding and cytotoxic properties of the complexes. Some of these complexes, in view of their unique mode of binding with DNA, were found to affect the viability of cancer cells by bringing about specific modes of cell death, namely,

A. Riyasdeen
Department of Animal Science, Bharathidasan University, Tiruchirappalli 620 024, Tamil Nadu, India

R. Loganathan • M. Palaniandavar (✉)
Department of Chemistry, Central University of Tamil Nadu, Thiruvarur 610 004, Tamil Nadu, India
e-mail: palaniandavar@cutn.ac.in; palaniandavarm@gmail.com

M.A. Akbarsha (✉)
Mahatma Gandhi-Doerenkamp Center, Bharathidasan University, Tiruchirappalli 620 024, Tamil Nadu, India
e-mail: akbarbdu@yahoo.com; mgdcaua@yahoo.in

P.R. Sudhakaran (ed.), *Perspectives in Cancer Prevention – Translational Cancer Research*, DOI 10.1007/978-81-322-1533-2_11, © Springer India 2014

apoptosis, necrosis, and/or necroptosis, with or without generation of reactive oxygen species. This review summarizes the salient outcomes of our systematic study and the potential leads these cytotoxic complexes provide.

Keywords
Apoptosis • Cobalt(II) • Copper(II) • Iron(II) • Medicinal Chemistry • Necroptosis • Necrosis • Nickel(II) • Transition metals

11.1 Introduction

Medicinal applications of metals can be traced back to almost 5000 years (Bharti and Singh 2009). During the past three decades, the use of metal complexes as pharmaceuticals and chemotherapeutics has been increasing (Marzano et al. 2009). The discovery of cisplatin (*cis*-diamminedichloroplatinum(II)) as a cancer therapeutic has been a milestone in metallotherapeutics. Cisplatin is a well-known transition metal-based anticancer agent used as a highly effective therapeutic against almost all types of cancers and very specifically testicular, bladder, lung, gastrointestinal, and ovarian cancers (Zhang and Lippard 2003). Unfortunately, cisplatin is known to produce several side effects such as ototoxicity, neurotoxicity, and nephrotoxicity. The nephrotoxic effect of cisplatin renders it dose limiting. Since its mechanism of action in cancer therapy is its covalent binding with adenine and guanine bases in DNA, leading to adduction, the binding is irreversible including with DNA in normal tissues since this drug has low degree of selectivity. Second- and third-generation platinum-based compounds have come up for cancer therapy, some of them being carboplatin, oxaliplatin, nedaplatin, and lobaplatin, but these are also not totally exonerated of toxicity (Boulikas et al. 2007). More importantly, the cancers develop resistance to these drugs which further limit their use in cancer therapy.

These limitations in cisplatin-based metal drugs have necessitated an extensive search for more-efficacious, less toxic, and target-specific, non-covalently DNA-binding metal-based anticancer drugs. The variety of metal ion functions in biology has stimulated the development of new metallodrugs other than Pt drugs with the aim to obtain compounds acting via alternative mechanisms of action (Marzano et al. 2009). Transition metals represent the d-block element which includes groups 3–12 on the periodic table. Their d-electron shells are in the process of being filled. This property of transition metals led to the foundation of coordination complexes. A metal complex or coordination compound is a structure consisting of a central metal atom, bonded to a surrounding array of molecules or anions (Rafique et al. 2010). Transition metals exhibit different oxidation states and can interact with a number of biomolecules. This property of transition metals has encouraged the development of metal-based drugs with promising pharmacological application and may offer unique therapeutic opportunities. These trace metals are essential for the biological processes as about 30–40 % of all known proteins including metalloenzymes require metal cofactors (e.g., Fe, Cu, Zn, Ni, Mn) for their proper folding into an active three-dimensional (3-D) structure (Kastenholz 2006, 2007). Therefore, considerable effort has been now focused on the development of new anticancer drugs based on transition metal complexes, particularly biocompatible complexes, that bind to and cleave DNA under physiological conditions.

Our laboratories have been involved in synthesis, characterization, and studies on DNA binding, DNA cleavage, and anticancer property of transition metal complexes of iron(II), cobalt(II), nickel(II), and copper(II), metals which play biological roles and have physiological significance.

1 2 3 4

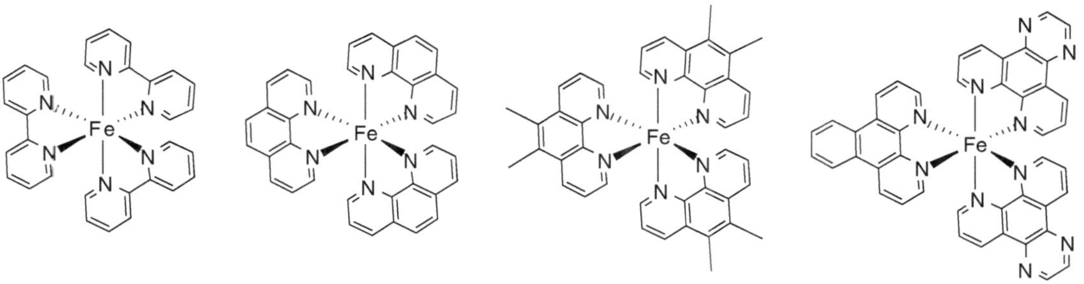

Scheme 11.1 Structures of *rac*-$[Fe(diimine)_3]^{2+}$ complexes

According to the classification of Zitka et al. (2012), all these metals are essential metals and occur in proteins. Herein we present a brief review of our recent work with special reference to DNA-binding and cleavage and anticancer properties.

11.1.1 Iron(II) Complexes

The trace element iron has important physiological roles in the body. It serves as an oxygen carrier from the lung to tissues by red blood cell hemoglobin, as a transport medium for electrons within cells, and as an integrated part of important enzyme systems in various tissues (Kastenholz 2007). Very recently, iron(II) chelators are emerging as a class of agents that show effective antitumor activity both in vitro and in vivo and can overcome resistance to standard chemotherapy (Torti et al. 1998; Bernhardt et al. 2003; Buss et al. 2004; Richardson 2005; Richardson et al. 2006; Kalinowski et al. 2007a, b). The anticancer properties of ferrocene-containing molecules have been studied (Fiorina et al. 1978). Iron(II) polypyridyl complexes cleave DNA by generating ROS in vitro (Wong et al. 2005). Recently, an iron(II) complex containing pentadentate pyridyl ligands has been found to exhibit a level of cytotoxicity higher than cisplatin (Wong et al. 2005).

Four mononuclear redox-active iron(II) complexes, namely, *rac*-$[Fe(diimine)_3]^{2+}$, where diimine = 2,2′-bipyridine (bpy) (**1**); 1,10-phenanthroline (phen) (**2**); 5,6-dimethyl-1,10-phenanthroline (5,6-dmp) (**3**); and dipyrido [3,2-*d*:2′,3′-*f*]quinoxaline (dpq) (**4**), have been synthesized in our laboratory (Scheme 11.1), and their DNA-binding and anticancer properties have been investigated (Ramakrishnan et al. 2011a). The use of 1,10-phenanthroline ligands in the complexes is of considerable interest because several ternary Ru(II) (Rajendiran et al. 2008) complexes of diimines strongly bind to DNA and exhibit prominent anticancer activities by inducing cell death. Also, substituted and modified 1,10-phenanthrolines, upon coordination to metal, play a vital role in DNA binding and in effecting conformational changes on DNA (Maheswari et al. 2006a; Ramakrishnan and Palaniandavar 2008).

All the four complexes have been screened against human breast carcinoma cell line (MCF-7) to understand the efficiency of these complexes in dealing with an ER-positive and p53-positive breast cancer. All the four iron(II) complexes were found to cleave pUC19 supercoiled DNA (SC DNA) in the presence of H_2O_2 as activator. These were active against MCF-7 breast carcinoma cell, but the 5,6-dmp complex **3** displayed prominent DNA binding through binding in the major groove of DNA and efficient DNA cleavage ability, which was higher than the other complexes even at low concentrations and in the presence of very low concentrations of H_2O_2. This complex exhibited cytotoxicity (IC_{50} at 24 h, 0.80 ± 0.04 μM; 48 h, 0.60 ± 0.03 μM) higher than the other complexes and also the widely used drug cisplatin, and induced apoptosis as

Scheme 11.2 Structures of *rac*-[Co(diimine)$_3$]$^{2+}$ complexes

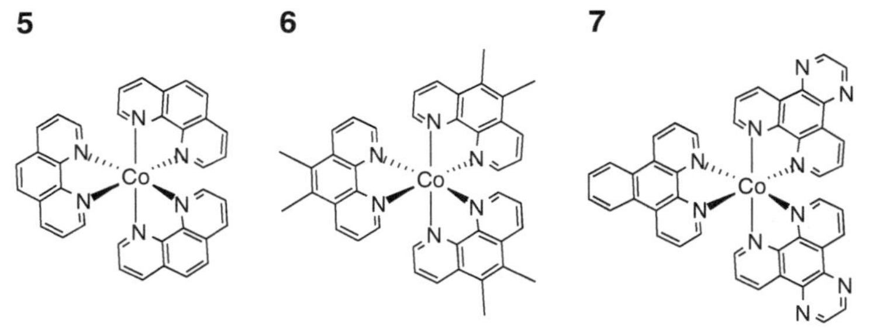

well as necroptosis, as revealed by morphological assessment data obtained by using AO/EB and Hoechst 33258 fluorescence staining methods. We suggest that the enhanced hydrophobicity conferred upon this complex by the 5,6-dmp co-ligand facilitates its transport through the cell membrane and its strong DNA binding as well as efficient DNA cleavage.

11.1.2 Cobalt(II) Complexes

Cobalt is recognized as an essential metal element widely distributed in the biological systems such as cells and body, and the interaction of cobalt(III) complexes of diimine (Barton and Raphael 1985; Tamilselvi and Palaniandavar 2002) and polypyridyl ligands with DNA has attracted considerable attention. The ability of a cobalt(II) complex to bind and nick plasmid DNA on photoactivation has been studied (Indumathy et al. 2008). The DNA-binding and photo-cleavage properties of certain Co(II) complexes have been recently reported (Sastri et al. 2003). We isolated three Co(II) complexes, namely, *rac*-[Co(diimine)$_3$]$^{2+}$, where diimine = 1,10-phenanthroline (phen) (**5**); 5,6-dimethyl-1,10-phenanthroline (5,6-dmp) (**6**); and dipyrido[3,2-*d*: 2′,3′-*f*]quinoxaline (dpq) (**7**) (Scheme 11.2), and characterized these complexes (Ramakrishnan et al. 2011b).

We investigated the role of diimine co-ligands on the mode and extent of DNA-binding and cleavage and cytotoxic properties of these complexes against breast carcinoma cell line MCF-7. The DNA-binding ability of *rac*-[Co(5,6-dmp)$_3$](ClO$_4$)$_2$ (**6**) was higher than the other two complexes. Interestingly, this complex binds to the major groove. Among the remaining two complexes, which bind to minor groove, the efficiency of *rac*-[Co(dpq)$_3$](ClO$_4$)$_2$ (**7**) was higher than *rac*-[Co(phen)$_3$](ClO$_4$)$_2$ (**5**). The DNA cleavage ability also follows the same order. The order of cytotoxicity of the complexes against breast carcinoma cell MCF-7 was **6** > **7** > **5**. All the three complexes induced cell death through both apoptosis and necrosis, but the complex *rac*-[Co(5,6-dmp)$_3$](ClO$_4$)$_2$ (**6**) was more aggressive than others, as revealed by morphological assessment data obtained by using AO/EB and Hoechst 33258 fluorescence staining methods.

11.1.3 Nickel(II) Complexes

Synthetic nickel(II) complexes have several potential applications in medicine, and very recently several nickel(II) complexes have been synthesized and tested for inhibition of cancer cell proliferation (Arguelles et al. 2004; Liang et al. 2004; Afrasiabi et al. 2005). Also, two closely related nickel(II) complexes have been shown to display different abilities toward DNA damage and cell viability (Matkar et al. 2006). Interestingly, nickel(II) complexes of the macrocyclic ligand [1,4,7] triazecan-9-ol act as potential antitumor agents (Liang et al. 2004). We isolated three tris(diimine)Ni(II) complexes, where diimine is 1,10-phenanthroline (phen) (**8**); 5,6-dimethyl-1,10-phenanthroline (5,6-dmp) (**9**); and dipyrido[3,2-*d*: 2′,3′-*f*]quinoxaline (dpq) (**10**) (Ramakrishnan et al. 2011b) (Scheme 11.3).

Scheme 11.3 Structures of *rac*-$[Ni(diimine)_3]^{2+}$ complexes

8 9 10

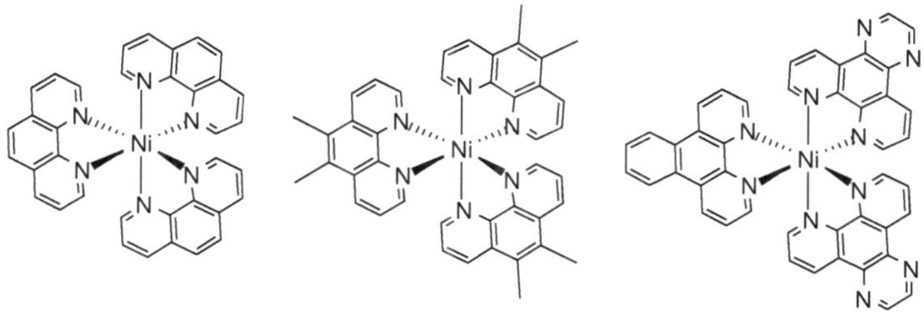

The role of diimine co-ligands on the mode and extent of DNA-binding and cleavage and anticancer activities of the complexes have been systematically investigated. The Ni(II) complexes displayed very strong DNA-binding activity. The binding ability of *rac*-$[Ni(5,6\text{-}dmp)_3](ClO_4)_2$ (**9**) is higher than other two complexes; among these two complexes, the binding of *rac*-$[Ni(dpq)_3](ClO_4)_2$ (**10**) is higher than *rac*-$[Ni(phen)_3](ClO_4)_2$ (**8**). The Ni(II) complexes **8**–**10** failed to cleave DNA as expected. Interestingly, Ni(II) complexes exhibited higher cytotoxicity (IC_{50} **8**, 8.0; **9**, 2.0; **10**, 2.0 μM at 48 h; IC_{50} **8**, 10.0; **9**, 3.0; **10**, 3.0 μM at 24 h) against human breast cancer (MCF 7) cell line than cisplatin. Also, the 5,6-dmp complex (**9**) showed cytotoxicity higher than the dpq complex (**10**) at 24 h incubation time, and all the compounds caused mostly apoptotic and to a certain extent necrotic modes of cell death.

11.1.4 Copper(II) Complexes

Copper(II) complexes are considered the best alternatives to cisplatin because copper is biocompatible and exhibits many significant roles in biological systems. Copper is found in all living organisms and is a crucial trace element in redox chemistry, growth, and development. It is important for the function of several enzymes and proteins involved in energy metabolism, respiration, and DNA synthesis, notably cytochrome oxidase, superoxide dismutase, ascorbate oxidase, and tyrosinase. The major functions of copper containing biological molecules involve oxidation-reduction reactions in which they react directly with molecular oxygen to produce free radicals (Tisato et al. 2010). Among non-Pt compounds, copper complexes are potentially attractive as anticancer agents. Actually, for many years a lot of researchers have actively investigated copper compounds based on the assumption that endogenous metals may be less toxic (Marzano et al. 2009). It has been established that the properties of copper-coordinated compounds are largely determined by the nature of ligands and donor atoms bound to the metal ion.

In recent years, several families of copper complexes have been studied as potential antitumor agents. Although only a little understanding of the molecular basis of their mechanism of action has been documented, copper complexes have attracted attention based on modes of action different from that of cisplatin (covalent binding to DNA). Therefore, copper complexes may provide a broader spectrum of antitumor activity (Marzano et al. 2009). Synthetic copper(II) complexes have been reported to act as pharmacological agents and as potential anticancer and cancer-inhibiting agents (Fernandes et al. 2006; Maheswari et al. 2006b). Very recently, certain mixed-ligand copper(II) complexes, which strongly bind and cleave DNA, have been shown to exhibit prominent anticancer activities and regulate apoptosis (Zhang et al. 2004).

11.1.4.1 Mononuclear Mixed-Ligand Copper(II) Complexes

a) Copper(II) Complexes of a Tridentate Phenolate Ligand

The new mononuclear copper(II) complexes $[Cu(L)(H_2O)_2]^+$ (**11**) and $[Cu(L)(diimine)]^+$ (**12**–**16**), where LH = 2-[(2-dimethylaminoethylimino)methyl]phenol and diimine = 2,2′-bipyridine (bpy) (**12**) or 1,10-phenanthroline

Scheme 11.4 Structures of copper(II) complexes of tridentate phenolate ligand

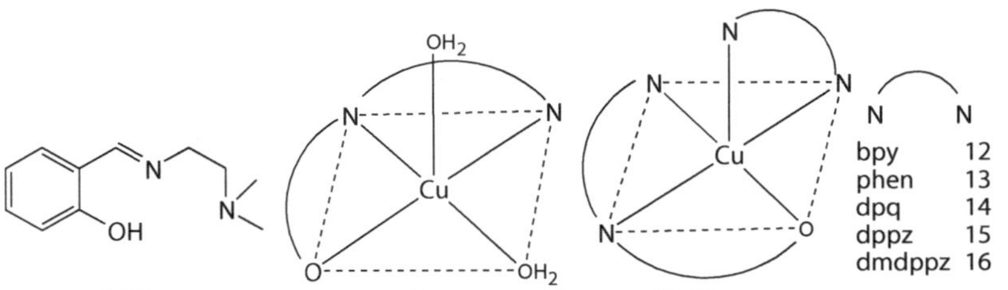

H(L) 11 12-16

Scheme 11.5 Structures of copper(II) complexes of tetradentate phenolate ligand

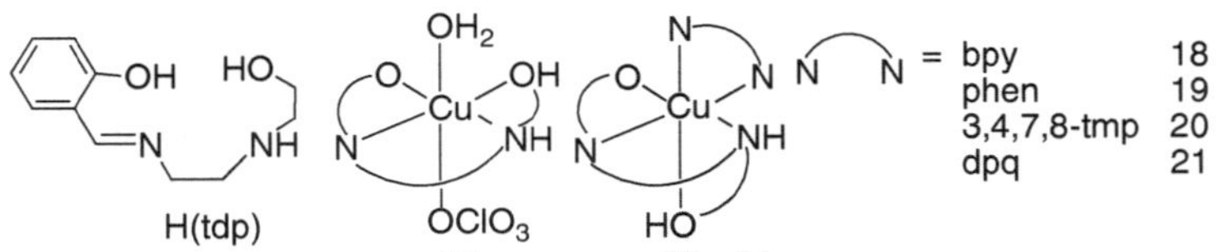

H(tdp) 17 18 - 21

(phen) (**13**) or dipyrido[3,2-*f*:2′,3′-*h*]quinoxaline (dpq) (**14**) or dipyrido[3,2-*a*:2′,3′-*c*]phenazine (dppz) (**15**) or 11,12-dimethyldipyrido[3,2-*a*:2′,3′-*c*]phenazine (dmdppz) (**16**) (Scheme 11.4), have been isolated and characterized (Jaividhya et al. 2012). All the complexes, except **12**, caused double-strand DNA cleavage of plasmid DNA and **15** cleaved plasmid DNA in the absence of a reductant at a concentration (40 μM) lower than **14**. It is remarkable that all the complexes displayed cytotoxicity against human breast cancer cell (MCF-7) and human cervical epidermoid carcinoma cell (ME 180) with potency higher than the currently used chemotherapeutic agent cisplatin and that **15** exhibited cytotoxicity higher than the other complexes.

b) Copper(II) Complexes of a Tetradentate Phenolate Ligand

The copper(II) complex [Cu(tdp)(ClO_4)] 0.5H_2O (**17**), where H(tdp) is the tetradentate ligand 2-[(2-(2-hydroxyethylamino)-ethylimino)methyl] phenol, and the mixed-ligand complexes [Cu(tdp)(diimine)]$^+$ (**18–21**), where diimine is 2,2′-bipyridine (bpy) (**18**); 1,10-phenanthroline (phen) (**19**); 3,4,7,8-tetramethyl-1, 10-phenanthroline (3,4,7,8-tmp) (**20**); and dipyrido[3,2-*d*: 2′,3′-*f*]quinoxaline (dpq) (**21**) (Scheme 11.5), have been isolated and characterized (Rajendiran et al. 2007).

All the complexes hydrolytically cleaved supercoiled DNA in the absence of an activating agent, and the cleavage efficiency was in the order **21** > **19** > **18** > **20** > **17**. The anticancer activity of the complexes on human cervical epidermoid carcinoma cell line (ME180) was examined. Interestingly, the observed IC_{50} values reveal that complex **20**, which caused conformational change on DNA and bound to bovine serum albumin (BSA) more strongly, exhibited cytotoxicity higher than other complexes. It also exhibited approximately 100 and 6 times more potency than cisplatin and mitomycin C for 24 and 48 h incubation times, respectively, suggesting that complex **20** can be explored further as a potential anticancer drug. Complexes **20** and **21** mediated the arrest of cells at S and G2/M phases in the cell cycle progression at 24 h harvesting time, where the cells progressed into apoptosis.

c) Copper(II) Complexes of L-tyrosine

The mononuclear mixed-ligand copper(II) complexes of the type [Cu(L-tyr)(diimine)](ClO_4), where L-tyr is L-tyrosine and diimine is 2,2′-bipyridine (bpy) (**22**); 1,10-phenanthroline (phen) (**23**); 5,6-dimethyl-1,10-phenanthroline (5,6-dmp) (**24**); and dipyrido[3,2-*d*:2′,3′-*f*] quinoxaline (dpq) (**25**) (Scheme 11.6), have been isolated and characterized (Ramakrishnan et al. 2009).

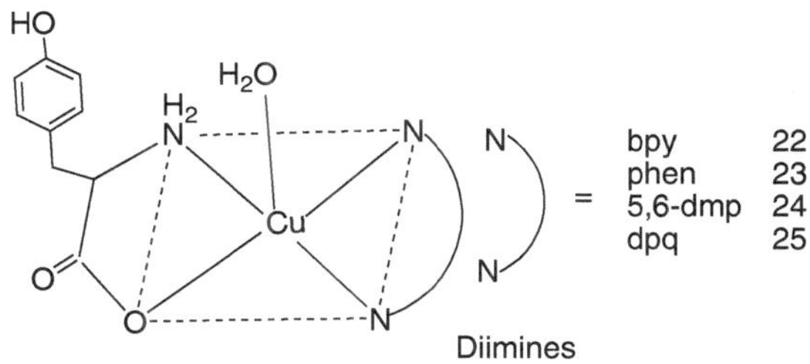

Scheme 11.6 Structures of copper(II) complexes of L-tyrosinate ligand

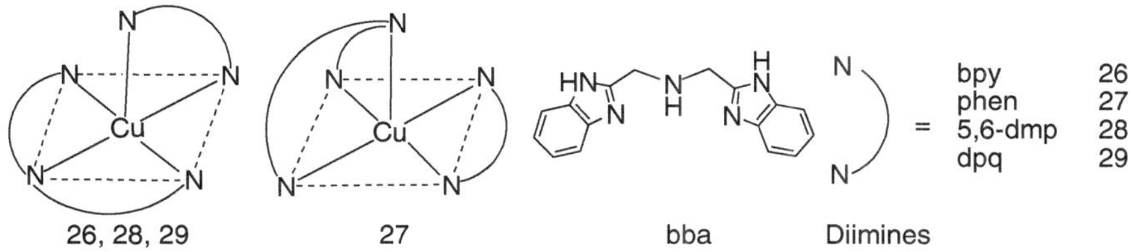

Scheme 11.7 Structures of copper(II) complexes of tridentate 3N donor ligand

All the complexes produced effective DNA (pUC19 DNA) cleavage at 100 μM concentration, and the order of DNA cleavage ability varied as **24** > **23** > **25** > **22**. Interestingly, complex **25** exhibited a DNA cleavage rate constant which was higher than that of the other complexes. Also, cytotoxicity studies on the non-small cell lung cancer (H-460) cell line showed that the IC_{50} values of **23**–**25** are more or less equal to cisplatin for the same cell line, indicating that they have the potential to act as very effective anticancer drugs in a time-dependent manner. The study of cytological changes revealed the higher induction of apoptosis and mitotic catastrophe for **25** and **24**, respectively. The alkaline single-cell gel electrophoresis (comet assay), DNA laddering, and AO/EB and Hoechst 33258 staining assays indicate that the DNA damage occurs to different extents. Flow cytometry analysis shows an increase in the percentage of cells with apoptotic morphological features in the sub-G0/G1 phase for **25**, while **24** shows mitotic catastrophe.

d) Copper(II) Complexes of *N,N*-Bis(Benzimidazol-2-Ylmethyl)Amine

Metal complexes containing benzimidazole (bzim) ligand moieties form an important class of biologically active compounds that can efficiently hydrolyze phosphodiester bond and cleave supercoiled pBR322 DNA (Tanious et al. 2004). Also, ligands incorporating bzim moieties selectively interact with a specific nucleotide sequence and bind to the minor groove of A–T tract duplex DNA (Teng et al. 1988; Pjura et al. 1987; Aymami et al. 1999; Parkinson et al. 1990), and a bzim unit provides a conformationally stable and appropriate platform on which to build further DNA sequence recognition (Wahnon et al. 1994). The design of a molecule, which can effect double-strand DNA cleavage, must include a reactivatable metal center like copper and also recognition elements that bind to duplex DNA and at nicked sites as well.

A series of mononuclear mixed-ligand copper(II) complexes $[Cu(bba)(diimine)](ClO_4)_2$ **26**–**29**, where bba is *N*,*N*-bis(benzimidazol-2-ylmethyl)amine and diimine is 2,2′-bipyridine (bpy) (**26**); 1,10-phenanthroline (phen) (**27**); 5,6-dimethyl-1,10-phenanthroline (5,6-dmp) (**28**); or dipyrido[3,2-*d*:2′,3′-*f*]-quinoxaline (dpq) (**29**) (Scheme 11.7), have been isolated by us and characterized (Loganathan et al. 2012).

Absorption spectral titrations with calf thymus (CT) DNA reveal that the intrinsic DNA-binding affinity of the complexes depends upon the diimine co-ligand, dpq (**29**) > 5,6-dmp (**28**) > phen (**27**) > bpy (**26**). All the complexes exhibited oxidative DNA cleavage ability, which varied as **29** > **28** > **27** > **26** (ascorbic acid) and **28** > **27** > **29** > **26** (H_2O_2). Also, the complexes

Scheme 11.8 Structures of dinuclear copper(II) complexes of benzamide ligand

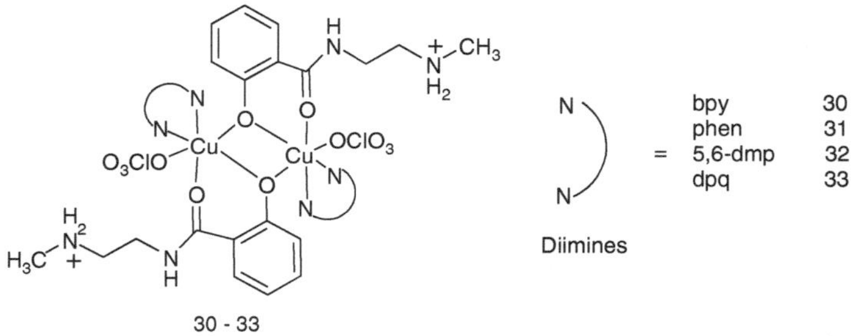

cleaved bovine serum albumin in the presence of H_2O_2 as an activator with the cleavage ability varying in the order **28** > **29** > **27** > **26**. The highest efficiency of **28** to cleave both DNA and protein in the presence of H_2O_2 is consistent with its strong hydrophobic interaction with the biopolymers. The IC_{50} values of complexes **26**–**29** against cervical cancer cell (SiHa) were almost equal to that of cisplatin, indicating that they have the potential to act as effective anticancer drugs in a time-dependent manner. The morphological assessment data obtained by using acridine orange/ethidium bromide (AO/EB) and Hoechst 33258 staining revealed that complex **28** induces apoptosis much more effectively than the other complexes. Also, the alkaline single-cell gel electrophoresis study (comet assay) suggests that the same complex induced DNA fragmentation more efficiently than others.

11.1.4.2 Dinuclear Mixed-Ligand Copper(II) Complexes

The copper centers in some multinuclear complexes act synergistically to cleave DNA with higher efficiency or selectivity (Humphreys et al. 2002; Alvarez et al. 2003; Li et al. 2005). Karlin and co-workers (Humpreys et al. 2002; Li et al. 2005) have shown that nuclearity is a crucial parameter in oxidative DNA cleavage, with the synergy between the metal ions contributing to the high nucleolytic efficiency of polynuclear copper(II) compounds. Therefore, designing suitable multinuclear copper complexes for DNA binding and cleavage under both oxidative and hydrolytic conditions, depending upon the recognition elements in the ligand, is of remarkable importance in considering the advantages of processes that produce fragments similar to those formed by restriction enzymes (Humphreys et al. 2002; Li et al. 2005). So, we synthesized four new copper(II) complexes (Scheme 11.8) and examined their cytotoxicity.

The dinuclear copper(II) complexes $[Cu_2(LH)_2(diimine)_2(ClO_4)_2](ClO_4)_2$ (**30**–**33**), where LH = 2-hydroxy-*N*-[2-(methylamino) ethyl] benzamide and diimine = 2,2′-bipyridine (bpy, **30**); 1,10-phenanthroline (phen, **31**); 5,6-dimethyl-1,10-phenanthroline (5,6-dmp, **32**); and dipyrido [3,2-*d*:2′,3′-*f*]quinoxaline (dpq, **33**) (Scheme 11.8), have been isolated and characterized (Ramakrishnan et al. 2010).

Complex **33** interacts with calf thymus DNA more strongly than all other complexes through strong partial intercalation of the extended planar ring (dpq) with a DNA base stack. Interestingly, **32** exhibited a DNA-binding affinity higher than **31**, suggesting the involvement in hydrophobic interaction of coordinated 5,6-dmp with the DNA surface. All the four complexes exhibited prominent DNA cleavage even at very low concentrations (nM) in the presence of H_2O_2 as an activator, with the order of cleavage efficiency being **32** > **31** > **33** > **30**. Studies on the anticancer activity toward HEp-2 human larynx cell line revealed that the ability of the complexes to kill the cancer cells varied as **32** > **33** > **31** > **30**. Also, interestingly, the IC_{50} value of **32** was lower than that of cisplatin, suggesting that the hydrophobicity of methyl groups on 5 and 6 positions of the complex enhances the anticancer activity. The mode of cell death brought about by the complex was explored by using various biochemical techniques like comet assay, mitochondrial membrane potency, and Western blotting. The 5,6-dmp complex was found to induce nuclear condensation and fragmentation in the cancer cell. Also, it triggered the activation of caspases by releasing cytochrome *c* from mitochondria to cytosol, suggesting that it induces apoptosis in cells via the mitochondrial pathway.

11.2 Conclusions

From a physiological point of view, biologically active metals can be divided into two groups: (1) essential metals, which are crucial for numerous biochemical processes, and (2) toxic metals, which are harmful to the body (Zitka et al. 2012). All the four essential metals we dealt with, namely, iron, cobalt, nickel, and copper, are expected to produce no or little side effect. The most efficacious complexes we studied, tris(diimine)metal(II), where metal = Fe, Ni, Co, Cu, can be considered as potential leads for further study to find the mechanism of entry into the cell, since study of metal ion transport in humans is the most intense one in the area of effects of metallodrugs on an organism, and the mechanism of action in bringing about the medicinal effect. The anticancer activity of the mixed-ligand complexes depends on both the primary and diimine co-ligands. This review brings out a very important finding that ligand hydrophobicity plays a vital role in the induction of cell death. Interestingly, among tris(diimine) metal(II) complexes and the mixed-ligand copper(II) complexes of the primary ligands tdp, L-tyr, bba, amide, and phenolate ligand, those with 5,6-dmp co-ligand show apoptotic activity higher than those with other co-ligands, irrespective of the cancer cell line used due to the enhanced permeability of the 5,6-dmp complex across the cell membrane. Also, it emerges from our present study that DNA cleavage activity is not a requisite for a drug to act as an anticancer agent, as the tris(diimine)Ni(II) complexes (**8–10**) exhibit more prominent cytotoxicity than their cobalt(II) analogues (**5–7**), but it does not show DNA cleavage activity.

Acknowledgments Professor M. A. Akbarsha is Gandhi-Gruber-Doerenkamp Chair of Doerenkamp-Zbinden Foundation (DZF), Switzerland, and also Visiting Professor to King Saud University, Kingdom of Saudi Arabia. Professor M. Palaniandavar is a recipient of Ramanna National Fellowship of the Department of Science and Technology (DST), Government of India, New Delhi (SR/S1/RFIC/01/2007-2010 and SR/S1/RFIC/01/2010-2013). A. Riyasdeen and R. Loganathan are Senior Research Fellows of the Council of Scientific and Industrial Research (CSIR), Government of India, New Delhi (CSIR/09/475(0163)/2010-EMR-1 and CSIR/09/475(0169)/2012-EMR-I, respectively). The financial assistance from these various sources/agencies is gratefully acknowledged.

References

Afrasiabi Z, Sinn E, Lin W, Ma Y, Campana C, Padhye S (2005) Nickel (II) complexes of naphthaquinone thiosemicarbazone and semicarbazone: synthesis, structure, spectroscopy, and biological activity. J Inorg Biochem 99:1526–1531

Alvarez MG, Alzuet G, Borras J, Macias B, Castineiras A (2003) Oxidative cleavage of DNA by a new ferromagnetic linear trinuclear copper(II) complex in the presence of H_2O_2/sodium ascorbate. Inorg Chem 42:2992–2998

Arguelles RMC, Ferrari MB, Biscegli F, Pellizi C, Pelosi G, Pinelli S, Sassi M (2004) Synthesis, characterization and biological activity of Ni, Cu and Zn complexes of isatin hydrazones. J Inorg Biochem 98: 313–321

Aymami J, Nunn CM, Neidle S (1999) DNA minor groove recognition of a non-self-complementary AT-rich sequence by a tris-benzimidazole ligand. Nucl Acid Res 27:2691–2698

Barton JK, Raphael A (1985) Site-specific cleavage of left-handed DNA in pBR322 by lambda-tris (diphenylphenanthroline) cobalt(III). Proc Natl Acad Sci USA 82:6460–6464

Bernhardt PV, Caldwell LM, Chaston TB, Chin P, Richardson DR (2003) Cytotoxic iron chelators: characterization of the structure, solution chemistry and redox activity of ligands and iron complexes of the di-2-pyridyl ketone isonicotinoyl hydrazone (HPKIH) analogues. J Biol Inorg Chem 8:866–880

Bharti SK, Singh SK (2009) Recent developments in the field of anticancer metallopharmaceuticals. Int J Pharm Tech Res 1:1406–1420

Boulikas T, Pantos A, Bellis E, Christofis P (2007) Designing platinum compounds in cancer: structures and mechanisms. Cancer Ther 5:537–583

Buss JL, Greene BT, Turner J, Torti FM, Torti SV (2004) Iron chelators in cancer chemotherapy. Curr Top Med Chem 4:1623–1635

Fernandes C, Parrilha GL, Lessa JA, Santiago LJM, Kanashiro MM, Boniolo FS, Bortoluzzi AJ, Vugman

NV, Herbst MH, Horn A (2006) Synthesis, crystal structure, nuclease and in vitro antitumor activities of a new mononuclear copper (II) complex containing a tripodal N30 ligand. J Inorg Chim Acta 359: 3167–3176

Fiorina VJ, Dubois RJ, Brynes S (1978) Ferrocenyl polyamines as agents for the chemoimmunotherapy of cancer. J Med Chem 21:393–395

Humphreys KJ, Karlin KD, Rokita SE (2002a) Efficient and specific strand scission of DNA by a dinuclear copper complex: comparative reactivity of complexes with linked tris(2-pyridylmethyl)amine moieties. J Am Chem Soc 124:6009–6019

Humpreys KJ, Hohnson AJ, Karlin KD, Rokita SE (2002) Oxidative strand scission of nucleic acids by a multinuclear copper II) complex. J Biol Inorg Chem 7: 835–842

Indumathy R, Kanthimathi M, Weyhermuller T, Nair BU (2008) Cobalt complexes of terpyridine ligands: crystal structure and nuclease activity. Polyhedron 27:3443–3450

Jaividhya P, Dhivya R, Akbarsha MA, Palaniandavar M (2012) Efficient DNA cleavage mediated by mononuclear mixed ligand copper (II) phenolate complexes: the role of co-ligand planarity on DNA binding and cleavage and anticancer activity. J Inorg Biochem 114:94–105

Kalinowski DS, Sharpe PC, Bernhardt PV, Richardson DR (2007a) Design, synthesis, and characterization of new iron chelators with anti-proliferative activity: structure-activity relationships of novel thiohydrazone analogues. J Med Chem 50: 6212–6225

Kalinowski DS, Yu Y, Sharpe PC, Islam M, Liao YT, Lovejoy DB, Kumar N, Bernhardt PV, Richardson DR (2007b) Design, synthesis, and characterization of novel iron chelators: structure-activity relationships of the 2-benzoylpyridine thiosemicarbazone series and their 3-nitrobenzoyl analogues as potent antitumor agents. J Med Chem 50:3716–3729

Kastenholz B (2006) Important contributions of a new quantitative preparative native continuous polyacrylamide gel electrophoresis (QPNC-PAGE) procedure for elucidating metal cofactor metabolisms in protein-misfolding diseases – a theory. Protein Peptide Lett 13:503–508

Kastenholz B (2007) New hope for the diagnosis and therapy of Alzheimer's disease. Protein Peptide Lett 14:389–393

Li L, Karlin KD, Rokita SE (2005) Changing selectivity of DNA oxidation from deoxyribose to guanine by ligand design and a new binuclear copper complex. J Am Chem Soc 127:520–521

Liang F, Wang P, Zhou X, Li T, Li Z, Lin H, Gao D, Zheng C, Wu C (2004) Nickel(II) and cobalt(II) complexes of hydroxyl-substituted triazamacrocyclic ligand as potential antitumor agents. Bioorg Med Chem Lett 14:1901–1904

Loganathan R, Ramakrishnan S, Suresh E, Riyasdeen A, Akbarsha MA, Palaniandavar M (2012) Mixed ligand copper(II) complexes of *N,N*-bis(benzimidazol-2-ylmethyl)amine (BBA) with diimine co-ligands: efficient chemical nuclease and protease activities and cytotoxicity. Inorg Chem 51:5512–5532

Maheswari PU, Rajendran V, Evans HS, Palaniandavar M (2006a) Interaction of *rac*-$[Ru(5,6\text{-dmp})_3]^{2+}$ with DNA: Enantiospecific DNA binding and ligand-promoted exciton coupling. Inorg Chem 45:37–50

Maheswari UP, Roy S, Dulk HD, Barends S, Wezel GV, Kozlevcar B, Gamez P, Reedijk JJ (2006b) The square-planar cytotoxic [Cu(II)(pyrimol)Cl] complex acts as an efficient DNA cleaver without reductant. J Am Chem Soc 128:710–711

Marzano C, Pellei M, Tisato F, Santini C (2009) Copper complexes as anticancer agents. Anti-Cancer Agent Med Chem 9:185–211

Matkar S, Wrischnik LA, Jones PR, Blumberg UH (2006) Two closely related nickel complexes have different effects on DNA damage and cell viability. Biochem Biophys Res Commun 343:754–761

Parkinson JA, Barber J, Douglas KT, Rosamond J, Sharples D (1990) Minor-groove recognition of the self-complementary duplex d(CGCGAATTCGCG)2 by Hoechst 33258: a high-field NMR study. Biochemistry 29:10181–10190

Pjura PE, Grzeskowiak K, Dickerson RE (1987) Binding of Hoechst 33258 to the minor groove of B-DNA. J Mol Biol 197:257–271

Rafique S, Idrees M, Nasim A, Akbar H, Athar A (2010) Transition metal complexes as potential therapeutic agents. Biotech Mol Bio Rev 5:38–45

Rajendiran V, Karthik R, Palaniandavar M, Evans HS, Periasamay VS, Akbarsha MA, Srinag BS, Krishnamurthy H (2007) Mixed-ligand copper(II)-phenolate complexes: effect of co-ligand on enhanced DNA and protein binding, DNA cleavage, and anticancer activity. Inorg Chem 46:8208–8221

Rajendiran V, Murali M, Suresh E, Palaniandavar M, Periasamy VS, Akbarsha MA (2008) Non-covalent DNA binding and cytotoxicity of certain mixed-ligand ruthenium(II) complexes of 2,2-dipyridylamine and diimines. Dalton Trans 28:2157–2170

Ramakrishnan S, Palaniandavar M (2008) Interaction of rac-$[Cu(diimine)_3]^{2+}$ and rac-$[Zn(diimine)_3]^{2+}$ complexes with CT DNA: effect of fluxional Cu(II) geometry on DNA binding, ligand-promoted exciton coupling and prominent DNA cleavage. Dalton Trans 29:3866–3878

Ramakrishnan S, Rajendiran V, Palaniandavar M, Periasamay VS, Akbarsha MA, Srinag BS, Krishnamurthy H (2009) Induction of cell death by ternary copper(II) complexes of L-tyrosine and diimines: role of coligands on DNA binding and cleavage and anticancer activity. Inorg Chem 48:1309–1322

Ramakrishnan S, Shakthipriya D, Suresh E, Periasamy VS, Akbarsha MA, Palaniandavar M (2010) Ternary dinuclear copper(II) complexes of a hydroxybenzamide ligand with diimine coligands: the 5,6-dmp ligand enhances DNA binding and cleavage and induces apoptosis. Inorg Chem 50:6458–6471

Ramakrishnan S, Suresh E, Riyasdeen A, Akbarsha MA, Palaniandavar M (2011a) DNA binding, prominent DNA cleavage and efficient anticancer activities of tris(diimine)iron(II) complexes. Dalton Trans 40:3524–3536

Ramakrishnan S, Suresh E, Riyasdeen A, Akbarsha MA, Palaniandavar M (2011b) Interaction of *rac*-$[M(diimine)_3]^{2+}$ ($M = Co$, Ni) complexes with CT DNA: role of 5,6-dmp ligand on DNA binding and cleavage and cytotoxicity. Dalton Trans 40:3245–3256

Richardson DR (2005) Molecular mechanisms of iron uptake by cells and the use of iron chelators for the treatment of cancer. Curr Med Chem 12:2711–2729

Richardson DR, Sharpe PC, Lovejoy DB, Senaratne D, Kalinowski DS, Islam M, Bernhardt PV (2006) Dipyridyl thiosemicarbazone chelators with potent and selective antitumor activity form iron complexes with redox activity. J Med Chem 49:6510–6521

Sastri CV, Eswaramoorthy D, Giribabu L, Maiya BG (2003) DNA interactions of new mixed-ligand complexes of cobalt(III) and nickel(II) that incorporate modified phenanthroline ligands. J Inorg Biochem 94:138–145

Tamilselvi P, Palaniandavar M (2002) Spectral, viscometric and electrochemical studies on mixed ligand cobalt(III) complexes of certain diimine ligands bound to calf thymus DNA. Inorg Chim Acta 337:420–428

Tanious FA, Hamelberg D, Bailly C, Czarny A, Boykin DW, Wilson WD (2004) DNA sequence dependent monomer-dimer binding modulation of asymmetric benzimidazole derivatives. J Am Chem Soc 126: 143–153

Teng MK, Usman N, Frederick CA, Wang AHJ (1988) The molecular structure of the complex of Hoechst 33258 and the DNA dodecamer d(CGCGAATTCGCG). Nucl Acid Res 16: 2671–2690

Tisato F, Marzano C, Porchia M, Pellei M, Santini C (2010) Copper in diseases and treatments, and copper-based anticancer strategies. Med Res Rev 30: 708–749

Torti SV, Torti FM, Whitman SP, Brechbiel MW, Park G, Planalp RP (1998) Tumor cell cytotoxicity of a novel metal chelator. Blood 92:1384–1389

Wahnon D, Hynes RC, Chin J (1994) Dramatic ligand effect in copper(II) complex promoted transesterification of a phosphate diester. J Chem Soc Chem Commun 12:1441–1442

Wong EL, Fang GS, Che CM, Zhu NY (2005) Highly cytotoxic iron(II) complexes with pentadentate pyridyl ligands as a new class of anti-tumor agents. Chem Commun 36:4578–4580

Zhang CX, Lippard SJ (2003) New metal complexes as potential therapeutics. Curr Opin Chem Biol 7: 481–489

Zhang S, Zhu Y, Tu C, Wei H, Yang Z, Lin L, Ding J, Zhang J, Guo Z (2004) A novel cytotoxic ternary copper(II) complex of 1,10-phenanthroline and L-threonine with DNA nuclease activity. J Inorg Biochem 98:2099–2106

Zitka O, Ryvolova M, Hubalek J, Eckschlager T, Adam V, Rene K (2012) From amino acids to proteins as targets for metal-based drugs. Curr Drug Metab 13: 306–320

12 Why Is Gallbladder Cancer Common in the Gangetic Belt?

Ruhi Dixit and V.K. Shukla

Abstract

Carcinoma of the gallbladder (CaGB) is the commonest malignancy of the biliary tract. There is wide variation in the incidence of carcinoma of the gallbladder in India ranging from 1.2 per 100,000 for males and 0.9 per 100,000 for females in southern India to 4.5 per 100,000 males and 10.6 per 100,000 females in northern India. The incidence is highest in eastern Uttar Pradesh and western Bihar regions of India. This wide geographical variation in the incidence of carcinoma of the gallbladder suggests that environmental factors might be playing an important role in its causation. Both these regions lie downstream of the river Ganges which is the main source of water for all uses such as drinking water and for irrigation. The river Ganges receives an extremely high load of pollutants in the form of untreated domestic sewage, industrial and agricultural effluents containing aromatic hydrocarbons, nitrosamines and chemicals such as nitrates and nitrites which are by-products from domestic sewage. Pesticides which are frequently used in agricultural industry can also play a role in CaGB. Typhoid infection is prevalent in this region which may also be associated with the gallbladder carcinogenesis. Lifestyle and smoking have also been correlated with the CaGB. Adulteration in our cooking oil (mustard) by sanguinarine and diethylnitrosamine has also been found to be linked with CaGB. It is possible that carcinoma of the gallbladder is the disease of multifactorial etiology.

Keywords

Gallbladder cancer • Gangetic belt • Cholelithiasis • Heavy metals

12.1 Introduction

Gallbladder cancer (GBC) is the third most common gastrointestinal neoplasm and it is mostly common in northern India (Shukla et al. 1985).

R. Dixit • V.K. Shukla (✉)
Department of General Surgery, Institute of Medical Sciences, Banaras Hindu University, Varanasi 221 005, India
e-mail: vkshuklabhu@gmail.com

P.R. Sudhakaran (ed.), *Perspectives in Cancer Prevention – Translational Cancer Research*, DOI 10.1007/978-81-322-1533-2_12, © Springer India 2014

A survey by the Indian Council of Medical Research (ICMR) described that the incidence of GBC in women in northern India is one of the highest in the world (National Cancer Registry Programme 2002). We can find a wide geographical variation in the incidence of GBC in India. It actually varies from 1.2 per 10,000 for males and 0.9 per 10,000 for females in northern India. Its occurrence is higher in the eastern UP and western Bihar regions of India. These regions are situated near the river Ganges. This river water might be an important factor for the GBC incidence in such areas only. River Ganges is the prime source of water in these areas for drinking water and irrigation. The river Ganges is highly polluted with industrial waste, domestic sewage and agriculture effluents. Such environmental factors also play a role in the gallbladder carcinogenesis in these regions. The Ganges water usually consists of pollutants like pesticides; heavy metals such as cadmium, chromium and lead; and industrial wastes having aromatic hydrocarbon and nitrosamines and chemicals (nitrates and nitrites) which are by-products from domestic sewage (Gupta et al. 2005a, b). Various factors play a role in GBC as it is mentioned in a study that there is no single agent for gallbladder carcinogenesis, but it is known to be a disease of multifactorial aetiology (Kowalewski and Todd 1971). Following are the factors which might be playing a role in gallbladder carcinogenesis.

12.1.1 Metallothionein

Metallothionein (MT) is the low molecular weight metal-binding protein mostly present in the liver, kidneys, heart, testes and brain. MT usually binds to heavy metals by making clusters of thiolate bonds. They store these MT ions in the liver and play a protective role against heavy metal toxicity (Kägi and Kojima 1987; Freedman and Peisach 1989; Frazier and Din 1987; Liu et al. 1990). It has been reported in experimental model that normal tissues which are deficient of MT are more prone to cadmium (Cd) carcinogens (Frazier and Din 1987; Liu et al. 1990). Therefore, we look for the expression of MT in GBC in comparison to cholelithiasis and normal gallbladder. The results of this study showed an increased expression of MT in GBC. It's overexpression has also been reported in breast, gastric and oesophageal cancers (Schmid et al. 1993; Monden et al. 1997; Hishikawa et al. 1997). Heavy metals like cadmium are excreted and concentrated by the hepatobiliary system. Those tissues which show low or no expression of MT were more susceptible to Cd carcinogenesis as MT prevents such tissues from heavy metal toxicity. Thus, we concluded from this study that high-level expression of MT in GBC cases may indirectly reflect the exposure to Cd and other heavy metal toxicity and their higher concentration in the gallbladder. Content of heavy metals like Cd found to be at a higher concentration in the potable water samples studied in Varanasi region (Krishnamurti and Vishwanathan 1990) has been reported, where GBC is so common, and, therefore, this may also be an aetiological factor of GBC in this part of India (Shukla et al. 1998a, b).

12.1.2 Heavy Metals and Gallbladder Cancer

Ganges receives domestic sewage and industrial agriculture effluent. High concentrations of certain heavy metals are found in sewage, irrigation and potable water. It has been reported that high concentration of cadmium and other heavy metals is found to be present in water from such region. These heavy metals have also been found to be implicated in cancer progression (Leonard 1983). We also tried to see the association of GBC with exposure to heavy metals. Cadmium, chromium and lead concentrations were estimated in GBC, cholelithiasis and healthy control. Their concentrations were significantly higher in carcinoma of the gallbladder in comparison to gallstones. These metals were also found in drinking water of such region which confirms the hypothesis. They are known as the chemical carcinogens; therefore, we reported that their high biliary concentration in GBC patients might be a causing factor of gallbladder cancer (Shukla et al. 1998a, b).

12.1.3 Micronutrients

Micronutrients can also be a factor modifying the multistage process of carcinogenesis. Various studies have shown that deficiency of micronutrients is found to be associated with cancer. Cases of gallbladder cancer (I), cholelithiasis (II) and healthy controls (III) were included in a study. Selenium (Se), zinc (Zn), copper (Cu), manganese (Mn), ascorbic acid (vitamin C) and alpha-tocopherol (vitamin E) concentrations were estimated in serum, bile and gallbladder tissue in groups I and II and only serum in group III. We have found low serum, biliary and tissue concentrations of Se, Zn and vitamin E in patients having GBC in comparison to cholelithiasis. Earlier study on heavy metals from one group has shown higher biliary concentrations of cadmium (Cd), chromium (Cr) and lead (Pb) in carcinoma of the gallbladder. They are known chemical carcinogen. This, when associated with the reduced levels of protective micronutrients like Se, Zn and vitamin E, is involved in preventing damage to membrane lipids, protein and nucleic acids by acting as free radical scavenger; this could further promote the multistage process of carcinogenesis (Shukla et al. 2003).

Other than micronutrients, there exist some other trace elements such as copper (Cu) and zinc (Zn) which can play a role in carcinogenesis. An elevated serum copper and low zinc levels have been found in various cancers like in breast cancer (Garofalo et al. 1980; Gupta et al. 1991), gastrointestinal tract cancer (Inutsuka and Araki 1978; Gupta et al. 1993) and lymphomas (Margerison and Mann 1985). In a similar way, zinc serum levels have been found to be decreased in different malignancies (Garofalo et al. 1980; Gupta et al. 1991, 1993, 2005a, b; Inutsuka and Araki 1978; Margerison and Mann 1985; Gray et al. 1982). Therefore, we have demonstrated alteration in the serum, biliary and tissue levels of Cu and Zn in patients with GBC and cholelithiasis. We concluded that patients with GBC show alterations in the Cu and Zn levels of serum and tissue. Thus, Cu/Zn ratio could also be a factor for the prevalence of this gallbladder disease in northern part of India.

12.1.4 Nitrate and Nitrite

India is an agriculture-based country. In recent years, use of nitrate-based fertilizers has been increased. Thus, it leads to high intake of nitrate through drinking water and vegetables. We found a higher biliary concentration of nitrate in GBC patients in comparison to cholelithiasis in our study. Similar results have also been shown in gastric cancer, brain tumours and hepatocellular carcinoma (Fraser et al. 1980). The high nitrate content in bile may be converted to nitrite and in turn nitrosamine which is known to be carcinogenic and could initiate gallbladder carcinogenesis (Shukla et al. 2004).

12.1.5 Pesticides

Pesticides in crop protection are used in excessive quantity, and it all ultimately mixes with the Ganges water, and water is frequently used in the daily requirements like for drinking and irrigation. It has already been demonstrated by various studies that pesticides play a crucial role in carcinogenesis (Nayak et al. 1995; Rehana et al. 1996); it can even cause liver cell carcinogenesis in experimental model (Ito et al. 1995; Kolaja et al. 1996). Another research was conducted by our earlier work was done to look at the pesticides presence in the causation of gallbladder cancer. A total of sixty patients of gallbladder diseases have been collected, of which 30 have GBC and 30 have cholelithiasis. Bile and blood samples were collected to estimate the pesticides' concentration. Organochlorine pesticides have shown earlier an association with the oesophageal and stomach cancers (Ditraglia et al. 1981). We also evaluated the concentration of some pesticides in gallbladder cancer patients. The estimated results have shown significantly higher concentration of BHC and DDT in gallbladder cancer patients when compared with cholelithiasis. Thus, it can also be an important factor in gallbladder carcinogenesis in our region (Shukla et al. 2001).

12.1.6 Bile and Bacteria

Bacterial presence can also be a causative factor for the gallbladder carcinogenesis. Primary bile acids change to secondary bile acids, due to the chronic bacterial infection which leads to the development of tumour (Hill 1986). In our earlier study in 2007, we tried to see the association of gallbladder cancer with chronic bacterial infection. We observed higher bile culture positivity in GBC in comparison to cholelithiasis and control (Sharma et al. 2007). Another study concluded that concentration of biliary deoxycholate was higher in GBC as compared to cholelithiasis (Shukla et al. 1993). In a previous study, we demonstrated the role of bacterial degradation of primary bile acids in GBC, and the study reported that the bacterial degradation of primary bile acids could also be a factor for gallbladder cancer (Pandey et al. 1995). Typhoid and paratyphoid can also correlate with the incidence of GBC in North India as these two are very common in such parts (Shukla et al. 1985). It is also concluded that approximately 2.5 % of total number of enteric fever cases is known to associate with the biliary system which leads to a chronic carrier state (Old 1990). Gallbladder diseases, including carcinoma, are common in the northern part of India and so are *Salmonella typhi* infection and typhoid carrier state. The typhoid carrier state may be one of the possible mechanisms of gallbladder carcinogenesis. There is 8.47 times more risk of developing carcinoma of the gallbladder in culture-positive typhoid carriers than the noncarriers (Welton et al. 1979; Nath et al. 1997, 2008; Shukla et al. 2000).

12.1.7 Dietary Factors

Other factors which may also correlate with the gallbladder carcinogenesis are dietary factors. Various studies concluded from their observation that intake of animal proteins, fats and oily food increases the risk of GBC, whereas intake of vegetables and fruits decreases the risk in patients for developing GBC (Kato et al. 1989). Another work also stated that ingestion of vegetables, fibre, vitamin C and vitamin E showed a lower risk of GBC but a higher risk is associated with the addition of sugar in desserts with the causation of biliary tract cancer (Moerman et al. 1995). We also (2002) evaluated the role of diet in gallbladder carcinogenesis. Significant odds ratios were seen with the consumption of radish (OR 0.4, 95 % CI 0.17–0.94), green chilies (OR 0.45, 95 % CI 0.21–0.94) and sweet potato (OR 0.33, 95 % CI 0.13–0.83) among vegetables and mango (OR 0.4, 95 % CI 0.16–0.93), melon (OR 0.3, 95 % CI 0.14–0.64) and papaya (OR 0.44, 95 % CI 0.2–0.64) among fruits. We concluded that vegetables and fruits showed a protective effect on gallbladder carcinogenesis but red meat (beef and muffin) was found to be associated with increased risk of gallbladder cancer (Pandey and Shukla 2002).

12.1.8 Mustard Oil

Mustard oil is frequently used as cooking medium in this part of country. It is already reported that mustard oil has an inflammatory response (Shukla and Arora 2003; Shukla et al. 2003). They were reported to have a tumorigenic response on consumption of mustard oil. Edible mustard oil is usually adulterated with argemone oil because argemone seeds closely resemble with the mustard seeds and colour of both the oils are the same (Ghosh et al. 2005). Sanguinarine and diethylnitrosamine are found to be present in the adulterated and fried mustard oil. Sanguinarine is an alkaloid of argemone oil. Recent studies have shown that argemone oil and isolated sanguinarine possess genotoxic and carcinogenic potential which is implicated in DNA damage in the blood of dropsy patients (Das et al. 2005). Similarly, diethylnitrosamine has also been reported to induce hepatocarcinogenesis (Bhosale et al. 2002). We also investigated the association of mustard oil as cooking medium with gallbladder cancer in northern

India. Concentration of sanguinarine and diethylnitrosamine were estimated in gallbladder cancer and cholelithiasis patients, and it was reported that sanguinarine and diethylnitrosamine concentrations in the gallbladder tissue increased in patients with gallbladder cancer compared to patients with cholelithiasis. We reported that there is an association between mustard oil and GBC (Dixit et al. 2013).

12.2 Lifestyle, Reproduction Factors and Risk of GBC

We also evaluated the risk of gallbladder cancer association with the lifestyle, parity, menstrual and reproductive factors. Sixty-four newly diagnosed GBC cases were included in the study and the detailed information regarding smoking, chewing habits, alcohol drinking and parity, menstrual and reproductive factors were collected in a pro forma. We stated that tobacco and chewing were associated with increased odds of gallbladder cancer. Similarly early menarche, late menopause, multiple pregnancies and childbirth increased the risk of gallbladder cancer (Pandey and Shukla 2003). A recent study also described a higher risk of developing gallbladder diseases in older, multiparous women and men with diabetes. They also showed an increased risk of gallbladder diseases by the intake of chickpeas and unsafe water and in villages having heavy water pollution (Unisa et al. 2011). Cigarette smoking is an important health hazard and nicotine is one of the main carcinogens known. Nicotine is found to be involved in DNA damage, genetic instability and inhibition of apoptosis (Campain et al. 2004). Our recent study was aimed to assess the role of nicotine in gallbladder carcinoma. A significant higher value of tissue nicotine concentration was observed in the gallbladder carcinoma group. These elevated nicotine concentration in tissue samples from gallbladder cancer is indicative of its strong association with the disease (Basu et al. 2012).

From the above discussion, we can conclude that multiple factors are playing a role in gallbladder carcinogenesis. So, it might be possible that such environmental factors are associated with the development of gallbladder cancer in the Gangetic plane.

References

Basu SP, Priya R, Singh TB, Srivastava P, Mishra PK, Shukla VK (2012) Role of nicotine in carcinoma of the gallbladder: a preliminary report. J Dig Dis 13: 536–540

Bhosale P, Motiwale L, Ignle AD, Gadre RV, Rao KVK (2002) Protective effect of Rhodotorula glutinisNCIM3353 on the development of hepatic preneoplastic lesions. Curr Sci 83:303–308

Campain JA (2004) Nicotine: potentially a multifunctional carcinogen? Toxicol Sci 79:1–3

Das M, Ansari KM, Dhawan A, Shukla Y, Khanna SK (2005) Correlation of DNA damage in epidemic dropsy patients to carcinogenic potential of argemone oil and isolated sanguinarine alkaloid in mice. Int J Cancer 117:709–717

Ditraglia D, Brown DP, Namekata T, Iverson N (1981) Mortality study of workers employed at organochlorine pesticide manufacturing plants. Scand J Work Environ Health Suppl 4:140–146

Dixit R, Srivastava P, Basu SP, Srivastava P, Mishra PK, Shukla VK (2013) Association of mustard oil as cooking media with gallbladder cancer. J Gastrointest Cancer 44:177–181

Fraser P, Chilvers C, Beral V, Hill MJ (1980) Nitrate and human cancer: a review of the evidence. Int J Epidemiol 9:3–11

Frazier JM, Din WS (1987) Role of metallothionein in induced resistance to cadmium toxicity in isolated rat hepatocytes. Experientia Suppl 52:619–626

Freedman JH, Peisach J (1989) Resistance of cultured hepatoma cells to copper toxicity. Purification and characterization of the hepatoma metallothionein. Biochim Biophys Acta 992:145–154

Garofalo JA, Ashikari H, Lesser ML, Menendez-Botet C, Cunningham-Rundles S, Schwartz MK, Good RA (1980) Serum zinc, copper, and the Cu/Zn ratio in patients with benign and malignant breast lesions. Cancer 46:2682–2685

Ghosh P, Krishna Reddy MM, Sashidhar RB (2005) Quantitative evaluation of sanguinarine as an index of argemone oil adulteration in edible mustard oil by high performance thin layer chromatography. Food Chem 91:757–764

Gray BN, Walker C, Barnard R (1982) Use of serum copper/zinc ratio in patients with large bowel cancer. J Surg Oncol 21:230–232

Gupta SK, Shukla VK, Vaidya MP, Roy SK, Gupta S (1991) Serum trace elements and Cu/Zn ratio in breast cancer patients. J Surg Oncol 46:178–181

Gupta SK, Shukla VK, Vaidya MP, Roy SK, Gupta S (1993) Serum and tissue trace elements in colorectal cancer. J Surg Oncol 52:172–175

Gupta SK, Ansari MA, Shukla VK (2005a) What makes the Gangetic belt a fertile ground for gallbladder cancers? J Surg Oncol 91:143–144

Gupta SK, Singh SP, Shukla VK (2005b) Copper, zinc, and Cu/Zn ratio in carcinoma of the gallbladder. J Surg Oncol 91:204–208

Hill MJ (1986) Microbes and human carcinogenesis. Edward Arnold, London

Hishikawa Y, Abe S, Kinugasa S, Yoshimura H, Monden N, Igarashi M, Tachibana M, Nagasue N (1997) Overexpression of metallothionein correlates with chemoresistance to cisplatin and prognosis in esophageal cancer. Oncology 54:342–347

Inutsuka S, Araki S (1978) Plasma copper and zinc levels in patients with malignant tumors of digestive organs: clinical evaluation of the C1/Zn ratio. Cancer 42: 626–631

Ito N, Hasegawa R, Imaida K, Kurata Y, Hagiwara A, Shirai T (1995) Effect of ingestion of 20 pesticides in combination at acceptable daily intake levels on rat liver carcinogenesis. Food Chem Toxicol 33:159–163

Kägi JH, Kojima Y (1987) Chemistry and biochemistry of metallothionein. Experientia Supp 52:25–61

Kato K, Akai S, Tominaga S, Kato I (1989) A case-control study of biliary tract cancer in Niigata Prefecture, Japan. Jpn J Cancer Res 80:932–938

Kolaja KL, Stevenson DE, Walborg EF Jr, Klaunig JE (1996) Selective dieldrin promotion of hepatic focal lesions in mice. Carcinogenesis 17:1243–1250

Kowalewski K, Todd EF (1971) Carcinoma of the gallbladder induced in hamsters by insertion of cholesterol pellets and feeding dimethylnitrosamine. Proc Soc Exp Biol Med 136:482–486

Krishnamurti CR, Vishwanathan P (1990) Toxic metals in Indian environment. Tata McGraw Hill Publishing Company Ltd., New Delhi

Leonard A (1983) The mutagenic and genotoxic effect of heavy metals. In: Proceeding of an international conference on heavy metals in the environment. Edinburgh: CEP consultant 700

Liu J, Kershaw WC, Klaassen CD (1990) Rat primary hepatocyte cultures are a good model for examining metallothionein-induced tolerance to cadmium toxicity. In Vitro Cell Dev Biol 26:75–79

Margerison AC, Mann JR (1985) Serum copper, serum ceruloplasmin, and erythrocyte sedimentation rate measurements in children with Hodgkin's disease, non-Hodgkin's lymphoma, and nonmalignant lymphadenopathy. Cancer 55:1501–1506

Moerman CJ, Bueno de Mesquita HB, Smeets FW, Runia S (1995) Consumption of foods and micronutrients and the risk of cancer of the biliary tract. Prev Med 24:591–602

Monden N, Abe S, Sutoh I, Hishikawa Y, Kinugasa S, Nagasue N (1997) Prognostic significance of the expressions of metallothionein, glutathione-S-transferase-pi, and P-glycoprotein in curatively resected gastric cancer. Oncology 54:391–399

Nath G, Singh H, Shukla VK (1997) Chronic typhoid carriage and carcinoma of the gallbladder. Eur J Cancer Prev 6:557–559

Nath G, Singh YK, Kumar K, Gulati AK, Shukla VK, Khanna AK, Tripathi SK, Jain AK, Kumar M, Singh TB (2008) Association of carcinoma of the gallbladder with typhoid carriage in a typhoid endemic area using nested PCR. J Infect Dev Ctries 2:302–307

National Cancer Registry Programme (2002) Two-year report of the population based cancer registries 1997–1998. Indian Council of Medical Research, New Delhi

Nayak AK, Raha P, Das AK, Raha R (1995) Organochlorine pesticide residues in middle stream of the Ganga River, India. Bull Environ Contam Toxicol 54: 68–75

Old DC (1990) Salmonella. In: Parbet TA, Collier LH (eds) Topley and Wilson's. Principle of bacteriology, virology and immunity, 8th edn. Edward Arnold, London

Pandey M, Shukla VK (2002) Diet and gallbladder cancer: a case-control study. Eur J Cancer Prev 11:365–368

Pandey M, Shukla VK (2003) Lifestyle, parity, menstrual and reproductive factors and risk of gallbladder cancer. Eur J Cancer Prev 12:269–272

Pandey M, Vishwakarma RA, Khatri AK, Roy SK, Shukla VK (1995) Bile, bacteria, and gallbladder carcinogenesis. Surg Oncol 58:282–283

Rehana Z, Malik A, Ahmad M (1996) Genotoxicity of the Ganges water at Narora (U.P.), India. Mutat Res 367:187–193

Schmid KW, Ellis IO, Gee JM, Darke BM, Lees WE, Kay J, Cryer A, Stark JM, Hittmair A, Ofner D et al (1993) Presence and possible significance of immunocytochemically demonstrable metallothionein overexpression in primary invasive ductal carcinoma of the breast. Virchows Arch A Pathol Anat Histopathol 422:153–159

Sharma V, Chauhan VS, Nath G, Kumar A, Shukla VK (2007) Role of bile bacteria in gallbladder carcinoma. Hepatogastroenterology 54:1622–1625

Shukla Y, Arora A (2003) Enhancing effects of mustard oil on preneoplastic hepatic foci development in Wistar rats. Hum Exp Toxicol 22:51–55

Shukla VK, Khandelwal C, Roy SK, Vaidya MP (1985) Primary carcinoma of the gall bladder: a review of a 16-year period at the University Hospital. J Surg Oncol 28:32–35

Shukla VK, Tiwari SC, Roy SK (1993) Biliary bile acids in cholelithiasis and carcinoma of the gall bladder. Eur J Cancer Prev 2:155–160

Shukla VK, Aryya NC, Pitale A, Pandey M, Dixit VK, Reddy CD, Gautam A (1998a) Metallothionein expression in carcinoma of the gallbladder. Histopathology 33:154–157

Shukla VK, Prakash A, Tripathi BD, Reddy DC, Singh S (1998b) Biliary heavy metal concentrations in carcinoma of the gall bladder: case-control study. BMJ 317:1288–1289

Shukla VK, Singh H, Pandey M, Upadhyay SK, Nath G (2000) Carcinoma of the gallbladder – is it a sequel of typhoid. Dig Dis Sci 45:900–903

Shukla VK, Rastogi AN, Adukia TK, Raizada RB, Reddy DC, Singh S (2001) Organochlorine pesticides in carcinoma of the gallbladder: a case-control study. Eur J Cancer Prev 10:153–156

Shukla VK, Adukia TK, Singh SP, Mishra CP, Mishra RN (2003) Micronutrients, antioxidants, and carcinoma of the gallbladder. J Surg Oncol 84: 31–35

Shukla VK, Prakash A, Chauhan VS, Singh S, Puneet (2004) Biliary nitrate and risk of carcinoma of the gallbladder. Eur J Cancer Prev 13:355–356

Unisa S, Jagannath P, Dhir V, Khandelwal C, Sarangi L, Roy TK (2011) Population-based study to estimate prevalence and determine risk factors of gallbladder diseases in the rural Gangetic basin of North India. HPB (Oxford) 13:117–125

Welton JC, Marr JS, Friedman SM (1979) Association between hepatobiliary cancer and typhoid carrier state. Lancet 1:791–794

Stress and Cancer Risk: The Possible Role of Work Stress

13

Marcus James Fila

Abstract

Despite widespread public belief that stress may lead to cancer, research on this relationship remains inconclusive. However, recent work points to the possibility that hostile naturalistic settings may contribute to cancer risk. Within organizational research, work stress is thought to be one of the greatest sources of psychological stress in people's lives and is increasingly becoming a modern-day pandemic. Thus, this paper outlines the nature of stress, including how excessive and chronic stress negatively affects human health and may possibly lead to cancer; argues that a causal link between stress and cancer may exist, despite being frequently overlooked due to ethical and practical research difficulties; and presents an industrial/organizational psychologist's viewpoint of workplace stress by outlining two prominent models used in the social sciences. Finally, the author suggests that future collaboration between experimental cancer researchers and workplace psychologists may help further address the possible link between work stress and cancer.

Keywords

Stress • Cancer • Work • Workplace • Strain

13.1 Stress and Cancer Risk: The Possible Role of Work Stress

It is widely acknowledged in organizational research within the social sciences that work stress is becoming a modern-world pandemic and may be many people's biggest stressor (Sulsky and Smith 2005). Moreover, excessive and chronic stress has been implicated in a number of

M.J. Fila, PgDip, MBA, MS (✉)
Department of Economics, Management, and Accounting, Hope College, 141 E 12th St. Holland, MI 49423, USA
e-mail: fila@hope.edu

P.R. Sudhakaran (ed.), *Perspectives in Cancer Prevention – Translational Cancer Research*, DOI 10.1007/978-81-322-1533-2_13, © Springer India 2014

serious conditions, including depression (Hammen 2005; Monroe and Simons 1991), progression of HIV (Capitanio et al. 1998; Leserman et al. 2002), and cardiovascular disease (Krantz and McCeney 2002; Rozanski et al. 1995). As such, all sectors of society have become increasingly aware of work stress over the past generation, and decreasing work stress has become an international priority at personal, organizational, and societal levels (Griffin and Clarke 2011).

Given its established link to other serious forms of disease, there exists a widespread public belief that stress may be linked to cancer, through both *direct* effects (e.g., the body's physiological response to psychological stressors) and *indirect* pathways (e.g., unhealthy response behaviors, such as smoking and over eating) (Cohen et al. 2007; Sulsky and Smith 2005). However, research findings to date have been mixed (Duijts et al. 2003; Heffner et al. 2003; Lutgendorf et al. 1994; Turner-Cobb et al. 2001), with some concluding that stress is more likely to be attributable to cancer progression than to initiation (Cole et al. 2001). Additionally, stress can be difficult to prove beyond all reasonable doubt (Sulsky and Smith 2005), and to further complicate matters, the field of cancer research is fraught with ethical and practical issues that hinder much experimental research in field settings (Cohen et al. 2007). Because of these inherent difficulties, a possible link between pervasive levels of stress and development of cancers in naturalistic settings may be being overlooked. Recently, however, Abeysinghe and Gu (2010) recorded cancer data from a Shanghai-based population analyzed through an age period cohort technique, finding strong evidence that those whose mental health had suffered due to the stress of the Chinese social revolution were more likely to have been diagnosed with cancer than others.

Similarly, given the paramount economic, familial, social, and societal importance of work and the physical number of hours typically spent in work-related activities, efforts of organizational practitioners and scientists to identify and reduce stress have been motivated by a desire for improvements in employee quality of life and, ultimately, work performance (Griffin and Clarke 2011; Kahn and Byosiere 1992). For example, one survey illustrated that 48 % of workers react to their work-related stress by cutting corners, lying about sick days, and covering up incidents that should be reported (Boyd 1997). A more insidious reason to identify and reduce stress is the increasing number of lawsuits filed by workers claiming for stress-related injuries (Earnshaw and Cooper 1994). However, evidence of strong relationships between chronic stress and a host of life-threatening diseases, possibly including cancer (see Cohen et al. 2007), is perhaps the most pervasive reason to understand and mitigate workplace stress wherever possible. As such, the four aims of this paper are to outline the nature of stress, including how excessive and chronic stress negatively affects human health; to argue that a causal link between stress and cancer may exist, despite being frequently overlooked due to ethical and practical research difficulties; to present an industrial/organizational psychologist's viewpoint of workplace stress by outlining two prominent models used in the social sciences; and to suggest that future collaboration between experimental cancer researchers and workplace psychologists may help further address the possible link between work stress and cancer.

13.1.1 What Is Stress?

Most people are in agreement that stress is both an important and pervasive part of modern life (Kahn and Byosiere 1992). Moreover, excessive levels of stress may negatively affect physical and emotional health and detrimentally effect performance at work (Sulsky and Smith 2005). These concerns appear substantiated, with 60–90 % of visits to healthcare professionals being for potentially stress-related disorders, such as headaches, back pain, and cardiovascular disease (Cummings and VandenBos 1981). Moreover, 14 % of all insurance compensation claims are for stress-related illnesses and injuries (Pelletier and Lutz 1991), and it is estimated that the USA loses approximately 550 million work days annually to stress-related absenteeism (Danna and Griffin 1999).

Stress is not a single event, but a dynamic process involving appraisal, response, and attempts to cope with and manage stressors in order to meet goals (Sulsky and Smith 2005). Potential stressors initiate this process based on personal, group, and situational characteristics, how the individual appraises a potential stressor (i.e., whether or not it is viewed as a stressor) and how he/she responds to the stressor (e.g., physiological and/or psychological strains) (Kahn and Byosiere 1992; Lazarus and Folkman 1984). For most stressors, the perception of threat and severity of stress is based on a psychological appraisal which occurs prior to the physical stress response. Conditions appraised as stressful may then lead to acute reactions. Moreover, if persistent these short-term responses may lead to chronic longer-term strains, as well as behavioral coping mechanisms, which in some cases may contribute further to strain (Sulsky and Smith 2005).

13.1.2 Stress and Health

Studies of work stress in the health and social sciences generally focus on either the occurrence of environmental events that tax one's ability to cope; individual responses to events that are indicative of this overload, such as perceived stress and event-elicited negative affect; or both (Kahn and Byosiere 1992; Sulsky and Smith 2005). Stress is generally thought to influence the pathogenesis of physiological disease by inducing negative affective states (e.g., feelings of anxiety and depression), which exert direct effects on biological processes and/or behavioral patterns that influence disease risk (Cohen et al. 1995). Chronic stressors are generally considered to be the most toxic because they are more likely than most acute stressors to result in long-term or permanent changes in the emotional, physiological, and behavioral responses that influence susceptibility to and course of disease (Cohen et al. 1995; McEwen 1988).

The most direct pathway from stress to serious disease is through stressor-elicited endocrine responses. According to Cohen et al. (1995) and McEwen (1988), two endocrine response systems are particularly reactive to psychological stress: the hypothalamic-pituitary-adrenocortical axis (HPA) and the sympathetic-adrenal-medullary (SAM) system. Cortisol, the primary effector of HPA activation in humans, regulates a broad range of physiological processes, including anti-inflammatory responses; metabolism of carbohydrates, fats, and proteins; and gluconeogenesis. Similarly, catecholamines, which are released in response to SAM activation, work in concert with the autonomic nervous system to exert regulatory effects on the cardiovascular, pulmonary, hepatic, skeletal muscle, and immune systems. Prolonged or repeated activation of the HPA and SAM systems can interfere with their control of other physiological systems, resulting in increased risk for physical and psychiatric disorders (Cohen et al. 1995; McEwen 1988). The mediating effects of HPA and SAM systems on stress and disease are evidenced in animal and human studies demonstrating how a wide variety of stressful stimuli provoke activation of these systems. For example, stress has been linked to depression (Monroe and Simons 1991; Van Praag et al. 2004), the progression of HIV (Capitanio et al. 1998; Leserman et al. 2002), and cardiovascular disease (Kivimaki et al. 2006; Krantz and McCeney 2002; Rozanski et al. 1995).

13.1.3 Stress and Cancer Risk

In addition to the aforementioned diseases, experimental research in animals and some creatures has found that stress contributes to the initiation, growth, and metastasis of select tumors (Cohen et al. 2007; Wu et al. 2010). Moreover, mechanistic experiments in humans indicate that stress affects key pathogenic processes in cancer, such as antiviral defenses, DNA repair, and cellular aging (Antoni et al. 2006). The focus of many of these studies is basic biology, e.g., whether the experience of stress and changes in gene expression may be associated with tumor progression (Ross 2008). However, studies looked for associations between chronic psychological stress and the incidence or course of cancer in humans have yielded mixed and moderately controversial results (Duijts et al. 2003; Heffner et al. 2003; Lutgendorf et al. 1994; Turner-Cobb et al. 2001). For example, contrary to community beliefs, there has been no evident association between stress and breast cancer risk in large prospective cohort studies (see Kricker et al. 2009). Overall, despite some promising findings stress is presently thought to be more influential in the *progression* and *recurrence* of cancer than its initial onset (Cole et al. 2001). This extant literature on the relationship between stress and cancer in humans is summarized by Antoni et al. (2006), who outline possible multiple effects of stress on human tumor biology, including through impairment and enhancement of estrogen synthesis (Kricker et al. 2009).

13.1.4 Are We Overlooking a Causal Link?

The inconclusive evidence of direct effects of stress on cancer may be causing us to overlook its possible effects for several reasons. First, as already mentioned stress may contribute to cancer risk through indirect pathways, such as behavioral changes occurring as adaptations or coping responses to stressors including smoking, decreased exercise and sleep, and poorer adherence to medical regimens (Lutgendorf et al. 1994). Second, many cancers are diagnosed only after years of growth, making an association between stress and disease onset difficult to demonstrate (Cohen et al. 2007). Third, the field is fraught by ethical and practical difficulties in designing and implementing adequate studies. For example, studies frequently collapse groups of patients across various types of cancer to maximize power. However, cancer is a heterogeneous group of diseases with multiple etiologies, and the contribution of stress-related perturbations (e.g., HPA and SAM activation, diminished antiviral defenses) are likely to vary across sites and stages. Furthermore, effects of psychological stress are likely to be more pronounced in cancers facilitated by impairments in antiviral immunity and sustained activation of hormonal response (e.g., cervical cancer, hepatocarcinoma, and HIV-related tumors), than more common cancers, such as breast cancer (Cohen et al. 2007). Thus, smaller effect sizes could be overlooked even if causally validated.

An alternative viewpoint to the study of stress and cancer is that naturalistic settings may offer strong conclusions (although scientifically validating findings may be challenging). For example, Abeysinghe and Gu (2010) recently recorded cancer data from a Shanghai-based population analyzed through an age period cohort technique. The authors found strong evidence that those whose mental health had suffered due to the stress of the Chinese social revolution experienced significantly more incidents of cancer than others (Abeysinghe and Gu 2010). Moreover, they concluded that human history is replete with "experiments" that have caused enormous stress on some human populations, and that data on incidents of serious disease from such historical events, had it been recorded, may have provided rich sources of information to examine the link between stress and cancer.

Although evidence such as that found by Abeysinghe and Gu (2010) is presently rare within cancer research, it takes the first steps in suggesting that humans who are exposed to psychologically stressful conditions over a sustained period may be at a higher risk of cancer. Given the established link between stress and other diseases, perhaps the existential possibility of a stress-cancer relationship is more important than its falsifiability. For example, organizational research suggests that the modern world of work is gradually intensifying and becoming more demanding and stressful (Burchell 2002), with stress in the workplace now considered to be a modern-world pandemic (Sulsky and Smith 2005). As such, the possibility exists – and should thus be explored – that excessive and chronic workplace stress may be connected to cancer. Accomplishing this arguably requires marrying an understanding of work stress from a psychological standpoint with existing experimental methods in examining cancer. Therefore, the final section of this paper offers a brief overview of work stress from an industrial/organizational perspective, and two prominent models of work stress are outlined, with the intention of stimulating future research.

13.2 Work Stress: A View from Industrial/Organizational Psychology

Over the past 40 years, a considerable body of stress-related theory and practice has developed, encompassing research from many fields including psychology, sociology, medicine, public health, engineering, and economics (Griffin and Clarke 2011). Within the field of psychology, stress research has been identified mainly in the clinical, medical, and occupational/organizational disciplines (Beehr and Franz 1987). From a work perspective, conventional wisdom suggests that workers in highly developed countries should experience the greatest levels of psychological well-being (including happiness, peace, and fulfillment), because they are among the world's highest-paid employees. However, beyond the very lowest income levels, the earning-to-well-being relationship is not linear (Diener et al. 1995), and many of today's workers are experiencing elevated levels of stress, leading to a variety of physical and psychological strains which are detrimental to both their own well-being and that of the organization (Sulsky and Smith 2005).

Stress researchers have maintained for over a century that not all stress is harmful, and that a certain amount is actually beneficial to health and performance (Selye 1956; Yerkes and Dodson 1908). However, stress arising from unpleasant or aversive physiological or emotional states resulting from adverse experiences that are uncertain or beyond the employee's control can be detrimental to human health and functioning (Beehr and Bhagat 1985; Hart and Cooper 2001). More specifically, growing evidence in the health and social sciences implicates work stress in the development of a number of physical and psychological *strains*. Strains are adverse and potentially harmful reactions of an individual to stressful work (De Croon et al. 2004) and include adverse physiological changes, decrements in role performance, and psychological reactions (such as emotional tensions) (Karasek and Theorell 1990). For example, by directly damaging the physical and mental health of employees, overly stressful employment conditions may erode employee job satisfaction and commitment to the organization and contribute to intentions to quit the organization (Faragher et al. 2005; French et al. 1982; Siegrist 1996). Stress may lead to job-related worries, physical and/or emotional exhaustion, depression, psychological distress, psychiatric distress, affective disorder symptomatology, psychotic affective disorder, mild psychiatric morbidity, social dysfunction, tension, anxiety, irritability, state anger, trait anger, schizophrenia/delusion/hallucinations, need to recover after work, lack of identification, hostility, frustration, and burnout (Karasek and Theorell 1990). Furthermore, as previously mentioned, stress has been consistently linked to life-threatening health disorders such as cardiovascular disease and the progression of various cancers (Cohen et al. 2007).

In certain circumstances, the stressor may be identified before strains are apparent, or the resultant strains can be treated with the individual returning to normal (Sulsky and Smith 2005). However, treatment of strains attributed by the employee to an overly stressful work environment essentially put a "Band-Aid" on the problem, because the individual may perceive having little or no control over their presence or recurrence (Karasek and Theorell 1990). As such, these strains will likely persist unless the individual's perceptions of the environment change, or they leave the organization for reasons of job change or poor health (Sulsky and Smith 2005). Therefore, in accordance with Abeysinghe and Gu (2010), given the paramount economic, familial, social, and societal importance of work and the physical number of hours typically spent in work-related activities (Sulsky and Smith 2005), some workplaces may be more conducive to employee health-related problems than others, when controlling for expected variability in disease susceptibility between individuals. As such, responsibility for stress reduction at work lies not only with the individual but with the organization to ensure a healthy work environment that gives due attention to workplace characteristics (Diefendorff and Chandler 2011), such as how jobs are designed (Grant et al. 2011).

Myriad stress reduction and management programs have been outlined in the literature (e.g., Karasek and Theorell 1990; Sulsky and Smith 2005). However, perhaps the first step in understanding the possible role of work stress in cancer risk is an awareness of what social scientists have repeatedly evidenced to be stressors at work.

13.3 Two Classical Models of Work Stress: The Job Demands-Control-Support (JDC(S)) and Effort-Reward Imbalance (ERI) Models

The job demands-control-support (JDC(S)) (Karasek and Theorell 1990) and the effort-reward imbalance (ERI) models (Siegrist 1996) aim to capture characteristics of the psychosocial work environment by focusing on the work environment as the main locus of employee stress and strain. Moreover, both models provide practical recommendations for reducing stress and its deleterious outcomes by creating healthier work environments (Sulsky and Smith 2005). The JDC(S) model views work demands, control over working processes, and social support from within the workplace as integral to the stress process. Although underutilization can result in stress from boredom (Kahn and Byosiere 1992; Selye 1956), the main tenet of the JDC(S) model is that high demands can be stressful, especially if experienced in conjunction with a low control over how to manage them and inadequate support from proximal workplace constituents, such as coworkers and supervisor(s). As such, an employee's perception of fit with the work environment centers on demands being manageable and the availability of control and support resources (Kain and Jex 2010). Moreover, control and support are thought to both reduce stress directly and mitigate the stress of high perceived demands (Hausser et al. 2010; Karasek and Theorell 1990).

Demands are physical, social, or organizational aspects of the job that require sustained physical or mental effort (Demerouti et al. 2001). Examples of demands include deadlines, number of "widgets" made per hour, and number of reports due per week. Job control (also termed decision latitude) refers to control over work activities (Van der Doef and Maes 1999) and plays a central role in many organizational stress theories (for reviews see Frese 1989; Ganster 1989). Hackman and Oldham (1975) defined control as how much substantial freedom, independence, and discretion are provided by the job to the individual to schedule work and in determining the procedures to be used in carrying it out. The original demands-control model was extended by integrating workplace social support as a third dimension (Johnson and Hall 1988). Diverse mechanisms now exhibit how workplace support can affect psychological well-being, for example, as a buffering mechanism between psychological stressors and adverse physiological and psychological outcomes (Karasek et al. 1987); through basic physiological processes important to both acquisition of new knowledge and maintenance of long-term health (Henry and Stephens 1977); by facilitating active coping patterns and productive behavior – thus affecting health through second-order effects (Pearlin and Schooler 1978); and through positive sense of identity, based on socially confirmed values of contributions to collective goals (Stryker and Burke 2000).

In their recent review of organizational stress literature, Griffin and Clarke (2011) concluded that the most effective ways for organizations to minimize job stress are to (1) make reasonable demands of employees, (2) afford them sufficient control over how to meet demands, and (3) ensure provision of adequate support within the workplace. Moreover, because "many jobs are characterized by high demands, where the nature of the demands cannot be changed," control and support are particularly important to stress minimization (Griffin and Clarke 2011, p. 382). These concepts pervade the above and many other work stress theories in some form. However, the JDC(S)

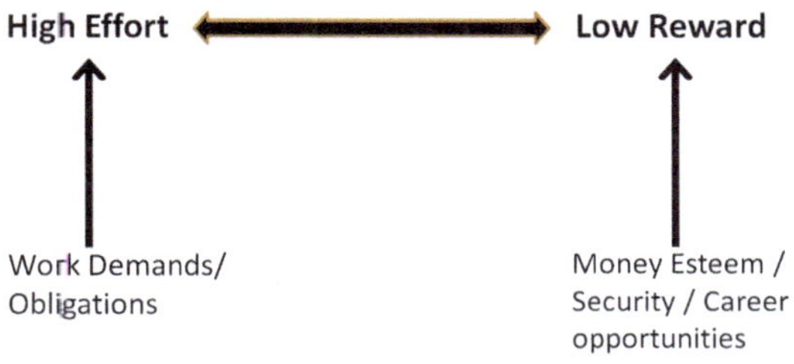

Fig. 13.1 The effort-reward imbalance model, taken from Siegrist (1996)

model offers a direct examination of how employees perceive these workplace characteristics.

The ERI model is grounded in equity theory (Adams 1965; Greenberg 1982), assuming a distributive justice institutional perspective, in which the labor contract is a reciprocal exchange of the fulfillment of work demands (effort) in return for income, job security, social mobility, and esteem (Siegrist 1996). Distributive justice refers to the fairness of these outcome distributions or allocations (Guillermina 1980), and in the USA, the merit or equity norm that those who work the hardest and/or are most productive should get the greatest rewards is the most common foundation for defining distributive justice (Greenberg 1982). The ERI model is designed to measure the symmetry/asymmetry of this effort-reward, equity-driven relationship (Siegrist 1996). Walster et al. (1973) summarized the key prediction of equity theory as being when individuals become distressed when they find themselves participating in inequitable relationships, and that distress increases with the degree of inequity. A more recent review by Mowday and Colwell (2003, p. 68) summarizes even more succinctly: "Inequitable treatment causes tension or distress, and people are motivated to do something about it." Thus, inequity, as represented in the ERI model, represents a stress mechanism triggered by a perception of distributive injustice (Greenberg 1984). This is depicted is Fig. 13.1.

Injustice as a stressor is relatively new within stress research, and the extent to which fairness perceptions provide unique insights into the relationship between justice and job strain is as yet underrepresented in organizational research (Rodwell et al. 2009). In one study, De Boer and colleagues (2002) explored the influence of organizational justice variables with the original JDC model and found that justice contributed to the explanation of job strain more than perceptions of demands or control. However, they concluded that further justice research with the JDC(S) model (i.e., including the social support dimension) is necessary to determine whether a greater prediction of strain can be achieved. Some studies have examined the effects of perceived demands, control, and support when augmented with perceptions of justice and, in particular, distributive justice as defined by the effort-reward relationship (e.g., Fillion et al. 2007; Rodwell et al. 2009; Rydstedt et al. 2007).

13.4 The Potential Role of Social Science Work Stress Models in Cancer Research

Psychological models of work stress such as the JDC(S) and ERI models may help predict risk of cancer by evidencing the circumstances under which employees are most likely to be stressed (direct path) and to perform response-driven coping behaviors to stress (indirect paths). For example, studies show that those employees experiencing high demands and low control in the workplace are more likely to smoke cigarettes than other employees (Lindstrom 2004). Similarly, Kouvonen et al. (2005) evidenced a relationship between effort-reward imbalance and smoking behaviors. Although some other studies to date have failed to find a more direct relationship between work stress and cancer (e.g., Schernhammer et al. 2004), there is arguably a role for social scientists to augment the methodologies and findings of cancer researchers. For example, by drawing on their knowledge of work settings, industrial and organizational psychologists could help design field experiments that overcome some of the ethical issues in exploring the possible work stress and cancer relationship. Additionally, awareness of established causal relationships between work conditions and employee stress may further assist cancer researchers in designing laboratory experiments that, as far as is possible, recapture the stressors experienced at work, thus promoting both internal and external validity.

The relationship between work stress and cancer remains shrouded in ambiguity. However this is arguably as much due to ethical and practical boundaries of experimental design as a credible scientific reason to doubt a relationship. As the field of cancer research continues to broaden, it may further include the perspective of social scientists who, with their awareness of the effects of psychosocial aspects of life situations (such as work) on human stressors, strains, and resultant coping behaviors, may offer alternative ways to address familiar questions surrounding the causes of cancer. Firmer answers to questions regarding the potential role of work stress on cancer may be just around the corner.

References

Abeysinghe T, Gu J (2010) The cultural revolution, stress and cancer. Resource Document. SCAPE Police Research Working Paper. http://ideas.repec.org/p/eab/microe/23118.html

Adams JS (1965) Inequity in social exchange. Adv Exp Soc Psychol 2:267–299

Antoni MH, Lutgendorf SK, Cole SW (2006) The influence of bio-behavioral factors on tumor biology: pathways and mechanisms. Natl Rev Cancer 6(3):240–248

Beehr TA, Bhagat RS (1985) Human stress and cognition in organizations: an integrated perspective. Wiley, New York

Beehr TA, Franz TM (1987) The current debate about the meaning of job stress. In: Ivancevich JM, Ganster DC (eds) Job stress, from theory to suggestions. Haworth Press, New York, pp 5–18

Boyd A (1997) Employee traps—corruption in the workplace. Manag Rev 86:9

Burchell B (2002) The prevalence and redistribution of job insecurity and work intensification. In: Burchell B, Lapido D, Wilkinson F (eds) Job insecurity and work intensification. Routledge, London, pp 61–76

Capitanio JP, Mendoza SP, Lerche NW, Mason WA (1998) Social stress results in altered glucocorticoid regulation and shorter survival in simian acquired immune deficiency syndrome. Proc Natl Acad Sci USA 95(8):4714–4719

Cohen S, Kessler RC, Gordon UL (1995) Strategies for measuring stress in studies of psychiatric and physical disorder. In: Cohen S, Kessler RC, Gordon UL (eds) Measuring stress: a guide for health and social scientists. Oxford University Press, New York, pp 3–26

Cohen S, Janicki-Deverts D, Miller DE (2007) Psychological stress and disease. JAMA 298(14): 1685–1687

Cole SW, Naliboff BD, Kemeny ME, Griswalk MP, Fahey JL, Zack JA (2001) Impaired response to HAART in HIV infected individuals with high autonomic nervous system activity. Proc Natl Acad Sci USA 98:12695–12700

Cummings N, VandenBos G (1981) The twenty-year Kaiser-Permanente experience with psychotherapy and medical utilization. Health Policy Q 2(1):159–175

Danna K, Griffin RW (1999) Health and well-being in the workplace. J Manag 25:357–384

De Boer EM, Bakker AB, Syroit JE, Schaufeli WB (2002) Unfairness at work as a predictor of absenteeism. J Organ Behav 23:181–197

De Croon EM, Blonk RWB, Broersen JPJ, Frings-Dresen MHW (2004) Stressful work, psychological job strain, and turnover: a 2-year prospective cohort study of truck drivers. J Appl Psychol 89(3):442–454

Demerouti E, Bakker AB, Nachreiner F, Schaufeli WB (2001) The job demands-resources model of burnout. J Appl Psychol 86:499–512

Diefendorff JM, Chandler MM (2011) Motivating employees. In: Zedeck S (ed) APA handbook of Industrial and Organizational Psychology, vol 3, Maintaining, expanding, and contracting the organization. American Psychological Association, Washington, DC, pp 65–135

Diener E, Diener M, Diener C (1995) Factors predicting the subjective well-being of nations. J Personal Soc Psychol 69:851–864

Duijts SFA, Zeegers MPA, Borne BV (2003) The association between stressful life events and breast cancer risk: a meta-analysis. Int J Cancer 107(6):1023–1029

Earnshaw J, Cooper CL (1994) Employee stress litigation: the UK experience. Work Stress 8:287–295

Faragher EB, Cass M, Cooper CL (2005) The relationship between job satisfaction and health: a meta-analysis. Occup Environ Med 62:105–112

Fillion L, Tremblay I, Manon T, Cote D, Struthers CW, Dupuis R (2007) Job satisfaction and emotional distress among nurses providing palliative care: empirical evidence for an integrative occupational stress-model. Int J Stress Manag 14(1):1–25

French JRP, Caplan RD, Harrison RV (1982) The mechanisms of job stress and strain. Wiley, London

Frese M (1989) Theoretical models of control and health. In: Sauter SL, Hurrell JJ, Cooper CC (eds) Job control and worker health. Wiley, New York

Ganster D (1989) Worker control and well-being: a review of research in the workplace. In: Sauter SL, Hurrell JJ, Cooper CC (eds) Job control and worker health. Wiley, New York

Grant AM, Fried Y, Juillerat T (2011) Work matters: job design in classic and contemporary perspectives. In: Zedeck S (ed) APA handbook of industrial and organizational psychology, vol. 1: Building and developing the organization, vol 1. American Psychological Association, Washington, DC, pp 417–453

Greenberg J (1982) Approaching equity and avoiding inequity in groups and organizations. In: Greenberg J, Cohen RL (eds) Equity and justice in social behavior. Academic Press, New York, pp 389–435

Greenberg J (1984) On the apocryphal nature of inequity distress. In: Folger R (ed) The sense of injustice: Social psychological perspectives. Plenum Press, New York, pp 167–186

Griffin MA, Clarke S (2011) Stress and well-being at work. In: Zedeck S (ed) APA handbook of industrial and organizational psychology. American Psychological Association, Washington, DC, pp 359–397

Guillermina J (1980) A new theory of Distributive Justice. Am Sociol Rev 45(2):3–32

Hackman JR, Oldham GR (1975) Development of the job diagnostic survey. J Appl Psychol 60:159–170

Hammen C (2005) Stress and depression. Annu Rev Clin Psychol 1:293–319

Hart PM, Cooper CL (2001) Occupational stress: toward a more integrated framework. In: Anderson N, Ones DS, Sinangil HK, Viswesvaran C (eds) Handbook of industrial, work, and organizational psychology, vol 2. Sage, Thousand Oaks, pp 93–114

Husser JA, Mojzisch A, Niesel M, Schulz-Hardt S (2010) Ten years on: a review of recent research on the job demand-control (−support) model and psychological well-being. Work Stress 24(1):1–35

Heffner KL, Loving TJ, Robles TF, Kiecolt-Glaser JK (2003) Examining psychosocial factors related to cancer incidence and progression: in search of the silver lining. Brain Behav Immun 17:S109–S111

Henry JP, Stephens PM (1977) The social environment and essential hypertension in mice: possible role of innervation of the adrenal cortex. Prog Brain Res 47:263–275

Johnson JV, Hall EM (1988) Job strain, work place social support, and cardiovascular disease: a cross-sectional study of a random sample of the Swedish working population. Am J Public Health 78: 1336–1342

Kahn RL, Byosiere P (1992) Stress in organizations. In: Dunnette MD, Hough LM (eds) Handbook of industrial and organizational psychology, vol 3, (pp. Consulting Psychologists Press, Palo Alto, pp 571–650

Kain K, Jex S (2010) Karasek's (1979) job demands-control model: a summary of current issues and recommendations for future research. In: Perrewe PL, Ganster DC (eds) New developments in theoretical and conceptual approaches to job stress. Emerald Group Publishing Limited, Bingley, pp 237–268

Karasek RA, Theorell T (1990) Healthy work: Stress, productivity, and the Reconstruction of working life. Basic Books, New York

Karasek RA, Gardell B, Lindell J (1987) Work and non-work correlates of illness and behavior in male and female Swedish white-collar workers. J Occup Behav 8:187–207

Kivimaki M, Virtanen M, Elovainio M, Kouvonen A, Vaananen A, Vahtera J (2006) Work stress in the etiology of coronary heart disease—a meta-analysis. Scand J Work Environ Heal 32(6):431–442

Kouvonen A, Kivimaki M, Virtanen M, Pentti J, Vahtera J (2005) Work stress, smoking status, and smoking intensity: an observational study of 46,190 employees. J Epidemiol Community Health 59:63–69

Krantz DS, McCeney MK (2002) Effects of psychological and social factors on organic disease: a critical assessment of research on coronary heart disease. Annu Rev Psychol 53:341–369

Kricker A, Price M, Butow P, Goumas C, Armes JE, Armstrong BK (2009) Effects of life event stress and social support on the odds of a 2cm breast cancer. Cancer Causes Control 20:437–447

Lazarus RS, Folkman S (1984) Stress, appraisal, and coping. Springer, New York

Leserman J, Petitto JM, Gu H et al (2002) Progression to AIDS, a clinical AIDS condition and mortality: psychosocial and physiological predictors. Psychol Med 32(6):1059–1073

Lindstrom M (2004) Psychosocial work conditions, social capital, and daily smoking: a population based study. Tob Control 13(3):289–295

Lutgendorf S, Antoni MH, Schneiderman N, Fletcher MA (1994) Psychosocial counseling to improve quality of life in HIV-infected gay men. Pat Educ Counsel 24:217–235

McEwen BS (1988) Protective and damaging effects of stress mediators. N Engl J Med 338(3):171–179

Monroe SM, Simons AD (1991) Diathesis-stress theories in the context of life stress research: implications for depressive disorders. Psychol Bull 110(3): 406–425

Mowday RT, Colwell KA (2003) Employee reactions to unfair outcomes in the workplace: the contributions of Adams' equity theory to understanding work motivation. In: Porter L, Bigley G, Steers RM (eds) Motivation and work behavior, 7th edn. McGraw-Hill, Burr Ridge, pp 222–254

Pearlin LI, Schooler C (1978) The structure of coping. J Organ Behav 19:2–21

Pelletier KR, Lutz RW (1991) Healthy people – healthy business: a critical review of stress management programs in the workplace. In: Weiss SM, Fielding JE, Baum A (eds) Perspectives in behavioral medicine: health at work. Erlbaum, Hillsdale, pp 189–204

Rodwell JJ, Noblet AJ, Demir D, Steane P (2009) Predictors of the attitudinal and health outcomes of aged care nurses. Presented at the 8th annual Australian Industrial & Organizational Psychology Conference, Sydney, 25–28 June, 2009

Ross K (2008) Mapping pathways from stress to cancer progression. J Natl Cancer Inst 100(13):914–917

Rozanski A, Blumenthal JA, Kaplan J (1995) Impact of psychological factors on the pathogenesis of cardiovascular disease and implications for therapy. Circulation 99(16):2192–2217

Rydstedt LW, Devereux J, Sverke M (2007) Comparing and combining the demand-control-support model and the effort-reward imbalance model to predict long-term strain. Euro J Work Organ Psychol 16(3): 261–278

Schernhammer ES, Hankinson SE, Rosner B, Kroenke CH, Willett WC, Colditz GA, Kawachi I (2004) Job stress and breast cancer: the nurses' health study. Am J Epidemiol 160(11):1079–1086

Selye H (1956) The stress of life. McGraw-Hill, New York

Siegrist J (1996) Adverse health effects of high effort/low reward conditions. J Occup Heal Psychol 1(1):27

Stryker S, Burke PJ (2000) The past, present, and future of an identity theory. Soc Psychol Q 63: 284–297

Sulsky LM, Smith CS (2005) Work stress. Thomson Wadsworth, Belmont

Turner-Cobb JM, Sephton SE, Speigel D (2001) Psychosocial effects on immune function and disease progression in cancer: human studies. In: Ader R, Felten DL, Cohen N (eds) Psychoneuroimmunology, 3rd edn. Academic Press, New York, pp 565–582

Van der Doef M, Maes S (1999) The job demand-control (−support) model and psychological well-being: a review of 20 years of empirical research. Work Stress 13(2):87–114

Van Praag HM, De Koet ER, Van Os J (2004) Stress, the brain and depression. Cambridge University Press, Cambridge

Walster E, Berscheid E, Walster GW (1973) New directions in equity research. J Personal Soc Psychol 25:151–176

Wu M, Pasta-Pereja JC, Xu T (2010) Interaction between Ras^{V12} and scribbled clones induces tumor growth and invasion. Nat Lett 463:545–548

Yerkes RM, Dodson JD (1908) The relation of strength of stimulus to rapidity of habit formation. J Comp Neurol Psychol 18:459–482

About the Editors

Prof. Oommen V. Oommen's research contributions on comparative endocrinology in nonmammalian vertebrates led to establish a somewhat identical pattern in these vertebrates as in homeotherms. He has published several papers on ecology and molecular phylogenetics of caecilians in collaboration with Natural History Museum, London, including a paper in *Science*. A new species (*Gegeneophis primus*) of caecilian and an extensive taxonomic revision of a hitherto poorly known rainforest caecilian species *Ichthyophis longicephalus* are his recent works. Scientists from Natural History Museum, London, honored him by naming a caecilian after him (*Ureaotyphlus oommeni*). He has strong research link with MD Anderson Cancer Center, USA, on plant products in cancer research which saw three International Symposia on Translational Research with Dr. Oommen as the Organizing Secretary, and the first of it was inaugurated by the President of India. His group demonstrated that melanin has a role beyond pigmentation functions in the thyroid-mediated effects and had a serendipitous finding of a commonly used antioxidant functioning as a thyroid mimetic, triggering metamorphosis. Dr. Oommen is active in science popularization as the President of Kerala Academy of Sciences. He also championed interdisciplinary research in the University of Kerala through founding Centre for Bioinformatics. Currently, Prof. Oommen V. Oommen is the Chairman, Kerala State Biodiversity Board; Emeritus scientist (CSIR), University of Kerala; and also an Adjunct Professor in Central University, Kasaragod.

Prof. M. Radhakrishna Pillai is the Director of the Rajiv Gandhi Centre for Biotechnology, a national research institute of the Government of India in Thiruvananthapuram, Kerala, India. Professor Pillai is one of India's well-known cancer biologists. A fellow of both the Science and Medical academies of India and the Royal College of Pathologists, London, Professor Pillai has been able to provide one of the most elaborate databases of cellular and molecular processes occurring during epithelial tumor progression, especially the roles of human papillomavirus and programmed cell death. His work on cellular manifestations of human papillomavirus infection, particularly p53 gene inactivation, defective apoptosis, and angiogenesis, culminated in the description of a "condemned mucosa syndrome," which was well received in the scientific community. He has also provided the first data from India on the existence of various HPV 16 subtypes showing how they are associated with various grades of cervical disease. Dr. Pillai currently coordinates a major European Union-funded program on HPV in the development of oropharyngeal cancers and an International Agency for Research on Cancer (IARC) program on efficacy of different doses of the HPV vaccine. Dr. Pillai has over 180 international peer-reviewed research publications.

Prof. Perumana R. Sudhakaran is a renowned biochemist who has made significant contribution in the area of vascular biology. His major areas of research include cell matrix interaction and cell signaling in both physiological and pathological

P.R. Sudhakaran (ed.), *Perspectives in Cancer Prevention – Translational Cancer Research*, DOI 10.1007/978-81-322-1533-2, © Springer India 2014

conditions including atherosclerosis angiogenesis and cancer. He has held key positions in academic and administrative capacity including the Head of the Department of Biochemistry; Dean, Faculty of Science and Director of Research, University of Kerala Thiruvananthapuram, Kerala, India; and Dean, School of Biological Sciences, Central University of Kerala, Kasaragod, India, and is presently the Director of Kerala State Biotechnology Commission. Dr. Sudhakaran has published over 130 original research articles in peer-reviewed international journals and is a fellow of the National Academy of Medical Sciences (India).

Author Index

A
Annapoorna, K., 121, 125
Anto, N.P., 21
Anto, R.J., 21–23, 36
Aruldhas, M.M., 121, 124, 125
Athira, A.P., 113
Awasthi, Y.C., 103

B
Banu, S.K., 121
Bava, S.V., 21–23, 26, 27, 36, 41

C
Chandel, M., 61
Chandrasekaran, M., 121
Cheriyan, V.T., 21

D
Dixit, R., 145, 149

F
Fila, M.J., 153

J
Jaiswal, S., 103
Jayakumar, J., 121

K
Kaur, S., 61
Kiran, M.S., 113, 115, 117
Kumar, A.P., 73
Kumar, N., 61

L
Li, F., 73

M
Menon, S.G., 21

N
Nachiyappan, A., 73
Nagini, S., 45, 47, 50, 53
Neelamohan, R., 121

P
Perumal, E., 73
Puliyappadamba, V.T., 21

R
Radhakrishna Pillai, M., 9
Rashid, A., 1
Ravichandran, S.D., 21

S
Sah, M., 103
Santhosh Kumar, T.R., 9
Sethi, G., 73
Shanmugam, M.K., 73
Sharma, A., 103, 105, 106
Sharma, R., 103
Sharma, U., 61
Sharmila, S., 121
Shukla, V.K., 145–149
Singh, B., 61
Sreekanth, C.N., 21
Srinivasan, N., 121
Stanley, J.A., 121
Subramaniam, A., 73–77, 80–82
Sudhakaran, P.R., 113
Suthagar, E., 121

T
Tan, B.K.H., 73
Thulasidasan, A.K.T., 21
Trivedi, S., 89

V
Vidya Priyadarsini, R., 45, 50–53, 55

P.R. Sudhakaran (ed.), *Perspectives in Cancer Prevention – Translational Cancer Research*, DOI 10.1007/978-81-322-1533-2, © Springer India 2014

Subject Index

A

Akt, 22, 23, 25–29, 33–41, 54, 77, 81
Aktpathway, 28, 41, 117
Angiogenesis, 4, 5, 33, 41, 53, 56, 76, 81–82, 105, 106, 113–119, 165, 166
Anthocephalus cadamba, 61–71
Anticancer, 2, 22, 32, 40, 41, 45–56, 104–105, 134, 135, 137–141
Anticancer drugs, 9–18, 56, 134, 138
Antigenotoxicity, 61–71
Antioxidant activity, 62–64, 69, 71
Apoptosis, 4, 5, 12, 17, 22, 23, 26, 27, 35–37, 39, 40, 47, 52–54, 77, 79–81, 104–106, 108, 128, 135–141, 149, 165
Azadirachtin, 46–55

B

Beta catenin, 81, 117
Breast cancer, 3, 4, 7, 11, 12, 14, 17, 18, 22, 50, 52, 94, 98, 135, 137, 147, 156

C

Carcinogenesis, 1, 31, 32, 37, 40, 50, 53, 104, 146–149
Carotenoids, 4–6
Caspase, 10–14, 16–18, 23, 28, 33, 36, 41, 46, 52, 53, 82, 106, 108, 141
Cell adhesion molecules, 41, 116, 117
Cell cycle, 10, 11, 14–16, 18, 40, 41, 51–52, 56, 76, 78, 81, 89–100, 106, 107, 138
Cell lines, 10–14, 17, 35, 40, 49, 50, 54, 77–80, 82, 83, 104, 105, 124, 125, 128, 135–141
Cervical tumors, 24, 29–31, 33, 35–37, 40
Checkpoint, 90–92, 94
Chemoprevention, 71, 104
Cholelithiasis, 146–149
Colorectal cancer, 6, 97, 98
Curcumin, 5, 21–41, 83, 115, 117

D

Disease, 3, 4, 46, 47, 62, 77, 80, 98, 104, 114, 122, 123, 126, 146–149, 154–157, 165
Drug resistance, 10

E

Estradiol, 124, 125

F

Flanking sequences, 89–100

G

Gallbladder cancer, 145–149
Gangetic belt, 145–149
Genotoxicity, 51, 65, 67

H

HCC. *See* Hepatocellular carcinoma (HCC)
Heavy metals, 146, 147
Hepatocellular carcinoma (HCC), 50, 73–84, 98
4-Hydroxynonenal, 105–108

L

Leukemia, 76, 107
Limonoids, 45–56
Lipid peroxidation, 62, 105
Lung cancer, 6, 17

M

MAPKs. *See* Mitogen-activated protein kinases (MAPKs)
Matrix metalloproteinases, 53, 113–119
Metastasis, 10, 33, 36, 53, 77, 80, 82, 114, 115, 126, 155
Microsatellites, 90
Mitogen-activated protein kinases (MAPKs), 22, 29, 31, 33–35, 37, 39–41, 54, 83, 118
Mitogenic effect, 124
MMP 2, 23, 33, 82, 115–118
MMP 9, 23, 33, 115, 117, 118

N

Neem, 45–56
NF-κB, 34
Nimbolide, 47, 50–55
Nutrition, 1–7

P.R. Sudhakaran (ed.), *Perspectives in Cancer Prevention – Translational Cancer Research*, DOI 10.1007/978-81-322-1533-2, © Springer India 2014

O
Oncogenesis, 52, 75

P
Paclitaxel, 21–41
Papillary thyroid carcinoma (PTC), 122–128
Pericellular proteolysis, 116
Phosphatidylserine, 26, 27
Phytochemicals, 1, 2, 4, 22, 40, 47, 48, 55, 56, 104
Prostate cancer, 6, 12, 49, 50, 98, 107
Protooncogene, 35, 83
PTC. *See* Papillary thyroid carcinoma (PTC)

R
Reactive oxygen species (ROS), 10–12, 18, 51, 52, 54, 62, 70, 83, 105–107, 135
Recombination, 52, 90, 91, 94
Repair, 1, 2, 5, 51–52, 56, 75, 90, 91, 94, 155
Replication, 14, 52, 90, 91, 94
ROS. *See* Reactive oxygen species (ROS)

S
Sanguinarine, 148, 149
Selectin, 116, 117
Senescence, 10, 14–16, 18, 62
Side population cells, 11–14, 16, 18
Signal transducer, 75
Simple sequence repeats (SSRs), 89–100
Soy isoflavones, 4
SSRs. *See* Simple sequence repeats (SSRs)
STAT3, 73–84
Stem cells, 9–14, 16–18, 82
Strain, 47, 62–63, 68, 69, 76, 155, 157–160
Stress, 7, 15, 41, 51, 62, 69, 83, 105–108, 153–160
Sulforaphane, 103–108
Synergism, 22, 26–27, 29, 31, 37, 39–41

T
Testosterone, 6, 124–129
Thyroid cancer, 121–129
Transcription, 4, 5, 23, 29, 31–33, 39, 53–54, 73–84, 90, 91, 94, 99, 106, 108, 116, 125–128
Transition, 10, 12, 14, 81, 90–92, 94, 114, 117, 134
Tumor, 2, 4–7, 22, 24, 26, 29–41, 74, 75, 77, 78, 80–83, 90, 98, 114–116, 122–129, 155, 156, 165
Tumorigenesis, 22, 31, 41, 76, 90, 124, 126

U
Ursolic acid, 83, 117

V
Vascular endothelial growth factor (VEGF), 23, 33, 41, 53, 82, 115, 117
VE-cadherin, 113–119
VEGF. *See* Vascular endothelial growth factor (VEGF)

W
Workplace, 154, 156–159